**CARDIOLOGY RESEARCH AND CLINICAL DEVELOPMENTS**

# OFF-PUMP CORONARY ARTERY BYPASS GRAFTING

# EVOLUTION, TECHNIQUES AND TECHNOLOGY

# CARDIOLOGY RESEARCH AND CLINICAL DEVELOPMENTS

Additional books in this series can be found on Nova's website under the Series tab.

Additional E-books in this series can be found on Nova's website under the E-book tab.

CARDIOLOGY RESEARCH AND CLINICAL DEVELOPMENTS

# OFF-PUMP CORONARY ARTERY BYPASS GRAFTING

# EVOLUTION, TECHNIQUES AND TECHNOLOGY

SHAHZAD G. RAJA
AND
MOHAMED AMRANI
EDITORS

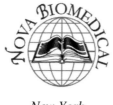

*New York*

Copyright © 2012 by Nova Science Publishers, Inc.

**All rights reserved.** No part of this book may be reproduced, stored in a retrieval system or transmitted in any form or by any means: electronic, electrostatic, magnetic, tape, mechanical photocopying, recording or otherwise without the written permission of the Publisher.

For permission to use material from this book please contact us:
Telephone 631-231-7269; Fax 631-231-8175
Web Site: http://www.novapublishers.com

### NOTICE TO THE READER

The Publisher has taken reasonable care in the preparation of this book, but makes no expressed or implied warranty of any kind and assumes no responsibility for any errors or omissions. No liability is assumed for incidental or consequential damages in connection with or arising out of information contained in this book. The Publisher shall not be liable for any special, consequential, or exemplary damages resulting, in whole or in part, from the readers' use of, or reliance upon, this material. Any parts of this book based on government reports are so indicated and copyright is claimed for those parts to the extent applicable to compilations of such works.

Independent verification should be sought for any data, advice or recommendations contained in this book. In addition, no responsibility is assumed by the publisher for any injury and/or damage to persons or property arising from any methods, products, instructions, ideas or otherwise contained in this publication.

This publication is designed to provide accurate and authoritative information with regard to the subject matter covered herein. It is sold with the clear understanding that the Publisher is not engaged in rendering legal or any other professional services. If legal or any other expert assistance is required, the services of a competent person should be sought. FROM A DECLARATION OF PARTICIPANTS JOINTLY ADOPTED BY A COMMITTEE OF THE AMERICAN BAR ASSOCIATION AND A COMMITTEE OF PUBLISHERS.

Additional color graphics may be available in the e-book version of this book.

**Library of Congress Cataloging-in-Publication Data**

Library of Congress Control Number: 2012935713

ISBN: 978-1-62081-549-6

*Published by Nova Science Publishers, Inc. † New York*

# Contents

| | | |
|---|---|---|
| **Section 1. Evolution** | | 1 |
| **Chapter I** | History of Coronary Artery Bypass Grafting<br>*Stephen Westaby* | 3 |
| **Chapter II** | History of Off-Pump Coronary Artery Bypass Grafting<br>*Fhilipe O. Prybicz, Joao C. C. Pereira<br>and Paulo R. Soltoski* | 27 |
| **Section 2. Techniques and Technology** | | 37 |
| **Chapter III** | Hemodynamic Changes during Off-Pump Coronary Artery Bypass Grafting<br>*Zachary Edgerton and James R. Edgerto* | 39 |
| **Chapter IV** | Techniques of Myocardial Stabilization and Coronary Artery Exposure in Off-pump Coronary Artery Bypass Grafting<br>*Fabiano Porta and Piet W. Boonstra* | 47 |
| **Chapter V** | Conduits for Coronary Artery Bypass Grafting<br>*Guo-Wei He* | 55 |
| **Chapter VI** | Techniques of Conduit Harvesting for Coronary Artery Bypass Grafting<br>*David O. Moore, Lonnie J. Ginn and Michael J. Mack* | 77 |
| **Chapter VII** | Technique of Off-Pump Multivessel Coronary Artery Bypass Grafting through Median Sternotomy<br>*Bryon J. Boulton and John D. Puskas* | 97 |
| **Chapter VIII** | Technique of Minimally Invasive Direct Coronary Artery Bypass (MIDCAB) Grafting<br>*Piroze M. Davierwala, David M. Holzhey and Friedrich W. Mohr* | 109 |
| **Chapter IX** | Technique of Totally Endoscopic Robot-Assisted Off-Pump Coronary Artery Bypass Grafting<br>*Eric J. Lehr, W. Randolph Chitwood Jr. and Johannes Bonatti* | 123 |

| | | |
|---|---|---:|
| **Chapter X** | Technique of Reoperative Off-pump Coronary Artery Bypass Grafting<br>*Shahzad G. Raja and Mohamed Amrani* | **145** |
| **Chapter XI** | Technique of Hybrid Coronary Revascularization<br>*Shahzad G. Raja and Charles D. Ilsley* | **165** |
| **Chapter XII** | Technique of Awake Off-pump Coronary Artery Bypass Grafting<br>*Kaan Kırali* | **175** |
| **Chapter XIII** | On-pump Beating-Heart Coronary Artery Bypass Grafting<br>*Ken Miyahara* | **213** |
| **Chapter XIV** | Anesthesia for Off-pump Coronary Artery Bypass Grafting<br>*Daniel Bainbridge* | **225** |
| **Chapter XV** | Verification of Graft Patency in Off-pump Coronary Artery Bypass Grafting<br>*Ramanan Umakanthan, Marzia Leacche, Christopher R. Byrne and John G. Byrne* | **243** |
| **Chapter XVI** | Atrial Pacing for Off-pump Coronary Artery Bypass Grafting<br>*Vassilios S. Gulielmos, Emmanouela G. Dalamanga and Pavlos G. Papoulidis* | **257** |
| **Index** | | **261** |

# Section 1. Evolution

In: Off-Pump Coronary Artery Bypass Grafting
Editors: Shahzad G. Raja and Mohamed Amrani

ISBN: 978-1- 62081-549-6
© 2012 Nova Science Publishers, Inc.

*Chapter I*

# History of Coronary Artery Bypass Grafting

*Stephen Westaby*
Distinguished Ralph Cicerone Professor, University of California Irvine
and Consultant Cardiac Surgeon
John Radcliffe Hospital, Oxford, United Kingdom

## Abstract

For centuries the heart has been recognized as the repository of soul and the seat of the emotions. Despite been known as vital for sustaining life for a long time the ability to successfully operate on the living beating heart was not achieved until the 1950s and 1960s. Coronary artery bypass grafting over the past five decades has become the most frequently performed cardiac operation with major improvements in the technique, technology, and perioperative management. This chapter provides a brief overview of the development of cardiac surgery and focuses on the evolution of surgery for myocardial revascularization.

## Setting the Stage for Cardiac Surgery

Cardiac surgery has a colourful and awe inspiring history. Perhaps the most significant step in the development of surgery as a science was the advent of anesthetics. Since prehistoric times, alcohol made from fermented fruit juice or grain was used as a sedative to relieve pain. During the Napoleonic wars anesthetics other than alcohol were essentially unknown, but Napoleon's own great surgeon Baron Dominique Jean Larrey noticed that during severe winter campaigns intense cold seemed to numb the limbs of those needing amputation. In 1839 Alfred Velpeau wrote "the avoidance of pain during operations is a fantasy that should not be indulged in. Cutting instruments and pain are inextricably associated with each other in the mind of patients". In 1776 Joseph Priestly, a gentleman farmer and chemist, discovered carbon dioxide and nitrous oxide gases. In 1799 Humphrey

Davey, a Cornish apothecary, investigated the properties of various gases by self application. Inhaled nitrous oxide produced a feeling of well being followed by persistent migraine but the pain of a broken tooth disappeared. There was no practical application of this finding until 1844 when in Hertford Connecticut, a fairground entertainment included "men who could not stop laughing". This stemmed from the fact that humans who inhaled nitrous oxide burst into spontaneous uncontrollable laughter. One man fell of the platform sustaining a fracture but remained unaware of the pain. The dentist Horace Wells then tested nitric oxide on himself during a tooth extraction and two years later William Morton another Boston dentist, found ether to be an affective anesthetic. Ether anesthetic became popular in the United States (U.S.) and was introduced into Europe successfully in Paris in 1846. In 1847 chloroform was employed by James Young Simpson, the Professor of Obstetrics at Edinburgh University. During 1853 whilst Queen Victoria was pregnant with her $8^{th}$ child, Prince Albert solicited a chloroform anesthetic for the birth of Prince Leopold. The Queen remained largely unconscious and free from pain. Chloroform soon became the most popular anesthetic particularly in Europe where French and English ambulance teams used it to treat soldiers at the siege of Sebastopol. An American physician Oliver Wendal Holmes coined the term anesthetic from the Greek word no feeling. However chloroform caused a number of fatalities. A 15 year old girl called Anna Greener died in Newcastle whilst having a toenail removed in January 1848. The danger of chloroform syncope became a popular subject for discussion in the medical journals but stimulated the evolution of techniques for cardiac resuscitation. Opinion was divided over the cause of deaths from chloroform syncope. John Snow, Queen Victoria's physician, regarded heart failure from too high a concentration of the vapour as the likely explanation, whereas Simpson and Lister considered respiratory failure to be important. Probably the first surgeon to attempt cardiac massage on a patient was Niehous of Bern, whose patient, a 40 year old man, died during chloroform administration for a goitre removal in 1880. He performed a left thoracotomy and began rhythmically compressing the heart whilst the anaesthetist continued with artificial respiration. The patient died. The first successful cardiac massage was achieved by Igelsrud of Tronsolm Norway at the turn of the century, when a 43 year old woman undergoing hysterectomy suffered cardiac arrest. After an unsuccessful attempt at artificial respiration, Igelsrud performed a left thoracotomy and massaged the heart using strong rhythmical manual compression for about 1 minute. The heart began to beat and the patient survived with complete recovery. The first recorded attempt to suture the heart came in 1895 when the Norwegian surgeon Axel Cappelen operated on a 24 year old man who had been stabbed through the fourth intercostal space on the left. Cappelen opened the chest by removing the fourth rib and found a one inch wound of the left ventricle. Sutures closed the wound and a lacerated coronary artery was ligated. An injection of saline was given to improve the patient's condition but he died 2 days later. Autopsy showed the patient to have died as a result of ligation of the myocardial blood supply. In 1896 Guiddo Farena of Rome operated on a 30 year old man with a 7mm stab wound of the right ventricle. This was easily closed with sutures but the patient died 3 days later with bronchopneumonia. Again the cardiac wound was already healing satisfactorily. Farena was refused permission to keep the heart following autopsy and did not publish his findings. The first clinical success came several months later in September 1896 when Ludwig Rehn of Frankfurt operated on a 22 year old man stabbed during a drunken brawl. Rehn operated to relieve cardiac tamponade and closed a 1.5cm laceration of the right ventricle with 3 interrupted sutures. He then packed the pericardial cavity with iodoform gauze as a precaution against infection. The man was known to be alive 10 years later. The first cardiac operation reported in the U.S. took place on 14 September 1902 when Luther Hill of Montgomery Alabama was called to the home of a 13 year old boy who had been stabbed 5 times in the chest. The boy was dyspnoeic, restless and in shock with a barely palpable pulse and inaudible heart sounds. Recognising cardiac tamponade, Hill proceeded to perform a thoracotomy by the light of oil lamps on the kitchen table. Hill had trained with Joseph Lister in England and christened his son Lister Hill.

In 1895 Willhelm Konrad Roentgen, Professor of Physics at the University of Wurtsberg discovered x-rays. This provided an enormous stimulus for many developments in medicine and surgery by opening up an entirely new field of diagnosis and study of disease. Roentgen was awarded the first Nobel Prize for physics. The first time x-rays were used for diagnosis was in 1896 when a drunken sailor was admitted to a London hospital with a stab wound in the back. He was paraplegic and x-rays of the spine showed the tip of a knife blade wedged between two vertebrae and encroaching on the spinal canal. Surgery to remove the blade resulted in resolution of the paraplegia. In 1903 Tuffier used x-rays to locate a bullet in the chest of a wounded soldier. The x-rays appeared to demonstrate a bullet in the region of the left atrium, so Tuffier explored the pericardial cavity. He located the bullet within fibrinous adhesions and removed it after which the patient made an uneventful recovery. The second half of the 19th century saw a tremendous amount of work on the heart and circulation with the eventual evolution of medical specialisation. In 1889 Augustus Waller, a general physician in Kensington London attempted to measure the electrical impulses created by the heart but his equipment was insufficiently sensitive to give an accurate record. Willhelm Einthoven of Leiden adapted a string galvanometer for the purpose and connected this to electrodes on the chest wall. His apparatus was extremely cumbersome with the subject sitting with his or her feet in a tub of salt solution. Nevertheless he identified the P, Q, R and S waves in 1903 and published many basic clinical observations. He was awarded a Nobel Prize in 1924 after which electrocardiography became a standard cardiological investigation. In 1919 James Herrick first described the electrocardiogram after coronary thrombosis confirmed by autopsy. The ECG in angina was first noted by Bousfield in 1918 and in 1920 Harold Pardee described a survivor of acute myocardial infarction with ECG records.

The development of angiography began surprisingly soon after Roentgen's description of x-rays. Experimental catheterisation of the heart had been undertaken as early as 1855 by Chauveau and Marey in France. They sought to study the pressures inside the heart and discover whether all the chambers contracted together or not. The great French physiologist Claude Bernard also catheterised the heart and measured cardiac output by chemical and temperature measurements of the blood. He succeeded in passing catheters retrogradely through the aortic valve via the carotid artery. After achieving right atrial catheterisation with a ureteric catheter in a cavader, the German urologist Forssmann engaged the aid of an assistant to catheterise himself. The assistant never failed and Forssmann cut down on a vein in his own left elbow and threaded the ureteric catheter through a wide bore needle into the vein. With a mirror arranged so that he could see the x-ray screen, he manipulated the catheter into the right heart then walked upstairs to the x-ray department to confirm his achievement radiographically. Despite significant advances in diagnostic cardiology, the problem of acute ventilatory disturbance when the chest was opened, mitigated against developments in thoracic surgery. Positive pressure ventilation emerged after the Glasgow surgeon Sir William MacEwen invented a flexible brass tube to be introduced into the upper airway of the unconscious patient. In 1885, the New York ear, nose and throat surgeon Joseph O'Dwyer devised a tube to be passed through the larynx and into the trachea of patients with diphtheria. Two years later George Fell of Buffalo designed bellows for giving artificial respiration to patients with opium poisoning. The bellows system was combined with O'Dwyer's tube to become the Fell-O'Dwyer apparatus which was used by Rudolph Matass for administering endotracheal anesthesia in 1899. Bellows provided positive pressure to keep the lungs inflated with the chest open. Other events then contributed to an environment to support cardiac surgery. In 1915 the medical student Maclean discovered heparin whilst working on thromboplastins in the laboratory of Howell. The development of antibiotics occurred more by accident than design but changed the face of modern surgery. Penicillin was discovered by chance in 1928 when Alexander Fleming, a Scottish bacteriologist working at St Mary's Hospital London, was growing staphylococci on petrie dishes. These were left on a work bench whilst he and his staff left for a three week holiday, during which the dishes became contaminated with a mysterious mould. When Fleming returned he noted that the colonies of bacteria in contact with the mould had been killed. Between the Great Wars there were few forays into the realms of cardiac surgery with the notable exceptions of Doyen's attempted mitral valvotomy in 1913, Tuffier's aborted aortic valvotomy the same year and Elliott Cutler's mitral valvotomy in 1923. By the end of the 1930s experimental work that would prove to be the foundation of modern cardiac surgery was just beginning. The first indication of future developments came in March 1937 when John Streider attempted to close a patent ductus arteriosus in a young woman with bacterial endocarditis. This patient died but Robert Gross then successfully closed a patent ductus in a 7 year old girl in 1938. Prior to World War I there were about 380 operations recorded for cardiac wounds with a mortality rate of 50%. World War I added about 60 more to the list. Most operations had been performed by French surgeons often with a substantial interval between wounding and operation. There were 6 recorded operations on the heart by British military surgeons with 3 successes. John Fraser, a captain in the Royal Air Force Medical Corps had observed 2 deaths from cardiac tamponade and realised that there was often enough time for surgical intervention. He decided to operate immediately on the next case where physical signs suggested a cardiac injury. His opportunity came in 1917 in a solider with multiple wounds of face, arms and chest. When Fraser opened the chest he found a perforation of the right atrium which he repaired. With appropriate management of the other wounds, the soldier made an excellent recovery. In 1917 Ballance operating on the evacuated casualties from Greece, operated on a solider with a bullet lodged in the wall of the left ventricle. The solider lost a considerable amount of blood and was transfused directly from a donor until the donor systolic pressure fell below 90 mmHg. The patient initially survived but died from infection 4 weeks later.

The beginning of World War II saw the development of penicillin by Howard Florey and Norman Healey in Oxford and the beginnings of a blood transfusion service. At the Thoracic Centre of the 160th General Hospital of the U.S. Army situated in England, Dwight Harken of Boston operated on 134 patients with retained missiles in the mediastinum without losing a single patient. Thirteen of these foreign bodies were within cardiac chambers. When Harken read a paper on his operations in 1947, Miscall of New York recounted that his Unit in the North of England had also removed 39 foreign bodied from the heart or pericardium without mortality. Two other significant cardiological events were reported in 1947. These were the pioneering work on electrical defibrillation by Kouwen Hoven. The first successful treatment of cardiac arrest by cardiac massage was by McKendry at St Anne's Military Hospital

Montreal. In 1949 Callaghan of Toronto used an electrode catheter to electrically stimulate a dog's heart. Paul Zoll then built on this information to construct a transthoracic pacemaker for patients in 1952.

At the end of World War II and the beginning of the 1950s the stage was set for great advances in cardiovascular surgery. Surgeons such as Harken and Biggalo returned to the U.S. with ideas and experience which would provide the stimulus for future developments. Closed cardiac operations had already caught the imagination of ambitious young men such as Walton Lillehei, John Kirklan, Denton Cooley, Donald Ross, Viking Bork, Brian Boyes and others who would mould cardiac surgery into a specialty. By this time John Gibbon was already working towards development of the pump oxygenator which would eventually prove the key to direct vision cardiac repair. Key areas of support such as safe anesthesia, cardiac catheterization, electrocardiography and defibrillation were now established as were antibiotics and anticoagulants.

## The Recognition of Coronary Artery Disease

The relationship between coronary atheroma and the symptom angina was not easily defined. Coronary artery disease was often found at post mortem in patients who had never complained of angina. The Irish physician, Dominic Corrigan, maintained that angina was due to disease in the aorta itself, since many patients with syphilis, died during an anginal attack but had no coronary occlusive disease. In 1772 William Heberden published his description of angina pectoris in the literary magazine Critical Review (II, 203-204). A 51 year old male reader recognised his own symptoms and wrote to Heberden, "I have never troubled myself much about the cause of it, but attributed it to an obstruction of the circulation or a species of rheumatism". In the event of sudden death he gave permission for an autopsy to establish the cause. Less than three weeks later his premonition was fulfilled and Heberden engaged the experienced anatomist John Hunter to open the body. Allegedly nothing was found to account for the death and Heberden concluded that angina was not due to an organic illness.

Hunter's first resident student, Edward Jenner attended the necropsy and was troubled by the negative outcome. Years later after Jenner had ascribed the anginal symptom to coronary obstruction he wrote that "almost certainly the coronary arteries were not examined". Hunter's extensive necropsy records certainly held clues to the association. In one case of cerebral embolus from a left ventricular thrombus Hunter noted (1770) "when I cut into the right ventricle I found the coronary artery as it goes between the auricle and ventricle, ossified". On 13 March 1775, Mr Rook, a 54 year old man with angina pectoris died "in a sudden and violent transport of anger". The eminent physician John Fothergill suspected angina and heart failure and asked Hunter to perform the autopsy. Hunter found calcific aortic and mitral stenosis and that the coronary arteries "from their origin to many of their ramifications upon the heart were become one piece of bone". Although Hunter's notes indicate that Rook "felt frequent pain in the arms" still "there was nothing very remarkable in the case worth taking notice of". Hunter's own anginal symptoms began in 1773 with an attack of severe epigastric pain accompanied by pallor ("the appearance of a dead man"). The pain lasted for 45 minutes and he was "perfectly recovered in two hours". In 1777 with worsening angina he was advised to go to Bath for spa therapy. Here Jenner made the correct diagnosis, recognised the relationship between angina and coronary disease but did not inform Hunter because he did not want to disturb his friend. In 1783 Hunter described three cases of congenital heart disease, one of which was Tetralogy of Fallot and in 1793, the year of his death, he identified bacterial endocarditis in a six year old boy. Despite unstable and nocturnal angina from 1789 onwards, Hunter failed to make the important pathological association. Hunter's autopsy confirmed Jenner's prediction that coronary atheroma would be found but Hunter's wish that his heart should be preserved was disregarded.

The first physician to establish the diagnosis of coronary thrombus in a living patient was Adam Hammer of St Louis (1876). He correctly reasons that the onset and rapid progression of anginal pain could be attributed to interruption of the coronary supply and that myocardial ischemia occurred through thrombotic occlusion of "at least one of the coronary arteries". In Hammer's own words, "I mentioned my convictions to my colleague at the bedside. He, however, had a nonplussed expression and burst out, "I have never heard of such a diagnosis in my life" and I answered, "Nor I also". Nevertheless, a carefully conducted post-mortem proved Hammer to be correct.

The range of symptoms and cardiac events attributable to coronary artery disease were defined by James Herrick of Chicago in 1912. Differentiation between a prolonged anginal attack and acute myocardial infarction was difficult, until electrocardiography came into general use in the 1920s and 1930s. After that, it was possible to recognize the electrical changes of myocardial ischemia and distinguish them from the permanent changes of infarction. Having identified the association between angina pectoris and coronary artery disease, the next step was to define an appropriate method of treatment.

## T Lauder Brunton and Amyl Nitrate

"Few things are more distressing to a physician than to stand beside the suffering patient, who is anxiously looking to him for that relief of pain which he feels utterly unable to afford. Perhaps there is no class of case in which such occurrences as this take place frequently as in some kinds of cardiac disease in which angina pectoris forms at once the post prominent and most painful and distressing symptom".

These were the words of T Lauder Brunton from his manuscript, "On the use of nitrate of amyl in anginal pectoris", published in the Lancet in 1867. Brunton was the first physician to achieve effective relief of angina by inhalation of amyl nitrate. This treatment provided the mainstay of anginal therapy in the early 1900s but was of limited value. Consequently, early consideration was given to the possibility of surgical intervention. Three different approaches were considered. The first efforts to relieve angina were by blocking the nervous innervation of the heart. Second, it seemed logical to reduce the metabolic requirements of the myocardium by reducing workload. Finally, it seemed logical to increase the blood supply to ischemic areas.

Charles Emile Francois-Frank first suggested thoracocervical sympathectomy for angina in 1899. His reasoning was indirect, in that sympathectomy was used for the treatment of thyrotoxicosis and some of Francois-Frank's thyrotoxic patients also had aortitis and angina. It was probably Charles Mayo (one of the Mayo brothers who, together with their father, founded the Mayo Clinic) who first performed cervical sympathectomy for angina in a U.S. Army major (1913). In 1916, the Bucharest surgeon, Thomas Jonnesco, who devoted most of his career to the surgery of the sympathetic nervous systems, operated on a 20 year old man with angina due to syphilitic aortitis. Jonnesco removed the lasts two cervical ganglia and the first two thoracic ganglia on the left side, and wanted to follow with right sided sympathectomy.

However the patient was so much improved that he declined the second operation. When seen 4 years later, he was completely asymptomatic and able to do heavy work.

An alternative method was proposed by the physicians Gastineau Earle and Strickland Goodall. They suggested that the sensory roots would be cut from the cardiac plexus at the point where they entered the spinal cord (posterior rhizotomy). In 1913, they persuaded Sampson Handley, their surgical colleague at the Middlesex Hospital to attempt the operation experimentally. Although he was able to section the second, third and fourth thoracic nerve roots on a cadaver, they collectively decided that injection of alcohol or novocaine into the nerve roots would be simpler and just as effective.

The concept of posterior nerve root section was resurrected 10 years later, when Danielopolu (Director of the Second Medical Clinic at the University of Bucharest) criticized the Jonnesco-type sympathectomy on the grounds that it produced an irreversible deterioration in cardiac function. He therefore directed his surgical colleague, Hristide, to cut the posterior roots of the upper thoracic spinal nerves which divided only sensory fibres. Danielopolu later declared cervicothoracic sympathectomy to be disastrous, from the therapeutic point of view, and concluded that removal of the stellate ganglion for angina was incompatible with life. In the 1920s many forms of sympathectomy were undertaken and alcohol was injected into the upper thoracic sympathetic ganglia or nerve roots. About two thirds of patients were relieved of their anginal pain, though the natural history of coronary artery disease progressed inexorably.

## Elliot Cutler and Thyroidectomy

Efforts to reduce cardiac workload were made by lowering the metabolic rate. This reduced requirements in those areas of limited myocardial perfusion. The concept of creating thyroid underactivity as a treatment for angina came in stages. Thyroidectomy was commonplace in the early part of the century, and occasionally, patients with congestive cardiac failure were seen to improve after remission from thyrotoxicosis. In 1927 Elliott Cutler in Boston saw a 61 year old woman with severe heart failure, who was thought to be suffering from latent hyperthyroidism. At operation the thyroid gland appeared normal, but the surgeon pressed on with the thyroidectomy regardless. Despite normal thyroid histology, the patient was greatly improved from the cardiac standpoint. On 15 June 1932 Cutler carried out the first subtotal thyroidectomy with the specific objective of relieving angina. This patient was symptomatically improved, as were several others. Total thyroidectomy was then undertaken to induce myxoedema, which in turn moderated the cardiovascular response to adrenaline. Eventually the operation was reduced to simple ligation of the superior and inferior thyroid arteries in order to preserve the recurrent laryngeal nerves and parathyroid glands.

Thyroidectomy was said to provide symptomatic relief in 80% of patients although they were often transformed physiologically and psychologically into a vegetative existence. Within a decade thyroidectomy fell into disrepute, partly because surgeons such as Singer (who performed section of the posterior nerve roots) and Rainey (who advised surgical division of the upper thoracic pre-ganglionic fibres) were achieving satisfactory results without the disadvantage of myxoedema. Some physicians, such as Sir James McKenzie also felt that the anginal syndrome should be preserved to prevent unduly severe exertion and ventricular fibrillation.

## Early Attempts to Increase Myocardial Blood Supply

An increased understanding of the pathophysiology of angina spawned efforts to increase myocardial blood supply. The initial attempts were indirect. In 1932, Claude Beck, Professor of Neurosurgery at the Western Reserve School of Medicine, Cleveland, sought to increase myocardial blood flow by creating collateral circulation within the pericardium. Beck's colleague, Alan Mortiz, drew attention to a report from Thorel (1903) where at post mortem a patient was found to have longstanding complete obstruction of both main coronary arteries. There were diffuse vascular adhesions around the heart and Thorel suggested that these must have supplied the myocardium with blood. Beck suggested that it might be possible to imitate this situation by creating adhesions between epicardium and pericardium. After a great deal of experimental work, he operated on his first patient, a 48 year old man, on 13 February 1935. He roughened the inside of the pericardial sac with a burr and denuded the epicardium. Between the two raw surfaces he grafted part of the pectoralis major muscle on its vascular pedicle. Within a year, the patient was asymptomatic. Beck then used pericardial fat and omentum as a source of vascularity and showed that after promoting adhesions, experimental animals could survive almost complete occlusion of the native coronaries.

In Britain, Laurence O'Shaughnessy used a pedicle of greater omentum to wrap the thoracic oesophagus after oesophagogastrectomy. This rapidly enhanced vascularity in the area of the anastomosis. In April 1933, he began to apply omental grafts to the epicardium and vascular anastomoses were soon formed with the epicardial blood vessels. O'Shaughnessy then sought to test his method in greyhounds, who are prone to heart failure. The dogs on which he performed coronary occlusion followed by omental grafts recovered and were able to return to the track. In 1936 he used the technique on a 64 year old man at Lewisham Hospital. The patient survived, but in later operations O'Shaughnessy avoided suturing the myocardium by applying omentum to the pericardium and using adhesive paste between the epicardium and the graft. In 1938 he reported symptomatic relief for all patients who had survived 6 months or more. Regrettably, O'Shaughnessy's work was truncated in World War II when he was killed at Dunkirk at the age of 40.

Other tissues, such as skin, jejunum and stomach were used experimentally as grafts during the 1950s, but the only satisfactory alternative to omentum appeared to be lung. This was used by the German surgeon Lezius in 1937. He created a pericardial window, painted acriflavine onto the epicardium and then sutured the lung to this area. In animals, he succeeded in demonstrating anastomoses between coronary and lung vessels radiographically.

This relatively simple approach was used on patients by several enthusiasts in the 1950s but the results were never impressive.

Another even simpler method to create adhesions was to stimulate chemical pericarditis. Thomas and Raisbeck, of New York, used sterile talc and instilled 2% novocaine on to the epicardium to prevent the irritant powder from producing ventricular fibrillation. Thomson used this technique extensively and 14 years later reported that most of his patients had been relieved of their symptoms. The operation only lasted about 20 minutes although four of the first 16 patients died in the post operative period. Other irritants included carborundum sand, powdered beef bone or asbestos, kaolin, iron filings, iodine, ether, alcohol, formaldehyde, cotton, human skin and water glass. In 1955, Harken used 95% carbolic acid to remove the epicardium and followed this by instilling powdered talc. Although many patients claimed to have fewer and less severe anginal attacks, experimental work gave no objective evidence of improved circulation to the myocardium. The alleged symptomatic improvement also occurred much too soon to be attributable to newly vascularised adhesions. Carbolic probably destroyed all the nerve endings.

## Revascularization through the Coronary Sinus

In 1935, Louis Grosse and Lester Blom at the Mount Sinai Hospital, New York observed that the severity of anginal pain was reduced if the patient developed right heart failure. They argued that the congested myocardium had a sluggish bloodflow from which more oxygen could be extracted. They then demonstrated that complete ligation of the coronary sinus (in dogs) could prevent death when a major coronary artery was occluded. After some time, the congestion disappeared due to collateral channels, but by that time intercoronary arteriolar connections had opened up. Mercier Fauteux, a Canadian working in Boston, attacked the problem from two different directions: first by removing the sympathetic nerves from around the coronary vessels (pericoronary neurectomy), and then by ligating the veins. He later switched to ligation of the great cardiac vein, which drains into the coronary sinus. Fauteux operated on humans in 1940 and by 1946, had a series of 16 patients, all with previous acute myocardial infarction confirmed by ECG. Eleven had been severely disabled by angina beforehand, but reported substantial clinical improvement. By 1941, Beck stopped using muscle grafts and resorted to venous ligation. He described the Beck I operation in 1945. This comprised of abrasion of the pericardium and epicardium, application of an inflammatory agent and partial occlusion of the coronary sinus. Mediastinal fat or pericardium were grafted to the surface of the myocardium.

If blood flow and oxygenation could be achieved by retrograde flow through the coronary sinus, it seemed logical that arterial blood should prove more satisfactory than venous blood. In 1943 Joseph Roberts (University of Texas Medical School, Galveston) showed by dye studies on dogs' hearts, that it was possible for Thebesius' veins to carry blood retrograde from the left ventricular cavity into the myocardium. This occurred when the pressure in the ventricle exceeded that in the coronary arteries. Of greater significance were experiments that showed that ischemic myocardium could be revascularised by joining a large artery to the coronary sinus or veins. When the brachiocephalic, subclavian or innominate artery was anastomosed to the coronary sinus via a glass cannula, the coronary veins became distended and pulsatile. The myocardium then continued to contract when the coronary arteries were ligated.

Beck followed this lead with his own experiments and on 27 January 1948 performed the first Beck II operation on a human patient. He excised a length of brachial artery and used this to join the descending aorta to the coronary sinus. The coronary sinus itself was ligated at its junction with the right atrium. This was a difficult operation and Beck soon changed to a two-stage procedure, whereby the graft was inserted first, and between 2 and 6 weeks later, the coronary sinus was partially ligated. The Beck II operation produced impressive, longstanding intercoronary connections, even though the graft tended to thrombose after a few weeks. However the operative mortality was 15-20% and this soon brought the procedure into disrepute.

## Vineberg and the Internal Mammary Artery

In 1939, the Italian physician, Fieschi suggested that bilateral ligation of the internal mammary arteries below their pericardiophrenic branches might increase myocardial blood flow. These branches normally give rise to small pericardial vessels, which in turn anastomose with other small arteries from the aorta. Fieschi persuaded his colleagues Zoja and Cesa-Bianchi to undertake this procedure on a patient with myocardial infarction. Bilateral ligation was performed under local anesthetic through an incision in the second intercostal space. Two years later, the patient remained well. The procedure was undertaken by others Italians, including Battezzati who reported 11 cases in 1955. The operation had the merit of being simple, with no operative mortality. It could be performed safely during recuperation from an acute myocardial infarction and was said to produce worthwhile results. Other investigators failed to demonstrate a significant increase in cardiac blood flow. When patients with angina were divided into two groups, one in which ligation was carried out and the other in which only the skin was incised (no ligation), the results showed patients in both groups to benefit equally. Such was the power of suggestion! The internal mammary artery was nevertheless destined to play an important part in the future of myocardial revascularization.

Arthur Vineberg began his experimental work at McGill University in 1946. He mobilised the left internal mammary artery, ligated the vessel distally and implanted the bleeding end into a tunnel in the left ventricular muscle close to the left anterior descending coronary artery. Remarkably no haematoma formed and he could later show that the artery formed anastomotic channels with neighbouring vessels. Why should this work? If a bleeding artery were to be implanted in any other muscle, it would simply result in a large haematoma. It appears that the myocardium has a potential sponge like quality. In early embryonic life, the sponge is soft and loose, deriving its oxygen from blood squeezed in and out of it. This is the method by which the hearts of many lower vertebrate animals, such as fish, obtain their nutrition. With further development of the human embryo, the sponge tightens and the coronary vessels and capillaries condense out of the spongy network. However, when intercoronary connections are opened under the stress of ischemia or a surgical procedure, there is a tendency to revert towards the sponge stage. This is the theoretical basis on which Vineberg based his procedure and in 1950, he operated on the first human patient. Three years later, he reported that the patient "from a condition of complete disability could walk 10 miles through the bush". Vineberg also used pads of pericardial fat, grafted to the surface of the left ventricle and in 1963 he employed a mesenteric graft. The greater omentum was detached completely from the fat and wrapped around the heart after denuding the epicardium.

In 1964, Vineberg reported 140 operations with 33% mortality, though for the decade 1954-63 the mortality was less than 2%. Of 109 surviving patients (1964) 91 had either no angina or slight pain on effort. In general clinical improvement was good, with a high percentage of patients able to return to work. Later, with the introduction of coronary arteriography by Sones, of the Cleveland Clinic, the Vineberg procedure was shown to produce worthwhile anastomoses with the native coronary circulation in 70-80% of internal mammary implants.

On 4 October 1955 Sidney Smith of Florida using a modification of the Vineberg procedure, harvested the long saphenous vein from the leg, anastomosed this proximally to the aorta and pulled the substance of the vein graft through the myocardium from base to apex. The 43 year old patient was asymptomatic 18 months later. Smith then abandoned the saphenous vein and used a perforated nylon prosthesis instead.

## Favaloro and Sones at the Cleveland Clinic

Just before Favaloro's arrival at the Cleveland clinic in 1962, two important events occurred. First, on 5 January 1962, Effler successfully operated on a severe obstruction at the left main coronary artery using the patch graft technique described by Senning. The first patch operations were performed using a pericardial graft to enlarge the lumen of the left main coronary artery. With increasing experience, longer patch reconstructions were performed. Sones' post operative angiograms showed that there was a direct relationship between the length of repair and post operative thrombosis; the longer the repair the greater the failure. Secondly, on 12 January 1962, Sones examined a patient operated on by Vineberg in Canada (1946). Using selective cannulation of the left internal mammary artery he showed that collateral circulation from the systemic artery implanted in to the myocardium was sufficient to diminish the myocardial perfusion deficit in the territory of an occluded left anterior descending coronary. As a result of these events Effler and the Cleveland Clinic were motivated towards a surgical solution to coronary artery disease.

At the Clinic Favaloro had difficulties with the authorities and could only be accepted as an observer without payment. Nevertheless Effler cut through the red tape and put Favaloro to work in his unit. At the time the Department of Thoracic Surgery consisted of Effler and his partner, Harry Groves, with a senior and junior resident. Most of the routine work was lung or oesophageal surgery. Only 3 or 4 open cardiac procedures were performed each week.

Favaloro was put to work in the intensive care unit and helped clean, siliconize and assemble the enormous heart-lung machine and Kay-Cross oxygenator. From the beginning Favaloro spent time with Sones and Shirey, who had by then performed hundreds of coronary angiograms with a degree of precision exclusive to the Cleveland Clinic. While the basic concepts of myocardial revascularization evolved, a lasting friendship developed between Sones and Favaloro. After a few months with Sones, it became clear to Favaloro that coronary patients fell in to groups: first those with diffuse disease that involved most of the coronary branches and second, those with localised obstructions occurring mainly at the proximal segments of the coronary arteries but with good distal run-off.

Favaloro passed the Educational Council Foreign Medical Graduate Examination and eventually became Chief Resident at the Cleveland Clinic in 1964. When median sternotomy became the standard approach for most heart operations, Favaloro had the idea that both internal mammary arteries might be implanted by the Vineberg method. He discussed the idea with Sones several times, but it was suggested that necrosis might occur if the sternum was deprived of that blood supply. Reviewing the anatomy he wrote "I thought it logical to think this a senseless warning". Finally in 1966 and by that time a staff member in the Department of Thoracic and Cardiovasclar Surgery, he dissected both mammaries and implanted them in the left ventricle. The right was implanted parallel to the left anterior descending coronary and the left on the lateral wall in a tunnel beneath the branches of the circumflex coronary. He went on to perform 38 consecutive bilateral implants without mortality or significant morbidity, possibly because the patients were selected very carefully.

The assistants at these operations soon grew tired of manually retracting the sternal edges, so Favaloro designed his self-retaining retractor. Late restudies of Favaloro's modification of the Vineberg procedure showed many patients existing on a well perfused coronary collateral system with both implants patent. A parallel series of patch graft operations on the left main stem carried substantial mortality (11 deaths in 14 patients) so much so that the kidney transplant team asked if they could cross match these patients as prospective donors before surgery.

## Evolution of Coronary Angiography

Without direct visualisation of the diseased coronary arteries, effective myocardial revascularization remained only a remote possibility. However, by the end of the 1950s, the development of microvascular techniques (for surgical reconstruction of blocked vessels) stimulated efforts towards a reproducible method for coronary angiography. The first deliberate experimental attempt to x-ray the coronary arteries was in 1933 when Peter Rousthoi, of Stockholm, injected contrast medium directly into the aorta or via the carotid artery. Interest waned until 1945 when Stig Radner of Lund, Sweden, injected contrast into the ascending aorta of patients via a puncture hole in the sternum. Opacification of the coronary arteries was only moderate and serious complications in two of five patients caused him to abandon the method. In 1948 Jorge Meneses Hoyos and Carlos Comgez del Campo of Mexico City, produced images of the thoracic aorta, its brachiocephalic branches and the coronary arteries. They used intra-aortic injection of 30 ml contrast medium through a needle inserted via the second intercostal space to the left of the sternum.

Retrograde transarterial catheterisation of the heart began in the 1940s, but was initially abandoned because of arterial spasm. In 1946 Pedro Farinas of Havana, catheterised the aorta via the femoral artery and obtained good contrast pictures of the abdominal aorta and iliac arteries. Retrograde arterial catheterisation was not widely adopted until Sven Seldinger of Stockholm published his technique for percutaneous catheterisation in 1953. Seldinger punctured the brachial or femoral artery with a hollow needle, then inserted a flexible guide wire through the needle and into the aorta. The catheter was threaded over the guide wire, which was withdrawn to allow the catheter to be manipulated safely to its destination. The advantage of this method was that catheters the size of a needle could be used to gain access to the cardiac chambers.

In 1952, the Italians, Lucio de Guglielmo and Mariano Guttadauro, working in Stockholm, passed a catheter through the radial artery into the ascending aorta. They then injected contrast, which they claimed would provide 100% imaging of the coronary arteries. At that time it was thought necessary to slow, or even stop, blood flow in the arteries whilst contrast was injected. Temporary cardiac arrest was induced by injection of acetyl choline and methods sought to block the aorta above the coronary arteries. An occlusive inflatable balloon catheter was used in an early attempt to obtain satisfactory opacifications of the coronaries.

In 1962, Sones and Shirey, of the Cleveland Clinic, achieved (by accident) direct and reproducible catheterisation of the coronary arteries. Using the brachial arterial approach under x-ray control, they manipulated a catheter into the coronary ostia and injected between 2 and 5 ml of contrast whilst watching the image intensifier. A permanent record was taken on cinefilm at 60 frames per second. By demonstrating the site of coronary occlusion, this method added a new dimension to coronary artery surgery and opened the way for direct arterial revascularization. To quote Floyd Loop, "Collectively, all of the cardiological advances in this century pale in comparison with this priceless achievement." In the early 1960s selective coronary angiography was carried out and if a major branch of the left coronary was occluded, a left internal mammary artery was implanted into the muscle of this territory. If a major branch of the right coronary was diseased, a right internal mammary artery implant was undertaken. If both vessels were occluded, bilateral Vineberg procedures were performed. When atheroma was localised to the coronary ostia, these were attacked directly through the aorta. If the patient had widespread coronary disease deemed unsuitable for internal mammary implants, thoracic sympathectomy was employed. However as a leading article in the British Medical Journal in 1967 concluded, "No operation has yet been shown to increase the patient's expectation of life". Inevitably, the results of this type of surgery were difficult to assess, as the natural history of coronary disease varied greatly. One patient might suffer acute myocardial infarction and die suddenly, with no previous history of angina. Another patient might have stable angina for many years or suffer an acute myocardial infarction and be alive, well and active 20 years later.

## Direct Myocardial Revascularization

It was only a matter of time before the suggestion arose to operate directly on the coronary arteries to achieve normal flow. Alexis Carrell (1910) had performed experimental vascular grafts between the descending aorta and left main coronary artery. He suggested that an operation of this nature might find a place in the treatment of angina when the ostia of the coronary arties were calcified; at this stage, the cause was usually syphilis. Direct vascular surgery remained primitive until 1945, when Gross and Crafoord independently described resection of coarctation of the aorta with end-to-end anastomosis. In 1953, Gordon Murray reported (at a congress in Lisbon) that he had resected the diseased part of the left anterior descending coronary artery in five patients and had replaced it with a vascular graft. This was done after experimental work on dogs, but without the benefit of coronary angiography. He used the internal mammary, the axillary or the carotid artery as the graft. In Russia, Vladimir Demikhov worked along similar lines, by joining the left internal mammary artery of dogs to their left anterior descending coronary a few millimetres beyond the origin. In 1955 he developed the operation further in experiments on human cadavers and live baboons. He then devised a three-way plastic tube to connect the internal mammary artery to two coronary branches beyond their obstruction. As usual, reports of Demikhov's pioneering work did not reach the West until after the initial clinical and experimental successes of Murray and Lillehei.

In 1956 Lillehei gave an account of two experimental procedures for coronary disease. On human cadavers he performed endarterectomy and on dogs he repeated Murray's type of anastomosis, using a plastic prosthetic tube to join the subvlavian artery to the circumflex branch of the left coronary. The latter method was largely unsuccessful due to thrombosis within the prosthetic graft. He therefore proceeded to attempt direct anastomosis between the left internal carotid or internal mammary artery to the circumflex coronary. Many of these grafts remained patent, but at the time Lillehei did not translate the work into clinical practice.

Angelo May working with Charles Bailey in Philadelphia, experimented with endarterectomy on human cadaver hearts. He passed a special instrument beyond the atheroma and pulled back to cut and remove the blockage. When he attempted to reproduce the procedure in dogs (by stripping off part of the vessel lining), all the animals developed thrombosis at the site of intervention. Soon afterwards, Bailey carried out the first human coronary endarterectomy (29 October 1956) by incising the coronary artery itself at a point beyond the blockage and passing a curette retrogradely through the vessel. The 51-year old patient was given heparin to prevent thrombosis and made a satisfactory recovery. Encouraged by this Bailey performed seven similar operations, with survival and symptomatic improvement in each case. Remarkably, these initial operations were undertaken without cardiopulmonary bypass. Because of the obvious technical limitations, Bailey subsequently changed to a direct approach through the aorta and coronary ostium using the Gibbon pump oxygenator. Without the benefit of coronary angiography, these procedures were largely based on the pathological principles outlined by Monroe Schlesinger of Beth Israel Hospital, Boston. In 1940 Schlesinger worked with cadaver hearts to characterise the zones of coronary occlusion by comparing radiographs with dissection. He found that most zones of coronary occlusion were less than 5 mm long and occurred within 3 mm of the ostia of the main coronary arteries. Bailey suggested that endarterectomy should be restricted to well localised short segments of coronary artery. In practice, this occurs in less than 20% of coronary artery patients.

Coronary endarterectomy or segmental excision with saphenous vein or internal mammary artery grafts were performed in the late 1950s before cardiopulmonary bypass came into widespread use. Longmire recalls the first direct anastomosis between the left internal mammary artery and the right coronary in 1958: "At the time we were doing the coronary thromboendarterectomy procedure and we also performed a couple of the earliest internal mammary to coronary anastomoses. We were forced into it when the coronary artery we were endarterectomising disintegrated and in desperation we anastomosed the left internal mammary artery to the distal end of the right coronary artery and later decided it was a good operation."

From Bailey's early work, it was apparent that when the endarterectomy passed across the mouth of a branch, the sheared-off atheroma detached from the main channel and tended to retract, form a clot and occlude. A death from this cause stimulated Senning to open the coronaries more extensively, peel out the diseased areas under direct vision and avoid the important side branches. The arteriotomy was then enlarged using a vein patch along the length of the incision. For this procedure, Senning used cardiopulmonary bypass at 23°C and closed the incisions with saphenous vein taken from the ankle.

For a short time, Bailey considered that emergency thromboendarterectomy might be used for treatment of acute myocardial infarction. He proposed that with cardiopulmonary bypass, the patient might undergo removal of the thrombus and endarterectomy of the atheromatous narrowing. He also reasoned that preoperative angiography was unnecessary, since the affected artery could be readily identified from the site of myocardial infarction. In 1963, George Nardi and Robert Shaw, of Harvard Medical School, reported four patients in whom they attempted this procedure. All died and the operation was never widely adopted.

Sabiston first employed aortocoronary saphenous vein bypass in 1962, during a re-operation. He made an end-to-end vein to right coronary artery anastomosis. Unfortunately, the patient died 3 days later of cerebral complications. Probably the first successful saphenous vein bypass graft was by Edward Garrett (1964) whilst he was working with DeBakey. He performed the bypass graft in order to wean a patient from cardiopulmonary bypass, and the long term result of the procedure was not reported until 10 years later.

It was the work of René Favaloro, at the Cleveland Clinic and Dudley Johnson in Milwaukee, beginning in 1967, that launched the widespread application of coronary artery surgery.

The possibility of studying the pathological anatomy of coronary arteries by cine-arteriography was the springboard for Favaloro's coronary bypass procedures. The idea of working directly on the coronary arteries in patients with severe localised proximal obstructions, but with good distal run-off encouraged Favaloro to attempt bypass of the obstruction. At first pericardial and venous-patch graft repairs in segmental localised obstructions were used. A single longitudinal incision was performed through the obstruction and the lumen of the artery enlarged by patch closure. Although occasionally successful in patients with a sharply localised obstruction of the right coronary artery, its application to the left coronary artery was seldom successful, with an operative mortality of 65%. In patients who needed long segmental reconstructions (2-4cm) the patch graft was a tedious task and the irregular surface left inside the artery produced turbulence and thrombosis.

Early experience with saphenous femoropopliteal bypasses and renal artery reconstruction, led Favaloro to think that if saphenous grafts worked in the distal circulation why not in the coronary arteries close to the ascending aorta, with high flow and high pressure! In May 1967 his colleague David Fergusson, referred a 51 year old woman who had had typical angina pectoris for 3 years. Selective cine-coronary angiography showed that the right coronary artery was totally occluded in the proximal third. The left coronary artery did not have significant occlusive disease and through collateral filling the distal portion of the right coronary artery appeared normal. Sones and Favaloro decided to begin with this patient with a completely occluded right coronary since failure of the reconstruction was unlikely to result in fatality. On 7 May, Favaloro resected the occluded portion of the artery and performed a saphenous vein interposition graft. Angiography eight days later showed excellent flow in the resected vessel. Recatheterised 10 years later, the graft and right coronary artery were patent. However, after a few operations using only interposed saphenous grafts, the technique showed certain limitations and he turned to the concept of aorto-coronary saphenous vein bypass grafts.

A bypass from the anterolateral wall of the aorta to the distal end of a resected segment using end to end anastomosis was attempted in 15 patients before this was changed to an end to side anastomosis with the coronary distal to the blockage. This was simpler and soon became the enduring technique.

After this initial success several substantial advances took place in 1968. Aorto-coronary bypass with saphenous vein was applied to the left coronary. The first operation was performed on a patient with obstruction of the left main stem but minimal distal disease in the left anterior descending or circumflex branches. A single vein graft to the proximal segment of the left anterior descending coronary showed excellent perfusion of the entire left coronary tree on postoperative angiography. Left main coronary obstruction could then be treated and coronary bypass was combined with left ventricular aneurysmectomy and valve replacement.

By the end of 1968, Favaloro had accumulated a series of 171 patients who had undergone direct myocardial revascularization. After that first full year, they knew that saphenous vein bypass grafts had a future. The concept of coronary artery bypass surgery developed by Favaloro was expanded from a single saphenous vein bypass of the right coronary artery to procedures involving the left coronary artery, to double and triple bypass procedures and mammary artery bypass procedures.

Although, as Mason Sones said, twentieth century cardiology could be divided into the pre-Favaloro and the post-Favaloro era, at the time it was difficult for Favaloro to persuade his colleagues. Nevertheless, he persisted in spite of their lack of confidence and disbelief expressed at different national meetings and at visits to hospitals. One of the main reasons for skepticism was that previous myocardial revascularization attempts had been performed in that "twilight zone" – where there was no objective demonstration that the surgeons' approach had changed the ischemic myocardium. In 1968, Favaloro already knew that this was an operation that could be performed efficiently with a well-defined technique, a very low mortality rate, and with excellent postoperative results. During the early days, some doctors simply did not believe the operative mortality – always below 5% - and their skepticism led them to doubt the truth of the statistics.

Direct anastomosis of the internal mammary artery to an obstructed coronary artery was described by Kolessov in 1967 and by George E. Green in 1968. Green worked on experimental microvascular suture anastomosis and demonstrated the potential for direct mammary artery to coronary artery anastomosis under the operating microscope. He recognised that suture of the internal mammary artery directly to a coronary arteriotomy should offer substantially more benefit than intramyocardial implantation. Green spent many hours examining hearts at the New York City Mortuary to convince himself and others that the distal segments of diseased coronary arteries were usually free from atheroma and greater than 1 mm in diameter. He practised mammary artery anastomosis to canine coronary arteries and demonstrated that these could sustain cardiac function. In February 1968, David Tice, Director of Surgery at the New York Veterans Administration Hospital, encouraged Green to proceed with a human bypass graft. The successful early operations were presented as footnotes to the experimental data published in Annals of Thoracic Surgery (May 1968).

Soon afterwards, it became clear that this new form of revascularization offered substantial benefits over previous therapeutic modalities, particularly for intractable angina.

When bypass grafting was performed in cases of angina that were unresponsive to medical management, symptoms were relieved in most cases. Widespread adoption of coronary revascularization came from 1968 onwards, with improvements in cardiopulmonary bypass and cardioplegic arrest. These facilitated the coronary anastomosis and provided the stimulus for a dramatic increase in the number and complexity of procedures.

Within a short time, following the experimental contributions of Cox and others, Favaloro proceeded to apply coronary bypass to acute myocardial infarction. On the first occasion a patient awaiting elective coronary surgery at the Bolton Square Hotel across the street from the clinic was reported to be suffering from severe, persistent central chest pain. The coronary angiogram had previously shown subtotal occlusion of the proximal left anterior descending coronary. Favaloro rushed to see the patient who was sweating, dyspnoeic and hypertensive. The electrocardiogram confirmed extensive anterolateral myocardial injury. Favaloro rapidly discussed the patient with Mason Sones and decided to proceed with emergency revascularization. This was performed uneventfully and the patient recovered function in the ischemic segment. The post operative left ventriculogram demonstrated only a small area of impaired wall motion and normal left ventricular end diastolic pressure. The graft was patent.

Within a year Favaloro and Sones had reported 18 impending myocardial infarctions and 11 acute infarctions treated by coronary bypass in the American Journal of Cardiology. They concluded that when surgery is performed within six hours of acute myocardial infarction most of the heart muscle can be preserved. The first double bypass to the right and left anterior descending coronaries was undertaken in December 1968, though a double interposition operation had been performed in March that year. These advances are summarised in the Journal of Thoracic and Cardiovascular Surgery as presented. Others soon adopted Favaloro's methods. In particular, Dudley Johnson of Milwaukee showed that grafts could be placed in distal segments of the coronary tree.

In 1970 endarterectomy was combined with coronary bypass either by the simple mechanical methods described by Groves, or by carbon dioxide gas endarterectomy as described by Soya. In the same year Favaloro began to use direct internal mammary to coronary artery anastomosis as developed by George Green of New York. By June 1970, 1086 bypasses had been performed with an overall mortality of 4.2%. Coronary anastomoses were performed with interrupted sutures, a method which has persisted at the Cleveland Clinic since that time.

Favaloro was invited to attend the 6th World Congress of Cardiology in London during 1970 and Donald Ross invited him to perform coronary surgery at the National Heart Hospital. During the first operating, after opening the right coronary and placing the first stitch, the scrub nurse accidentally pulled the vein off and tore the vessel. At least she did not drop the vein!

It was during the Congress in London that a large delegation from Argentina asked Favaloro to return home. Consequently in October 1970 Favaloro wrote a letter of resignation to Effler and pointed out that his work could be continued by the outstanding residents, Loop and Cheanvechai. Favaloro's decision to leave the Cleveland Clinic caused great sadness particularly to Mason Sones. Favaloro told his colleagues that he would leave at the beginning of July 1971 but he accepted an invitation to lecture in Boston in June and flew straight home to Argentina.

It transpired that Favaloro's first saphenous vein bypass operation was proceeded by that of Garrett in November 1964. Garrett was trying to perform a patch repair of a localised obstruction in the left anterior descending coronary and resorted to a vein graft for complications. Garrett eventually published this case in 1973 by which time thousands of operations had been performed in Cleveland and other centres in the United States. When Donald Effler left the Cleveland Clinic, Floyd Loop became Chief of Cardiac Surgery and with others (notably Delos Cosgrove and Bruce Lytle) created one of the largest cardiac surgical centres in the world, and certainly the best known for research and development in coronary artery surgery.

## Surgery of Left Ventricular Aneurysm

Bailey was the first surgeon to excise a post infarction left ventricular aneurysm. The 56 year old man was operated on 15 months after sustaining a large anterolateral myocardial infarction (15 April 1954). Bailey approached the pericardium through a left sixth interspace thoracotomy and dissected away the pericardial adhesions from "a smooth ovid bulge" involving the entire anterior wall of the left ventricle. Without cardiopulmonary bypass, he applied a large sideclamp to the aneurysm, which resulted in immediate improvement in cardiac ejection. He then applied a continuous suture beneath the clamp, followed by a series of interrupted mattress sutures. Then tentatively removing the clamp, the aneurysm was slowly cut away and the raw edges closed over with a third layer of sutures. The patient survived and remained in good health 3 years later.

In 1957, Bailey reported on nine patients after left ventricular aneurysmectomy; eight survived and were much improved. The single failure was due to thromboembolism and stroke, through dislodging clots in the aneurysm wall. Bailey learned to avoid damage to the mitral subvalvar apparatus by inserting a finger into the left ventricle. He also emphasised that it was unnecessary to attempt to remove all scar tissue and important to restore the left ventricle to as near normal size and shape as possible. Bailey's closed technique for ventricular aneurysm excision was soon superseded by the operation on cardiopulmonary bypass. On 17 January 1958, Cooley at Baylor, Houston used cardiopulmonary bypass to excise an aneurysm in a 50 year old male. This patient had sustained a myocardial infarction 3 months previously and his aneurysm was full of blood clot. For this patient there was a risk of massive embolus. The open technique allowed the thrombus to be removed, after which the aneurysm was excised and the ventricle repaired with a clear view of the internal structures. Lillehei followed with the same operation soon afterwards.

## The Early Clinical Trials

Although it is now known that 85% of patients with severe or unstable angina are relieved of symptoms, early and widespread acceptance of coronary bypass was delayed by clinical trails in stable angina that compared surgery with improving medical treatment. The trials were also designed to permit surgery in any individual who developed problematic angina, a situation that led to crossover in 25-40% of patients in the medial arms of most major trials. Another confounding factor was the rapid improvement in all aspects of management of coronary disease. Revascularization techniques improved dramatically after the late 1960s, with the development of cold potassium cardioplegia, oxygenated blood cardioplegia, retrograde cardioplegia, multiple dose cardioplegia, use of the internal mammary artery and intra-aortic balloon pumping for cardiac support. Medical treatment improved with the introduction of beta-receptor and calcium-channel blockers, documentation of the efficacy of nitrates and recognition of the importance of thrombotic occlusion and thrombolysis in ischemic heart disease. The best known cooperative studies (conducted in the 1970s and early 1980s) were the Veterans' Administration (VA) Cooperative study, the Coronary Artery Surgery Study (CASS) and the European Coronary Surgery Study. All were multicenter efforts to examine the efficacy of coronary artery bypass grafting versus medical treatment, in stable clinical situations.

## The Veterans' Administration Cooperative Study

The VA Cooperative Study screened more than 5000 patients between January 1970 and December 1974. Of these, 686 were entered into the final phase of the study. Ninety patients had severe left main coronary disease and 596 had multiple vessel disease. Patients were randomly assigned to medical or surgical management. The majority of all surgical patients received saphenous vein grafts and operative mortality was 5.6%. When patients were stratified according to the number of vessels grafted, operative mortality at 30 days was 0% for single vessel disease, 6.1% for two vessels and 7.3% for three vessels. Graft angiography in 84% of patients showed 69% of grafts to be patent at 10-15 months.

One of the most important findings of the VA Cooperative Study was that chronic stable angina in association with high-grade, left main coronary artery disease is a definite indication for coronary artery bypass grafting and that survival is clearly improved for this group of patients. In the 596 patients with coronary artery lesions in vessels other than the left main coronary artery, no clear short term (36 months) or long term (7 or 11 years) survival advantage was documented. At 36 months 87% of the medical group and 88% of the surgical group were alive; at 7 years 70% of the medical group and 77% of the surgical group were alive. Nevertheless, a statistically significant difference in survival was found for patients in two high-risk subgroups: patients with three vessel coronary artery disease and impaired left ventricular function; and those with prior myocardial infarction, hypertension or resting ST depression on the ECG. Only 52% of patients with three vessel disease and impaired ventricular function were alive at 7 years when treated medically, compared to 76% in those treated surgically; at 11 years, survival was 37% and 50% respectively. Survival at 7 years in those with two of the three clinical risk factors (hypertension, previously myocardial infarction and resting ST depression) was better if treated surgically than medically. Patients who fulfilled criteria for both high risk subgroups had the largest benefit from surgery (76% versus 36% survival at 7 years, and 54% versus 24% at 11 years)

# The CASS Study

CASS was a multicenter, North American investigation which enrolled patients from August 1975 to May 1979. It assessed the effects of coronary surgery on mortality and selected non-fatal endpoints. The register included 24,959 patients who underwent coronary angiography during the enrolment period. Of this group, 33% were recruited from study centres that did not participate in the final randomised study, or they were studied in a pilot trial only; 16,626 patients were screened for entry into the randomised trial. Subsequently, subjects were excluded from randomization if they had normal, minimal, or non-operable disease by angiography; class III or class IV angina; left main coronary artery disease; prior coronary bypass grafting; congestive heart failure; or were older than 65.

After all exclusions, only 780 patients were randomized to medical or surgical therapy. Not surprizingly mortality in both groups was low. Annual mortality rates in the surgical arm were 0.7%, 1.0% and 1.55% for patients with single, double and triple vessel disease, respectively. Mortality in the medial group was remarkably low, at 2.4%, 1.2% and 2.1% for single, double and triple vessel disease, indicating the rather benign nature of this type of coronary disease. No statistical difference was noted at 5 years between medical and surgical survival, although 5% of the medical group underwent coronary artery bypass grafting for amelioration of progressive symptoms. These patients remained in the medical group for data analysis. Of the 160 patients with ejection fractions of less than 0.5 and three vessel disease, survival was better (although not statistically) in the surgical arm at 7 years. Those with triple vessel disease and ejection fractions higher than 0.34 but lower than 0.50 also had an improved 7 year survival with surgery when compared with medical treatment (84% versus 70%).

Non-randomized patients from the CASS trial with either class I or class II angina (who refused randomization) and those patients with class III or class IV angina, who were excluded from the study by design, were also analyzed. This showed that medical treatment of patients with class III or class IV angina, three vessel disease and normal left ventricular function produced only a 74% 5 year survival, compared with 92% for surgical treatment. Comparison of those patients with class III and class IV angina, three-vessel disease and abnormal left ventricular function revealed a 5 year survival rate of 82% with surgery, but only 52% for those treated medically. In contrast, patients with class I or class II angina and normal left ventricular function had a 5 year survival in excess of 92% with medical or surgical treatment. These later results confirmed the superiority of surgical treatment for patients with severe angina, amidst considerable skepticism based on the earlier analyses.

Another purpose of the CASS study was to examine quality of life under the two different treatments. Patients treated surgically had significantly less chest pain, fewer activity limitations and required less therapy with nitrates or beta-blockers. At 5 years, surgically treated patients had significantly longer treadmill times, less exercise-induced angina and less ST segment elevation than medically treated patients. In the U.S., these improvements in physiological findings were not reflected by an increase in employment or recreational status. This led to the policy that patients who were moderately symptomatic after infarction, or had chronic, stable angina, should be managed medically first. If symptoms worsened, or the patient became dissatisfied with his or her lifestyle, coronary artery bypass grafting was recommended. At the same time, quality of life and work status studies in the UK demonstrated considerably better rehabilitation statistics. Westaby, at the Royal Postgraduate Medical School, reported a greater than 70% return to work and increase in physical activity in chronically disabled patients with angina, including those performing heavy manual work.

## The European Coronary Surgery Study

The third major randomized trial was the European Coronary Surgery Study. This multicenter prospective randomized trial studied 768 men under the age of 65 with mild to moderate angina, 50% or greater stenosis of at least two major coronary arteries and normal left ventricular function. Results showed that coronary artery bypass grafting improve survival overall, but especially in patients with severe three vessel disease or proximal left anterior descending lesions. Surprisingly, the subgroup with left main coronary artery disease did not have a statistically significant increase in survival after surgery when compared with medical treatment. However, the numbers with left main disease were small. Symptoms (including anginal attacks, use of beta-adrenergic blockers and nitrates, and poor exercise performance) were significantly ameliorated in the surgical group at 5 years. Operative mortality was 3.6%. For patients with three vessel disease, the 5 year survival was 94% in the surgical group and 90% in the medically treated group. When an important left anterior descending stenosis was present, a 5 year survival of 92.7% was achieved with surgery, whereas only 82% of medically treated patients were alive. Both findings were statistically significant. For patients with left ventricular dysfunction and ischemic ST segment depression of greater than 1.5mm, surgery improved survival to 91.7% at 5 years, compared to 79% without surgery.

In summary, the European study documented significantly improved survival in patients with proximal left anterior descending stenosis, associated with disease in one or two other vessels, and also in those with an ECG showing ST segment depression of greater than 1.5 mm at rest.

Patients with myocardial infarction and cardiogenic shock were an especially difficult group to treat, and consequently attracted the early interest of both medical and surgical teams. With the introduction of intra-aortic balloon counterpulsation, many of these patients could be stabilized. Inability to wean the intra-aortic balloon pump was a situation in which early angiography and coronary bypass surgery improved survival. By 1973, the Massachusetts General Hospital was able to report improved 1 year survival, from 20% with balloon pumping alone to 37% with intra-aortic balloon support plus early coronary bypass grafting.

Based on these major and sometimes contradictory landmark studies, controversies surrounding indications for coronary artery surgery were inevitable. Each study had problems when compensating for important improvements in treatment and crossover from medial to surgical groups. Differences in the types of patient enrolled, particularly the relatively benign class of patient, made comparisons between the studies difficult. Nevertheless, broad clinical indications for coronary artery surgery were agreed upon and summarised by Cohen. These were: class III angina that was unresponsive to medical therapy, unstable angina, left main coronary stenosis and symptomatic patients with triple vessel disease. Relative indications were high risk subgroups, post myocardial infarction (with positive stress test at low workload) and those in cardiogenic shock.

Later single centre studies of high risk patients confirmed clear superiority of surgery over medical treatment. For those with triple vessel disease and impaired left ventricular function, the difference in survival for medical versus surgical treatment was 53% versus 89%. Coronary bypass became the most frequently performed operation in the U.S. and heralded widespread expansion in cardiac surgical facilities to cope with the commonest cause of death in adult males.

The Cleveland clinic maintained its dominance in the field through the efforts of Loop, Cosgrove, Lytle and others who performed thousands of primary and re-operative procedures. Long term follow up of their patients has formed the basis for numerous publications to define the risks and benefits of coronary surgery.

## Evolution of Coronary Angioplasty

The notion of dilating narrowed blood vessels using a balloon catheter began with Dotter, who was the first to apply the concept to lesions of the peripheral arteries.

The idea arose when he inadvertently passed an angiography catheter retrogradely though an occluded iliac artery into the abdominal aorta. This stimulated the idea of purposely enlarging stenotic arterial segments by catheter techniques. In 1964, Dotter and Judkins reported the first successful transluminal dilatation of a popliteal artery stenosis. A co-axial catheter system was used, which involved placing a small guide catheter across the stenosis followed by dilating catheters of various sizes to enlarge the narrowed area.

The "Dotter technique" was never widely accepted and initial attempts to design a balloon catheter failed through lack of appropriate materials. However in 1974 Andreas Grüntzig in Zurich produced a polyvinyl chloride balloon catheter and used it to dilate peripheral arterial stenosis, with good results.

Encouraged by his initial success, he modified the system for use in the coronary arteries and experimented with this on dogs in the autopsy room. Grüntzig and Miller then inserted the small balloon catheter intraoperatively in patients undergoing coronary artery surgery, and demonstrated that human coronary narrowings could be enlarged in the same way. By 1977 the catheter system had been refined sufficiently to allow percutaneous use in humans, and on 16 September, the first percutaneous coronary artery dilatation was performed in Zurich. In 1978 Grüntzig published the results of the first five patients.

Clearly the prospect of dilating coronary atheroma by a percutaneous catheter method had widespread appeal for both the interventional cardiologist and the patient who might avoid surgery. Coronary angioplasty was adopted widely, particularly for the treatment of isolated single and then double vessel coronary stenosis.

Improvements in balloon technology and the developments of atherectomy (laser and mechanical) and intracoronary stents has greatly increased the scope of catheter techniques. As a result, coronary artery bypass surgery is now reserved for cases of increasing difficulty and an ever increasing number of patients requiring re-operation.

# The Resurrection of Less Invasive Coronary Bypass

There is seldom logic in sequence of scientific or surgical development, and significant advances are often recycled. Whilst improved operating conditions with cardioplegic arrest provided the stimulus for an explosion in surgical myocardial revascularization, recent years have witnessed a swing back to the so-called "less invasive" techniques. Coronary bypass is undertaken without opening a cardiac chamber, and consequently it is not necessary to divert blood from within the heart. With continued ventilation of the lungs and unimpaired blood flow there is no need for a pump oxygenator. The only technical requirement for coronary bypass is a bloodless anastomotic field, which can be achieved by temporary coronary occlusion whilst the circulation is supported through uninterrupted cardiac action.

When emerging technology stifled attempts to operate on the beating heart a few surgeons persisted. Ankeney (1972) described 143 patients in whom cardiopulmonary bypass was not used. Buffolo, from Saõ Paulo, Brazil reported coronary bypass by simple interruption of coronary flow (1985) and in the same year, Benetti from Buenos Aires, described 700 operations. Benetti's experience, which now includes more than 2000 cases, was stimulated by limited resources. In Argentina, non pump coronary surgery allowed a substantially greater throughput of patients than would otherwise have been possible. Post operative angiography showed no difference in graft patency between bypass and non bypass patients when the saphenous vein or the internal mammary artery were used.

Others followed the lead of Benetti and Buffolo in a range of selective, emergency and re-operative coronary operations. Pfister, of the Washing Hospital Centre, reported 220 operations without cardiopulmonary bypass, comparing the outcome with 220 conventional operations matched for number of grafts, left ventricular function and date of operation. He concluded that for selected patients with disease of the left anterior descending and right coronary arteries, coronary bypass could be performed successfully without extracorporeal circulation. Also, that left ventricular function was better preserved than after cold cardioplegic arrest.

The superior preservation of left ventricular function in non pump patients despite periods of unprotected regional ischemia is persuasive. Akins, from the Massachusetts General Hospital, performed a comparative study of coronary operations with and without cardiopulmonary bypass. He found that post operative septal wall motion was abnormal in all cardiopulmonary bypass patients with aortic cross clamping (global ischemia). Those operated without had either no change or an improvement in septal motion after revascularization. Benetti also investigated myocardial injury by performing intra-operative left ventricular biopsies and showed superior preservation of the mitochondria in non bypass patients. Collectively the data from these groups suggested that non-pump coronary operations were safe, avoided the damaging effects of cardiopulmonary bypass and were advantageous, particularly for those with impaired ventricular function or a wish to avoid blood transfusion. Increasing experience of non pump coronary bypass through a median sternotomy then led to the concept of minimally invasive coronary bypass. Benetti, Calafiore, Subramanian and others then achieved direct anastomosis between the left internal mammary artery and the left anterior descending coronary through a 10cm incision in the 4$^{th}$ left intercostal space. Fonger demonstrated the feasibility of the subxiphoid approach for anastomosis of the gasto-epiploic artery to the posterior descending branch of the right coronary. These procedures, whilst of limited use in routine coronary surgery, are useful for re-operations and in high risk patients where sternotomy and cardiopulmonary bypass are deleterious. Videoscopic harvest of the internal mammary artery, new types of instrument and chest wall retractors together with pharmacological slowing of cardiac action have been introduced to facilitate this new approach.

## Transmyocardial Laser Revascularization

The 1990s brought increased expectations from patients and a demand for treatment from those previously regarded as inoperable. With an increasingly elderly population, the number of patients with severe diffuse coronary disease or occluded vein grafts (but preserved left ventricular function) expanded rapidly. Transmyocardial laser revascularization (TMR) was introduced to treat patients with medically and surgically refractory angina and has been applied to cardiac transplant patients with severe diffuse graft atherosclerosis where conventional revascularization is untenable. The procedure involves firing a laser through the epicardial surface of the myocardium to drill channels and connect intra-myocardial sinusoids with the left ventricular cavity. Initial work by Frazier and Cooley at the Texas Heart Institute, and Cohn at Brigham and Women's Hospital, Boston provided anecdotal reports of dramatic relief of markedly debilitating angina. A multicentre trial sponsored by the Food and Drug Administration then demonstrated reproducible relief of angina, though experimental observations suggest that most laser channels occlude early and little myocardial blood flow originates from the left ventricle. Clinical improvement may reflect enhancement of coronary collateral circulation and the future role of the method remains to be defined.

## Reference

Westaby S. Landmarks in Cardiac Surgery. Isis Medical Media, Oxford.

In: Off-Pump Coronary Artery Bypass Grafting
Editors: Shahzad G. Raja and Mohamed Amrani

ISBN: 978-1- 62081-549-6
© 2012 Nova Science Publishers, Inc.

*Chapter II*

# History of Off-Pump Coronary Artery Bypass Grafting

*Fhilipe O. Prybicz[1], Joao C. C. Pereira[2] and Paulo R. Soltoski[2]*

[1]Hospital Universitário Evangélico de Curitiba
[2]Hospital Universitario Evangelico de Curitiba e Hospital de Clínicas da Universidade Federal do Paraná, Curitiba, Brazil

## Abstract

Surgical myocardial revascularization on the beating heart termed off-pump coronary artery bypass (OPCAB) grafting predated coronary artery grafting with the assistance of cardiopulmonary bypass. After the advent of the heart-lung machine, OPCAB operations were virtually abandoned, with a few exceptions. Over the past two decades OPCAB has been reinvented predominantly due to the realization that surgery on cardiopulmonary bypass may be associated with unwanted side effects that may result in suboptimal outcomes for the increasingly high-risk patient groups currently being referred for coronary artery bypass surgery. This chapter presents the historical background of the development of OPCAB.

## Introduction

The history of off-pump coronary artery bypass (OPCAB) grafting will take us back to the first Nobel Prize ever received by a scientist practicing in the United States. Alexis Carrell was honored with this prize in 1912 thanks to his magnificent contributions to cardiovascular and transplant surgery.

Since Carrell's experiments on vascular anastomosis, hundreds of surgeons around the world have engaged in the most exciting and evolving area of cardiovascular surgery, OPCAB grafting.

Goetz, Murray, Pronin, Sabiston, Kolesov, Favaloro and Green were only a few of the mentors of this advance in cardiac surgery since Gibbons' heart-lung machine.

OPCAB can be summarized as "one's search for the best method of myocardial revascularization while causing the least amount of adverse effects".

On-pump CABG, still considered as gold standard in many centers around the world, will soon become history! It will give place to a multidisciplinary initial approach, capable of offering coronary disease patients the best of all treatment modalities combined. Robotics, hybrid operating rooms and newer endoscopic materials are just some of the tools we will be utilizing in this new era of coronary artery disease treatment.

## Emergence and Evolution of Off-Pump Coronary Artery Bypass Grafting

Adam Hammer hypothesized that heart attacks could only occur if at least one coronary artery was obstructed, and in 1876 this German physician from Mannheim, living in Saint Louis, identified the role of coronary thrombosis in the causation of myocardial infarction [1].

Seminal reasonings such as in Hammer's own words "I mentioned my convictions to my colleague at the bedside. He, however, had a nonplussed expression and burst out, 'I have never heard of such a diagnosis in my live' and I answered, ' Nor I also'"; paved the initial steps for the diagnosis and treatment of myocardial ischemia [1].

History of myocardial revascularization goes back to the very beginning of the 20th century, when Alexis Carrell, attempting to perform an anastomosis between the descending aorta and a coronary artery of a dog, implanted a segment of carotid artery, and launched the search for methods of providing adequate blood flow to the ischemic heart. For his work on vessel transplantation and sutures, he was awarded the first Nobel Prize ever given to the United States, in 1912 [2].

Nearly twenty years later, in Cleveland, the Professor of Neurosurgery at the Western Reserve School of Medicine, Claude Beck, in an attempt to improve myocardial perfusion, suggested suturing different structures to the heart, such as pericardial fat, omentum or even the chest wall muscles to a scarified myocardium. His work was published in 1935 [3].

Beck's attempt to improve myocardial blood flow was based on a post-mortem report from Thorel (1903), in which a patient with longstanding proximal occlusion of both coronary arteries, was found to have dense vascular adhesions of tissues around his heartwhich were capable of keeping him alive [3].

Although Beck's operation was a genuine attempt towards myocardial revascularization, and was successfully performed on a 48-year-old man who became asymptomatic within one year of surgery. It would still take another decade for a different and yet successful procedure to be described [3].

Arthur Vineberg, in 1946, dissected and implanted the left internal mammary artery (LIMA) to a tunnel in the anterior left myocardial wall, and after several years of experimental work at McGill University, he finally performed this procedure in a man in 1950 [4,5].

His procedure, whose excellent patency was later demonstrated by coronary angiography by Sones, in 1962, is nowadays considered the first successful attempt at surgical revascularization of the heart [6].

The search for a better procedure continued with Gordon Murray in Canada and Vladimir P. Demikhov in Russia. These surgeons independently and almost simultaneously performed, in 1953, the first myocardial revascularizations anastomosing the LIMA to a coronary artery in dogs. These dogs remained alive for several months after these procedures [7,8].

In 1953, John Gibbon performed a successful closure of an atrial septal defect in an 18 year-old girl, utilizing the Model II, a cardiopulmonary bypass machine he had developed himself. The patient was Cecilia Bavolek, and this operation laid the foundation of modern cardiac surgery.

Dr. Gibbon's work of a lifetime was finally showing its clinical applications [9].

In 1960, Robert H. Goetz performed the world's first successful clinical CABG in humans, but this single case was only reported a year later as an addendum to a series of experimental procedures in dogs [10].

In 1962, David Sabiston performed a saphenous vein bypass to the right coronary artery (RCA), but unfortunately his patient suffered complications, surviving only a few days after surgery [11].

Also in 1962, Pronin performed successfully CABG in dogs using suture technique and a small device that would allow continuous coronary blood flow during the construction of the anastomosis. Pronin's principles of coronary perfusion are still applied today in OPCAB surgery [12].

Vasilii I. Kolesov, a careful observer of the experimental work of Demikhov, Murray, Goetz and Pronin, began his own experiments with myocardial revascularization in dogs [13].

His initial experience with dogs was not promising because a short occlusion of coronary flow would lead to ventricular fibrillation and death. Aware of the successful experimental work by Pronin, who used a collapsible cannula in dogs to provide continuous blood flow into a coronary artery, Kolesov constructed his own cannula, and his subsequent reports showed better results [14].

Eight dogs underwent follow-up for as long as 19 months, and the patency of the anastomoses was demonstrated in all animals. He performed Vineberg's procedures in some patients and also ligated both internal mammary arteries in others in an attempt to treat coronary insufficiency in those patients [15,16].

On 25 February 1964, Kolesov performed the first successful beating heart LIMA to left anterior descending artery, in Leningrad. He performed this procedure in several other patients, publishing his experience in Russia in 1965 and in the Journal of Thoracic and Cardiovascular Surgery in 1967 [14].

Garrett and DeBakey, also in 1964, performed a saphenous vein bypass to the left anterior descending (LAD) coronary artery, but would only report this case several years later, with good long term result [17].

Rene Favaloro, in November 1967, would perform his first myocardial revascularization as a variation of a planned right coronary artery endarterectomy. The procedure was a saphenous vein interposition graft to the right coronary artery, and although the cardiopulmonary bypass machine was installed, the procedure was performed on a beating heart [18].

At that moment, Favaloro, who had been a staff member at The Cleveland Clinic for two years, was performing a variation of Vineberg's procedure, dissecting and implanting both internal thoracic arteries to the left myocardium with good results, whereas patch graft repairs of coronary arteries, whose results were not as encouraging, were the current method of myocardial revascularization.

After Favaloro's coronary artery bypass with the saphenous vein, the patch graft procedures to the left main coronary proximal lesions were slowly being set aside since they carried significant mortality [19].

By this time, myocardial revascularization under cardiopulmonary bypass was steadily gaining worldwide utilization, and the very next year, 1968, Charles Bailey performed his first OPCAB operation in the United States, whereas George Green, in the same year, would perform his first on-pump CABG [20].

Kolesov was so ahead of his time, that from 1964 to 1974, his service was perhaps the only one performing routine off-pump myocardial revascularization. His understanding of the damage caused by the inflammatory reaction of cardiopulmonary bypass resulted in less than 18% of the patients being operated on pump by his group at that time [21,22].

Kolesov's device for continuous autoperfusion, devised for his experimental work with dogs would not be utilized in humans. He had noticed that the ischemic myocardium of humans was significantly more resilient to the brief ischemic period caused by coronary artery snaring for the procedure.

In 1967, Kolesov performed the first successful stapled anastomosis of the internal mammary artery to a coronary artery, and the patient was well after a three-year follow-up. His understanding of the need for better surgical techniques and instruments led to the creation of a coronary stapling device as well as very delicate scissors and magnifying glasses he utilized for CABG procedures [23].

Ankeney, in 1972, described 143 patients successfully operated on without cardiopulmonary bypass, but it was only after a latent period of approximately ten years that surgeons began to show some interest in the off-pump revascularization strategy [24].

In the early 1980s, two surgical groups independently started to perform routine off-pump myocardial revascularizations, Benetti's group in Argentina and Buffolo's in Brazil. Their procedures were performed mostly to the anteriorly located arteries of the heart, such as the LAD, the RCA and some diagonals.

From October 1980 to April 1983, Benetti had performed 30 coronary revascularizations off-pump. His selection criteria were good caliber vessels that were anteriorly located in the heart. No deaths or perioperative myocardial infarctions were observed in this series. But only 7% of Benetti's patients were candidates for off-pump surgery at the time [25].

Simultaneously and independently, Buffolo in Brazil collected 68 patients, from October 1981 to July 1982, and utilizing selection criteria similar to Benetti's, reported excellent results [26].

Buffolo, Benetti and several other surgeons worldwide demonstrated that off-pump revascularization was a promising procedure.

Off-pump CABG by avoiding cardiac arrest, introduction of cannulae into the ascending aortic arch and the heart-lung machine is regarded by several as the "ideal myocardial revascularization". However, the decade of the 1980's saw the proponents of OPCAB struggling to keep alive the "ideal myocardial revascularization" with several studies being published comparing the advantages and disadvantages of on and off-pump myocardial revascularization.

The inflammatory response, for instance, was one of the studied variables, and it was found to be reduced in off-pump coronary artery bypass considering there was less activation of inflammatory mediators and apparently reduced morbidity when compared to conventional CABG. Other areas of concern were the neurologic outcome, the pulmonary function, bleeding and blood requirement, differences in morbidity and mortality and in all these areas OPCAB showed some advantages over on-pump surgey [27-34].

As OPCAB matured as an established procedure, larger studies began to appear reporting more detailed outcomes with little differences found in the long term outcomes of on-pump and off-pump patients. The fact surgeons were able to observe in real time the myocardial contractility of the grafted area during off-pump surgery perhaps accounted for the lower incidence of perioperative myocardial infarctions in the off-pump revascularizations, since contractility deficits can be promptly identified and addressed, and myocardial necrosis markers confirm these findings [28].

## Technical Advances

One of the major limiting factors precluding the widespread utilization of off-pump CABG had always been the concern most surgeons had about the risks of incomplete revascularization.

Technical advances regarding exposure and stabilization allied to progressive confidence in the performance of procedure with tackling of learning curve have demonstrated that complete revascularization can be achieved in the majority of cases. The modern combination of robotics, computer enhanced endoscopic manipulation and anastomotic devices will simplify even more the future of complete revascularization as Balkthy has demonstrated in his 120 case-experience with excellent results utilizing the Flux A device [29].

The three limiting factors to an ideal surgical field in OPCAB are adequate exposure, blood flow and motion. Addressing each one separately simplifies the discussion of the off-pump cardiac surgery as we know today.

The first concern has been cardiac motion, as one would find it impossible to reproduce the same quality of anastomosis as that obtained on-pump if the target vessel is constantly moving.

The first devices utilized where in fact proximal and distal snares made of suture material that would be retracted and thus elevate the area to be grafted. Although feasible, this procedure could cause intimal fractures, particularly in severely atherosclerotic coronary vessels [26,35,36].

The medical industry invested heavily in the development of stabilization devices and several different models were tested. Initial prototypes applied a fork-like structure. When it was pressed against the area to be grafted, would make it motionless. Later versions substituted compression by suction, thereby resulting in less distortion of the heart and better hemodynamics.

Today we are facing endoscopic versions of the open-chest stabilizers, moving towards a fully endoscopic off-pump myocardial revascularization [37].

Once the motion issue was solved, another major concern was the adequate exposure of the posterior and lateral vessels of the heart. One of the landmarks for the adequate exposure of the heart was the posterior pericardial stitch, also called the Lima's stitch, responsible for anterior displacement of the heart and good access to the marginal and posterior arteries.

It has become clear over the years that complete myocardial revascularization would require not only surgical expertise, but a very coordinated team approach. The anesthesiologist would provide the surgeon with hemodynamic stability and optimal table positioning so that the posterior arteries of the heart could be adequately exposed with the stabilization device. One additional suction device, applied to the apex of the heart, would later substitute the pericardial stitch, allowing cardiac distraction out of the pericardial sac with minimal hemodynamic compromise [38,39].

The third element of the ideal off-pump CABG is a bloodless field. Since Murray's and Pronin's experimental work with dogs in the early fifties, the utilization of intraluminal stents has been considered very important, as it allows continuous blood flow throughout the construction of the anastomosis. The presence of the shunt has also served as a shield against inadvertent stitches to the posterior wall of the coronary arteries during anastomosis. There is some controversy regarding the utilization of intraluminal shunts since some studies have shown severe endothelial lesions associated with its use [40,41].

As the stabilization devices improve, motion has become lesser of an issue, and in several occasions there is no need for a stent. An alternative to keep a bloodless field is a mist blower, powered by a mixture of air or $CO_2$, this device gently "blows away" the blood from the field providing adequate view for suturing. The pioneers of OPCAB are currently reporting thousands of cases successfully treated, and as the procedure matures, we observe it is safe, it parallels on-pump revascularization in most aspects, and appears to be superior to conventional pump cases regarding a reduced perioperative myocardial damage, lower rates of renal dysfunction, atrial fibrillation and stroke, lower incidence of wound infection and lesser need for transfusion. It is also associated with reduction of postoperative intensive care unit and hospital stay and lower costs. Patients at a higher surgical risk appear to benefit the most from OPCAB [42-45].

## Future

"The future challenges" is what our mentor Prof. Tomas Salerno used to say during our surgical training in Bufallo, NY, just over a decade ago. At that time, minimally invasive did not mean to operate through small incisions, but rather without cardiopulmonary bypass. Today, and certainly in the near future, the next step will be how to perform complete myocardial revascularization off-pump through very small incisions.

Hybrid off-Pump CABG, in well-equipped operating rooms that allow coronary artery stenting combined with total arterial revascularization, and robotic technology, which associated with adequate lighting, practically eliminates the human limiting factors to the construction of adequate stapled coronary anastomosis, are just some of the new frontiers in the history of treatment of coronary artery disease.

# References

[1] Westaby S. Landmarks in Cardiac Surgery. Oxford: Isis Medical Media Ltd. 1997: 187.
[2] Westaby S. Landmarks in Cardiac Surgery. Oxford: Isis Medical Media Ltd. 1997: 229-230.
[3] Westaby S. Landmarks in Cardiac Surgery. Oxford: Isis Medical Media Ltd. 1997: 189-190.
[4] Vineberg AM. Development of an anastomosis between the coronary vessels and a transplanted internal mammary artery. *Can. Med. Assoc. J.* 1946;55:117-9.
[5] Vineberg A, Miller G. Internal mammary coronary anastomosis in the surgical treatment of coronary artery insufficiency. *Can. Med. Assoc. J.* 1951;64:204-10.
[6] Shrager JB. The Vineberg Procedure: The Immediate Forerunner of Coronary Artery Bypass Grafting. *Ann Thorac Surg* 1994;57:1354-64.
[7] Konstantinov IE. Vasilii I. Kolesov. A Surgeon to Remember. *Tex. Heart Inst J.* 2004;31:349-58.
[8] Murray G, Hilario J, Porcheron R, Roschlau W. Surgery of coronary heart disease. *Angiology* 1953;4:526-31.
[9] Westaby S. Landmarks in Cardiac Surgery. Oxford: Isis Medical Media ltd. 1997: 78.
[10] Goetz RH, Rohman M, Haller JD, Dee R, Rosenak SS. Internal mammary-coronary artery anastomosis. A nonsuture method employing tantalum rings. *J. Thorac. Cardiovasc. Surg.* 1961;41:378-86.
[11] Westaby S. Landmarks in Cardiac Surgery. Oxford: Isis Medical Media Ltd. 1997: 196.
[12] Pronin VI, Dobrova NB, Kurilovich JB. Revascularization of the heart by the method of anastomosis of the left thoracic and coronary arteries [in Russian]. *Grudn. Khir.* 1963;5:81-6.
[13] Kolesov VI, Potashov LV. Surgery of coronary arteries [in Russian]. *Eksp. Khir. Anesteziol.* 1965;10:3-8.
[14] Kolesov VI. Mammary artery-coronary artery anastomosis as method of treatment for angina pectoris. *J. Thorac. Cardiovasc. Surg.* 1967;54:535-44.
[15] Kolesov VI, Vishneevskaia IaN, Drevina AI, Tsalolikhina EIa. Treatment of coronary insufficiency by bilateral ligation of the internal mammary artery [in Russian].Vestn KhirIm I I Grek 1959;82:33-41.
[16] Kolesov VI. The physiological features and results of treatment of chronic coronary insufficiency with bilateral ligation of the internal mammary artery [in Russian]. *Klin. Med.* (Mosk) 1960;38:71-7.
[17] Garrett HE, Dennis EW, DeBakey ME.Aortocoronary bypass with saphenous vein graft. Seven-year follow-up. *JAMA* 1973;223:792-794.
[18] Favaloro RG. Saphenous vein autograft replacement of severe segmental coronary artery occlusion: operative technique. *Ann. Thorac. Surg.* 1968;5:334-9.
[19] Westaby S. Landmarks in Cardiac Surgery. Oxford: Isis Medical Media Ltd. 1997: 192.
[20] Green GE, Stertzer SH, Reppert EH. Coronary arterial bypass grafts. *Ann. Thorac. Surg.* 1968;5:443-50.
[21] Kolesov VI. Remote results of direct myocardial revascularization in atherosclerosis of coronary arteries [in Russian]. Khirurgiia (Mosk) 1977;7:17-21.

[22] Kolesov VI. Late results of a mammary-coronary anastomosis [in Russian].Vestn Khir Im I I Grek 1982;128:49-53.
[23] Kolesov VI, Kolesov EV. Twenty years' results with internal thoracic artery-coronary artery anastomosis. *J. Thorac. Cardiovasc. Surg.* 1991;101:360-1.
[24] Ankeney JL. To use or not to use the pump oxygenator in coronary bypass operation [editorial]. *Ann. Thorac. Surg.* 1975;19:108-9.
[25] Benetti FJ. Direct coronary surgery with saphenous vein bypass without either cardiopulmonary bypass or cardiac arrest. *J. Cardiovasc. Surg.* (Torino) 1985;26:217-22.
[26] Buffolo E, Andrade JCS, Succi JE, et al. Revascularizaçãodireta do miocárdiosemcirculaçãoextracorpórea: descrição da técnica e resultadosiniciais. *Arq. Bras. Cardiol.* 1982;38:365-73.
[27] Ascione R, Lloyd CT, Underwood MJ, et al. Inflammatory response after coronary revascularization with or without cardiopulmonary bypass. *Ann. Thorac. Surg.* 2000;69:1198-204.
[28] Calafiore AM, Di Mauro M, Canosa C, et al. Myocardial revascularization with and without cardiopulmonary bypass: advantages, disadvantages and similarities. *Eur. J. Cardiothorac. Surg.* 2003;24:953-60.
[29] Balkhy HH, Wann LS, Krienbring D, Arnsdorf SE. Integrating coronary anastomotic connectors and robotics toward a totally endoscopic beating heart approach: review of 120 cases. *Ann Thorac Surg* 2011;92:821-7.
[30] Puskas JD, Williams WH, Duke PG, et al. Off-pump coronary artery bypass grafting provides complete revascularization with reduced myocardial injury, transfusion requirements, and length of stay: a prospective randomized comparison of two hundred unselected patients undergoing off-pump versus conventional coronary artery bypass grafting. *Thorac. Cardiovasc. Surg.* 2003;125:797-808.
[31] Muneretto C, Bisleri G, Negri A, et al. Off-pump coronary artery bypass surgery technique for total arterial myocardial revascularization: a prospective randomized study. *Ann. Thorac. Surg.* 2003;76:778-82.
[32] vanDijk D, Nierich AP, Jansen EW, et al. Early outcome after off-pump versus on-pump coronary bypass surgery: results from a randomized study. *Circulation* 2001;104:1761-6.
[33] Covino E, Santise G, Di Lello F, et al.Surgical myocardial revascularization (CABG) in patients with pulmonary disease: beating heart versus cardiopulmonary bypass. *J. Cardiovasc. Surg.* (Torino) 2001;42:23-6.
[34] Nathoe HM, van Dijk D, Jansen EW, et al. A comparison of on-pump and off-pump coronary bypass surgery in low-risk patients. *N. Engl. J. Med.* 2003;348:394-402.
[35] Gerola LR, Moura LA, Leão LE, et al. Arterial wall damage caused by snaring of the coronary arteries during off-pump revascularization. *Heart Surg. Forum* 2000;3:103-6.
[36] Hangler H, Mueller L, Ruttmann E, et al. Shunt or snare: coronary endothelial damage due to hemostatic devices for beating heart coronary surgery. *Ann. Thorac. Surg.* 2008;86:1873-7.
[37] Gründeman PF, Budde R, Beck HM, et al. Endoscopic exposure and stabilization of posterior and inferior branches using the endo-starfish cardiac positioner and the endo-octopus stabilizer for closed-chest beating heart multivessel CABG: hemodynamic changes in the pig. *Circulation* 2003;108 Suppl 1:II34-8.

[38] Sepic J, Wee JO, Soltesz EG, et al. Cardiac positioning using an apical suction device maintains beating heart hemodynamics. *Heart Surg. Forum* 2002;5:279-84.

[39] Bergsland J, Karamanoukian HL, Soltoski PR, Salerno TA. "Single suture" for circumflex exposure in off-pump coronary artery bypass grafting. *Ann. Thorac. Surg.* 1999;68:1428-30.

[40] Wippermann J, Albes JM, Bruhin R, et al. Chronic ultrastructural effects of temporary intraluminal shunts in a porcine off-pump model. *Ann. Thorac. Surg.* 2004;78:543-8.

[41] Wippermann J, Albes JM, Brandes H, et al. Acute effects of tourniquet occlusion and intraluminal shunts in beating heart surgery. *Eur. J. Cardiothorac. Surg.* 2003;24:757-61.

[42] Diegeler A, Hirsch R, Schneider F, et al. Neuromonitoring and neurocognitive outcome in off-pump versus conventional coronary bypass operation. *Ann. Thorac. Surg.* 2000;69:1162-6.

[43] Onorati F, Olivito S, Mastroroberto P, et al. Perioperative patency of coronary artery bypass grafting is not influenced by off-pump technique. *Ann. Thorac. Surg.* 2005;80:2132-40.

[44] Peterson E. Off-Pump Bypass Surgery—Ready for the Big Dance? *JAMA* 2004; 291:1897-1899.

[45] Newman D. Longitudinal assessment of neurocognitive function after coronary artery bypass surgery. *N. Engl. J. Med.* 2001;344: 395-402.

# Section 2. Techniques and Technology

In: Off-Pump Coronary Artery Bypass Grafting
Editors: Shahzad G. Raja and Mohamed Amrani
ISBN: 978-1-62081-549-6
© 2012 Nova Science Publishers, Inc.

*Chapter III*

# Hemodynamic Changes during Off-Pump Coronary Artery Bypass Grafting

### Zachary Edgerton[1] and James R. Edgerton[2]
[1]Cardiopulmonary Research Science and Technology Institute
Dallas, Texas, US
[2]Heart Hospital Baylor Plano
Plano, Texas and
Cardiopulmonary Research Science and Technology Institute
Dallas, Texas, US

## Abstract

Displacement of the heart is necessary to expose the target vessel for distal anastomosis to achieve successful multivessel off-pump coronary artery bypass (OPCAB) grafting. Positioning for access to the coronary arteries leads to hemodynamic instability during OPCAB surgery. A number of mechanisms may be postulated to be the cause of hemodynamic disturbance during OPCAB, including coronary artery flow compromise, compression of the heart chambers, poor preload of the ventricles, and distortion of the cardiac valves. This chapter provides an insight in to the mechanisms and effects of hemodynamic changes during OPCAB grafting and strategies adopted to address these changes.

## Introduction

"Anyone who would attempt to operate on the heart should lose the respect of his colleagues" Christian Albert Theodor Billroth (1881) address to the Vienna Medical Society.
"Surgery of the heart has probably reached the limits set by nature to all surgery: no new method, and no new discovery, can overcome the natural difficulties that attend a wound of the heart." said Stephen Paget (son of Sir James Paget of Paget's disease) said in 1896 in his book "Surgery of the Chest."

And so it was until Gibbon's heart lung machine opened the heart to the surgeon's interventions. However, despite ever improving technological advancements the use of extracorporeal circulation and artificial oxygenators is attended by a host of morbidities. Seeking to reduce morbidity for their patients, surgeons have tried to develop techniques to operate on the surface of the beating heart without the aid of cardiopulmonary bypass (CPB). The major challenge to this is to obtain a still operative field and to have adequate visualization of the inferior and posterior vessels on the full beating heart. Initial efforts at pharmacologic stabilization failed. It takes the average surgeon two to four seconds to line up and complete a stitch through a coronary. Thus, in order to operate between heart beats, the heart rate would have to be lowered to 15 to 30 beats per minute which is incompatible with sustaining an adequate cardiac output.

Mechanical stabilizers have been developed to provide a near motionless field. However, lifting the heart to visualize the infero-posterior vessels is attended by marked hemodynamic derangement with hypotension and malperfusion. This chapter will examine the etiology of this hemodynamic decrement and methods to ameliorate it.

## Early Theories and Animal Work

In the preliminary stages of the development of the Utrecht Octopus® method, the reasons for hypotension when the heart is lifted were poorly understood. Five theories emerged:

1. Displacement of the heart obstructed inflow (superior vena cava and inferior vena cava) therefore eliminating pre-load of the muscle
2. Displacement of the heart caused valves to leak due to deformation
3. Displacement of the heart compressed the ventricles, decreasing mechanical efficiency
4. Displacement of the heart obstructed main outflow vessels (aorta)
5. Displacement of the heart obstructed coronary arteries causing decreased contractility of the heart

An examination of these theories was conducted in a series of animal studies conducted by Borst and Gründeman in the Utrecht. These studies employed the use of the Octopus® device, the first suction stabilizer. The initial study [1] utilized 8 pigs. The pigs were anesthetized and their hearts were then suspended in a pericardial cradle. Heart rate and rhythm were monitored by electrocardiogram. Right and left end ventricular pressures were monitored via catheter tip manometers inserted into the ventricles. Mean atrial pressures were monitored by fluid manometer lines inserted directly into each atrial appendage. Mean arterial pressure was monitored by a monometer placed in the femoral artery. Lastly, cardiac output was monitored by an ultrasound transit time flow probe placed around the aorta.

The hemodynamic variables were then simultaneous monitored as each pig advanced through the six consecutive phases of the experimental protocol: (1) Basal control position, (2) fixation of the Octopus®, (3) vertical displacement of the heart, (4) Trendelenburg maneuver, (5) return to horizontal position, and (6) after release of the Octopus®.

The first principle finding of the study was that vertical displacement of the porcine heart resulted in a nearly 50% reduction of stroke volume. The second finding was that this compromised status was reversed to an acceptable condition by performing the Trendelenburg maneuver.

During displacement of the heart, it was found that left ventricular stroke volume was nearly halved despite the fact that left ventricular preload was unchanged. They also found an elevated right ventricular preload. Gründeman et al. attributed these findings to mechanical interference with the heart's pumping action, noting that the right ventricular wall was visually crumpled against the surrounding tissue. It is also important to note that preliminary epicardial Doppler ultrasound observations showed no leakage of any of the cardiac valves and no evidence that there was any outflow obstruction due to kinking. It is believed that the efficacy of the Trendelenburg maneuver is due to increase in left and right ventricular filling and that the increased preload caused by the head-down position overcame the mechanical interference caused by displacement.

The findings of this study are limited for several reasons. The experiment was performed on healthy porcine hearts. It must be taken into account that the anatomical position of the heart is different in pigs than in humans. Furthermore, the hearts of patients undergoing surgery are expected to be in poor condition and may not tolerate displacement.

In a second study [2] Gründeman et al. created a second experiment, similar to their previously published work [1] in which they monitored the blood flow of the left anterior descending coronary artery, the right coronary artery, and the circumflex coronary artery using flow probes. This study reaffirmed the findings that displacement of the supine porcine heart caused severe decrease in stroke volume, mean arterial pressure, and coronary flow. It also found that the hemodynamic status was restored by the Trendelenburg maneuver and that coronary blood flow also returned to baseline values. It was therefore inferred that coronary blood flow is not mechanically obstructed by vertical displacement of the heart. The second study is subject to the same limitations as the first. Further investigation in human subjects would be required to overcome the limitations of these studies and obtain data consistent with real-world application.

## Human Work

Early human observations were published by Nierich [3] and Jansen [4]. They noted that moving the heart to reach the target site for anastomosis caused hemodynamic alteration, but did not characterize the etiology. They commented that the blood pressure could be returned to an acceptable range with fluid loading and inotropic agents.

It is difficult to extrapolate the Utrecht data collected from healthy animal hearts to diseased human hearts. Expanding on the findings of Gründeman et al., the seminal human study elucidating the etiology of the hemodynamic derangement was conducted in Dallas by Edgerton, Mack and associates[5]. This study instrumented 40 consecutive human hearts undergoing off pump coronary artery bypass grafting (OPCAB).

To obtain accurate measures of hemodynamic variables, several catheters were used. A Swan-Ganz catheter was inserted into the right internal jugular vein and a 20-guage catheter was inserted into the radial artery for pressure and blood gas monitoring. Two 18-guage catheters were introduced through the right pulmonary vein: the first into the left atrium, the second into the left ventricle. These were used to monitor left atrial pressure and left ventricular end-diastolic pressure. Right atrial pressure and right end-diastolic pressure as well as mixed venous oxygen saturation were monitored by means of the Swan-Ganz catheter. Cardiac output was measured via an ultrasound transit-time flow probe placed around the aorta.

Data was collected during positioning for circumflex anastomosis, posterior descending artery anastomosis, and left anterior descending artery anastomosis. A comparison of the three positions rendered these conclusions:

"Every positioning, even for the left anterior descending artery, caused an increase of right ventricular end-diastolic pressure. And the positioning for the posterior descending artery caused an increase of the left ventricular end-diastolic pressure, although it wasn't statistically significant. The positioning for the circumflex artery showed the largest increase of left and right ventricular end-diastolic pressures, resulting in the largest hemodynamic compromise. The positionings for the circumflex and the posterior descending arteries caused a larger increase of left and right atrial pressures than the positioning for the left anterior descending artery did [5]." *Thus, both the left and the right ventricular end diastolic pressures were increased in each of the positioning and the stroke volume was significantly decreased in each of the three positioning.*

Transesophageal echocardiography was performed. It showed *moderate to severe compression of both ventricles*, most severe in circumflex positioning. There did not appear to be significant outflow tract obstruction or valvular insufficiency contributing to the decrement in blood pressure.

The authors noted that their results were similar to the animal findings of Gründeman [1] with pressures in all four chambers elevated while blood pressure, cardiac output and stroke volume were decreased. *"However, in contrast to the animal studies, Trendelenburg positioning did not restore the mean arterial pressure, cardiac output, and stroke volume to normal"*. The authors concluded that the hemodynamic decrement of the displaced human heart is primarily due to biventricular compression, more marked on the thinner right ventricle. This theory explained the hemodynamic observations made in each positioning. Previous work by both Burfeind [6] and Jurmann [7] had suggested but not proven such an etiology.

## Strategies to Address Hemodynamic Compromise

To safely perform off pump coronary bypass grafting, the surgeon needs a thorough understanding of the hemodynamics of the displaced human heart. Armed with such knowledge, he can minimize the effects of biventricular compression, especially right ventricular compression.

Suction displacement devices in combination with regional suction immobilization devices are the tools to gain exposure. Although frequently placed on the apex, the suction displacement device is at times better utilized by placing the device off the apex for high circumflex vessels or on the acute margin for exposure of the right coronary artery in the atrioventricular groove.

Exposure of the left anterior descending and of the right coronary system is usually easily accomplished with simple gradual displacement. The surgeon usually encounters difficulty when exposing the circumflex and its branches. Knowing that right ventricular compression (and to a lesser degree, left ventricular compression) cause hypotension, the surgeon must create room for the right ventricle. This is the hallmark of successful exposure. Several maneuvers accomplish this. The pericardium is opened in an inverted T fashion. It is particularly helpful to open the pericardium along the diaphragm fully to the right. One can even extend this incision posteriorly, freeing right sided pericardium from the diaphragmatic pericardium. This allows the right pericardium to drift towards the right side un-tethered from the diaphragm. During this maneuver, care must be taken to avoid injury to the right phrenic nerve. Any pericardial stay sutures that are placed must be left loose so that the right ventricle can be free to move to the right, thus avoiding compression. Further room can be made for the right ventricle by elevating the right hemisternum. This is accomplished by angling the sternal retractor.

Having thus created room for the right ventricle, the surgeon next places the suction device just to the left of the apex. The heart is then slowly and gradually displaced. Use gravity to aid in exposure by rotating the table to the right and using Trendelenburg to augment right ventricular filling. When the target vessel is adequately visualized, the stabilizer foot is positioned around it and secured in this position. Once this is accomplished, if the hemodynamics are suboptimal, there is another maneuver the surgeon can employ. The suction displacement device can now be loosened and allowed to move a centimeter or two to the left. This further minimizes right ventricular compression and usually is attended by a 10 to 20 point elevation of the systolic blood pressure. Exposure of the target vessel is maintained by the stabilizer foot which has been locked into position. Essentially, the surgeon is trading right ventricular compression (which is poorly tolerated) for better tolerated left ventricular compression.

If the hemodynamics are still unacceptable, several steps should be followed:

- Patience. Initially unacceptable hemodynamics often improve with a little time and a little Trendelenburg
- Further elevate the right hemisternum
- Fully open the right pericardium into the right pleural space (again protecting the phrenic nerve
- Put the heart down and start again. Often subtle differences in the placement of the suction device or the angle of elevation can make a huge difference.
- Re-evaluate your grafting strategy. Do a different vessel first to relieve ischemia in the distribution of the right coronary artery or left anterior descending artery prior to approaching the circumflex.

Infrequently, the cause of the hypotension can be induced mitral insufficiency. The changed geometry of the displaced heart can increase the anteroposterior diameter of the mitral annulus resulting in central insufficiency. We have been able to successfully correct this by restoring the geometry of the mitral valve with external compression. First a deep pericardial retraction suture is placed in the posterior pericardium. Then a rolled up wet laparotomy pad is positioned along the coronary sinus and to the left. The heart is elevated.

Then, while watching the transesophageal echocardiogram, tension is placed on the deep pericardial retraction suture. This causes the laparotomy pad to push against the posterior mitral annulus restoring the geometry and relieving the insufficiency.

# Getting Started

## Build a Team

The key to being successful is realizing it is a *"different operation"* and not a *"new technique"* and training the *"team"* accordingly. When working without the aid of cardiopulmonary bypass issues of timing are even more critical. Team members must understand the concept and the goals. Team members must understand their individual roles and have a working knowledge of the equipment. Having a suction device fail in the middle of an anastomosis because it was attached to low pressure suction tubing can be tragic. Secure the buy in of the anesthesiologist. Anesthesia's active role is critical for a successful outcome. In contrast to arrested heart surgery, anastomoses cannot be performed without the anesthesiologist's active participation. Minute-to-minute monitoring of wall motion and hemodynamics is required. Success requires ongoing management of fluctuating hemodynamics associated with positional changes.

## Develop the Concept and Have a Grafting Strategy for Each Case

In conventional bypass surgery we deal with global ischemia and manage it by *decreasing myocardial oxygen demands*. In beating heart surgery we deal with *regional* ischemia and manage it by *minimizing the area of myocardial ischemia*. The grafting strategy is a design to minimize the area of regional myocardial ischemia during each anastomosis. In general:

- Collateralized vessels prior to collateralizing vessels
- Totally occluded prior to less occluded
- Minor vessels prior to major vessels
- Proximals prior to distals

## Stepwise Initiation of a Program

It is not necessary to hit a home run on day one. The prudent surgeon proceeds in a stepwise fashion, gaining skill and confidence. Start on cardiopulmonary bypass with the heart fully decompressed but beating. Then progress to partial cardiopulmonary bypass with the heart ejecting. Next do the LAD and RCA before turning on the pump and use pump assist while gaining skill exposing the circumflex vessels.

## Have a Bail-Out Plan

Avoid having to convert to cardiopulmonary bypass. Urgent conversion is attended by a high mortality [8]. Factors correlated with need to convert include: a surgeon early in his experience, congestive heart failure, and re-operations. The best way to get out of trouble is to avoid trouble. Early in your experience try to avoid: calcified vessels, small corkscrew vessels, the COPD patient with flattened diaphragms and a horizontal heart, pectus excavatum, left main stenosis, fresh infarcts, intramyocardial vessels, and patients with valvular insufficiency.

Further prudent measures include: keep the perfusionist in the room and prime the pump on high risk cases, place cannulation sutures if the patient is unstable, place pacing wires on the heart prior to initializing grafting, do proximal anastomoses first. In some high risk cases that are deemed to benefit from an off pump approach, the placement of an intra-aortic balloon pump can afford stabilization prior to grafting.

## Conclusion

Off pump coronary artery bypass grafting is an important technique that a well rounded surgeon should hold in his surgical tool box. To safely perform this technique, the surgeon must have a thorough understanding of the hemodynamic changes that occur during displacement of the heart. These changes are due to biventricular compression, and primarily due to right ventricular compression. The surgeon can take steps to minimize this compression during positioning as described. Certainly ischemia also plays some role [9] and the surgeon must minimize this by: having a grafting strategy to minimize the amount of regional ischemia, performing the anastomosis expeditiously, and judiciously using intravascular shunts. In some cases when the ventricular function is poor, placement of an intra-aortic balloon pump may facilitate the procedure [10]. In rare cases, right heart bypass may be considered [11] although this is a technique we have never found necessary.

## References

[1] Gründeman PF, Borst C, van Herwaarden JA, Mansvelt Beck HJ, Jansen EW. Hemodynamic changes during displacement of the beating heart by the Utrecht Octopus method. *Ann. Thorac. Surg.* 1997;63 (6 Suppl):S88-92.

[2] Gründeman PF. Vertical displacement of the beating heart by the Utrecht Octopus tissue stabilizer: effects on hemodynamics and coronary flow. *Perfusion* 1998;13:229-30.

[3] Nierich AP, Diephuis J, Jansen EW, et al. Embracing the heart: perioperative management of patients undergoing off-pump coronary artery bypass grafting using the octopus tissue stabilizer. *J. Cardiothorac. Vasc. Anesth.* 1999;13:123-9.

[4] Jansen E, Borst C, Lahpor JR, et al. Coronary artery bypass grafting without cardiopulmonary bypass using the octopus method: results in the first one hundred patients. *J. Thorac. Cardiovasc. Surg.* 1998;116:60-67.

[5] Mathison M, Edgerton JR, Horswell JL, Akin JJ, Mack MJ. Analysis of hemodynamic changes during beating heart surgical procedures. *Ann. Thorac. Surg.* 2000;70:1355-60.

[6] Burfeind WR, Duhaylongsod FG, Samuelson D, Leone BJ. The effects of mechanical cardiac stabilization on left ventricular performance. *Eur. J. Cardiothorac. Surg.* 1998;14:285-289.

[7] Jurmann MJ, Menon AK, Haeberle L, Salehi-Gilani S, Ziemer G. Left ventricular geometry and cardiac function during minimally invasive coronary artery bypass grafting. *Ann. Thorac. Surg.* 1998;66:1082-1086.

[8] Edgerton JR, Dewey TM, Magee MJ, et al. Conversion in Off-Pump coronary artery bypass grafting: an analysis of predictors and outcomes. *Ann. Thorac. Surg.* 2003;76:1138-1143.

[9] Yeatman M, Caputo M, Narayan P, et al. Intracoronary shunts reduce transient intraoperative myocardial dysfunction during off-pump coronary operations. *Ann. Thorac. Surg.* 2002;73:1411-1417.

[10] Suzuki T, Okabe M, Handa M, Yasuda F, Miyake Y. Usefulness of preoperative intraaortic balloon pump therapy during off-pump coronary artery bypass grafting in high-risk patients. *Ann. Thorac. Surg.* 2004;77:2056-2059.

[11] Gründeman PF, Borst C, Verlaan C, et al. Exposure of circumflex branches in the tilted, beating porcine heart: Echocardiographic evidence of right ventricular deformation and the effect of right or left heart bypass. *J. Thorac. Cardiovasc. Surg.* 1999;118:316-323.

In: Off-Pump Coronary Artery Bypass Grafting
Editors: Shahzad G. Raja and Mohamed Amrani

ISBN: 978-1- 62081-549-6
© 2012 Nova Science Publishers, Inc.

*Chapter IV*

# Techniques of Myocardial Stabilization and Coronary Artery Exposure in Off-pump Coronary Artery Bypass Grafting

*Fabiano Porta and Piet W. Boonstra*
Department of Cardiothoracic Surgery
Medical Center Leeuwarden
Leeuwarden, Netherlands

## Abstract

Although coronary artery bypass grafting without cardiopulmonary bypass was originally introduced nearly five decades ago, this technique was subsequently abandoned in favor of techniques of revascularization using cardiopulmonary bypass. It was not until the late 1980s that off-pump coronary artery bypass grafting was reintroduced. However, despite growing enthusiasm, this technique was used almost exclusively in patients with atherosclerotic disease limited to the left anterior descending coronary artery. For almost a decade after its rediscovery revascularization of other coronary territories remained elusive because of technical difficulties in exposing the lateral and inferior walls of the heart while preserving cardiac performance and hemodynamic stability. However, in recent years technical advances in coronary artery exposure and myocardial stabilization have resulted in a remarkable resurgence of interest for coronary artery bypass grafting without cardiopulmonary bypass, ultimately leading to the popularization of off-pump grafting of all coronary territories. The aim of this chapter is to describe strategies and techniques of coronary artery exposure and myocardial stabilization in off-pump coronary artery bypass grafting.

## Introduction

Off- pump coronary artery bypass (OPCAB) grafting is a technique whose origins can be traced back to the 1960s, when for the first time an internal mammary artery (IMA) was used for coronary grafting, as previously described by Kolesov and colleagues [1]. Starting from 1964 until 1974 they consistently performed OPCAB [2] with the use of ITA anastomosed to a coronary vessel [3]. They observed that the inflammatory response caused by blood contact with the cardiopulmonary bypass (CPB) circuit was too great to justify its use in coronary artery bypass grafting (CABG) patients. So they performed CABG on the beating heart, while elsewhere the use of CPB was developing as the golden standard for all heart surgery procedures. Their experience in OPCAB remained little known until the late 1980s, when Benetti [4] and Buffolo [5] independently presented the results of two large single center experiences in OPCAB, performed over a span of more than 10 years. These experiences opened the way to a dramatic increase in OPCAB worldwide and to the development of new techniques and devices to facilitate the exposure and stabilization of the coronary vessels during OPCAB.

## Exposing the Heart for OPCAB

Two practical aspects central to successful conduct of OPCAB include: exposure of the coronary vessel and stabilization of the moving area of the heart around that vessel. The key to success is to properly use exposure and stabilization techniques, without mixing them.

The first step in obtaining a perfect exposure of the target vessel begins with the opening of the pericardium via a large inverted T incision. On its caudal side this incision should be extended from the diaphragm laterally, avoiding damaging the phrenic nerve, on both right and left sides. The pleurae are not routinely opened. Cranially the pericardiotomy should reach the left brachiocephalic vein and then be extended downwards, until the junction between the superior vena cava and the left brachiocephalic vein. In order to improve the exposure further, stay sutures are applied in the pericardium in variable number, with a minimum of two sutures.

## Exposing the Anterior Wall

The stay sutures in the left side of the pericardium can be placed deeper in order to facilitate exposure of the anterior wall as well as parts of the lateral wall of the ventricle. However, inaccurate placing of the pericardial traction sutures can result in a large set of iatrogenic damage. Lesions of lung, phrenic nerve, thoracic aorta and esophagus are described [6].

The exposure of the lateral and inferior wall requires an important cardiac displacement rightwards, which can lead to deformation and compression of the right ventricle with subsequent hemodynamic deterioration. In order to avoid this complication, a right pleurotomy can be performed. This allows the heart to partially herniate into the right hemithorax [7,8]. Even a right ventricular assist device can be used during OPCAB [9]. In general, hemodynamic parameters will hardly be affected in case compression of the right side of the heart can be avoided.

During the initial clinical experiences with OPCAB, bradycardia was found advantageous, because it facilitated the surgeons' work "shooting on a moving target".

However, by using stabilizers bradycardia is no longer required. Moreover, bradycardia can lead to low cardiac output and hypotension due to a diminished stroke volume. In particular anastomosing the right coronary artery or one of its branches can lead to a temporary AV-block. So before tilting the heart and before starting to perform the anastomosis atrial pacing wires should be placed on the ventricle wall [10,11].

## Exposing the Lateral and Inferior Walls

A particularly useful method of exposing the lateral wall is the so called "single suture technique" described by Salerno et al [12]. This technique is the evolution of a previous method developed by Lima [13], who used to apply multiple sutures deeply in the posterior pericardium in order to expose the lateral wall. In this technique the surgeon should lift the heart with his left hand, while placing a heavy suture (usually no.1 silk) in the deepest point of the oblique sinus in the posterior pericardium. This maneuver can be facilitated by the surgeon's assistant who should gently lift the pericardium with a pair of forceps in that precise spot thus preventing the surgeon to accidentally damage the structures behind (thoracic aorta and esophagus). The hemodynamic changes due to this maneuver are transient and can be neutralized with a moderate Trendelenburg position of the patient. A well trained team can accomplish this maneuver in a few seconds. In another technique 15 inches vaginal tape is passed through the suture and snared down to the posterior pericardium using a regular tourniquet [14].

## Exposing Devices

Different kinds of vacuum exposing devices or apical suction devices are available. These devices can offer an alternative for, or can be additional to the single suture technique, with the advantage of avoiding injuries while placing the deep pericardial suture and a more precise and adjustable positioning. However, these devices cause epicardial hematoma, which are less traumatic than they look. The transient damage is caused by coronary vessel compression and microvascular collapse which extension depends on the amount of myocardium subject to vacuum and the pressure used [15,16,17,18].

## Stabilizing the Target Area

After completing the exposure of the target area it is necessary to stabilize the area around the target artery. This can be accomplished by means of a stabilizer, based on vacuum suction or mechanical pressure, or a 4cm x 4cm fenestrated piece of felt.

The current vacuum stabilizers work on the same principles and have in basic almost similar design and performances. The position of the stabilization arm is dependent on the surgeon's preference. The choice of the right or left blade of the sternal retractor for placing the stabilizer arm will be different for a right handed surgeon than for a left handed one. In either case or in the other, the arm of the stabilizer should not interfere with the visualization of the vessel as well as its suturing. It has been shown in studies on pig models that the amount of residual coronary artery excursion after stabilization was 1.5-2.4 mm with suction devices [19].

The stabilizers that are based on mechanical pressure share some similarities in design with the suction devices thus using local compression to stabilize the tissue in small area. Studies have been carried out to investigate the extent of the damage to the epicardial tissues due to mechanical compression [20,21]. Hematoxylin and eosin stained sections of tissue under the stabilizer foot showed in animal models intercellular edema, polymorphonuclear leukocytes infiltration and myocardial necrosis for 1 mm into the myocardium. Although detectable, the amount of injuries due to the stabilizer are considered negligible with no impairment of the regional ventricular motion.

Some authors described the use of a fenestrated piece of polytetrafluoroethylene (PTFE) felt of about 2.5 x 1.5 cm used as a cushion between a mechanical stabilizer and the epicardial surface thus preventing epicardial trauma [22]. Another method of mechanical stabilization is to cut a 4cm by 4 cm PTFE patch and adding a fenestration in its center large enough to accommodate the anastomotic site. The procedure consists in passing two 2-0 sutures proximally and distally under the target vessel deep into the myocardium. Then passing other two similar sutures parallel to the vessel on both sides and finally pass the adjacent sutures through the previously created patch. After suspending those sutures the final result is a local stabilization without keeping pressure on the target area and with no hemodynamic deterioration [23].

## Anterior Wall Revascularization

Starting with performing the anastomosis of the left anterior descending (LAD) or one of its branches, has the advantage of improving the perfusion of the anterior wall first. This is in particular important in case of a left main stem stenosis. Performing the anastomosis of the LIMA to the LAD as the first anastomosis, is not advised if the length of the LIMA is limited because the subsequent displacement of the heart rightwards, in case additional grafts have to be anastomosed to the lateral wall of the ventricle, will cause tension on the pedicle and eventually result in a damage of the anastomosis.

In order to get an optimal exposure of the LAD a moderate tilting of the heart is necessary. This can be achieved by placing one or more gauzes under the heart or by placing additional stay sutures (deeper) on the left side of the pericardium. Once a sufficient exposure has been achieved, a stabilizer can be placed. The anastomosis can then be performed in the usual fashion.

## Lateral Wall Revascularization

In order to expose the lateral wall of the ventricle, the apex of the heart has to be lifted out of the pericardium; a maneuver called "enucleation". Before beginning with the exposure of the lateral wall it is necessary to release all the pericardial exposing sutures in the right edge of the pericardium. In order to accommodate the right side of the heart especially in patients with moderate or severe chamber dilatation, a right pleurotomy can be performed, as described above. If the single suture technique is used, the surgeon can expose the lateral wall by pulling the two slings to the left, while directing the tourniquet of the deep stitch to the right side. During this process a moderate Trendelenburg position and a 30 degrees rotation of the table rightwards, will improve hemodynamics. After fixation of the slings and tourniquet, the region of the marginal obtuse branch should be adequately exposed. If the exposure is not sufficient, one or more gauzes can be placed in the region of the left pulmonary veins in order to further lift the heart. At this point it is possible to precisely place the stabilizer on the target vessel. Stabilizers can be conveniently placed on the right distal part of the sternal retractor's blade, although the best position may differ depending on the device's specific design.

## Inferior Wall Revascularization

Exposing the inferior wall is generally less challenging than the lateral one. An apical suction device can be placed both on the right or left proximal sternal retractor blade, according to the surgeon's preference. In case of single suture technique the surgeon has different choices for placing the slings and the tourniquet, mainly depending on the position of the target vessel. In order to expose the right coronary artery correctly, the slings should be pulled gently to the left and the tourniquet upward and towards the feet of the patient. This will lift the apex of the heart out of the pericardium and does partially rotate it to the left, thus exposing the right atrioventricular groove. A moderate Trendelenburg position can be applied and the table can be slightly rotated to the left. The stabilizer should be fixed on the right proximal retractor's blade in order to avoid the arm interfering with the surgical view of the vessel. This part of the right coronary artery usually runs in the epicardial fat tissue. In order to improve the view on the anastomotic site, an elastic tape or so called "vessel loop" with a blunt needle, should be passed underneath the coronary artery where after the coronary artery can be gently pulled upwards. To get exposure of the posterior descending coronary artery using the single suture technique, the slings should be placed alongside the target vessel and pulled upwards while the tourniquet will be pulled downwards, toward the feet of the patient. This will cause the apex to redirect to the ceiling. Additional gauzes can be placed to better accommodate the heart in this position. Again the stabilizer can be placed, for better comfort, on the right proximal retractor's blade. Anastomosis can be performed in the usual fashion.

## Conclusion

Although a variety of techniques have been introduced in an attempt to improve exposure and stabilization of coronary targets in OPCAB, total myocardial revascularization without CPB has remained elusive for many years. The main obstacle to total revascularization on the beating heart has been represented by the difficulty in exposing coronary targets located on the lateral and inferior wall of the heart while preserving hemodynamic stability. The techniques discussed in this chapter have proved to be safe and effective in accomplishing off-pump grafting of all coronary territories including those located in topographically difficult areas.

## References

[1] Olearchyk AS. Vasilii I. Kolesov. A pioneer of coronary revascularization by internal mammary-coronary artery grafting. *J. Thorac. Cardiovasc. Surg.* 1988;96:13-8.
[2] Kolesov VI, Potashov LV. Surgery of coronary arteries. *Eksp. Khir. Anesteziol.* 1965;10:3-8.
[3] Kolesov VI. Mammary artery-coronary artery anastomosis as a method of treatment for angina pectoris. *J. Thorac. Cardiovasc. Surg.* 1967;54:535-44.
[4] Benetti F, Naselli G, Wood M, Geffner L. Direct myocardial revascularization without extracorporeal circulation. Experience in 700 patients. *Chest* 1991;100:312-16.
[5] Buffolo E, Andrade JC, Branco JN, Aguiar LF, Ribeiro EE, Jatene AD. Seven year experience in 593 cases. *Eur. J. Cardiothorac. Surg.* 1990;4:504-7.
[6] Salerno TA. A word of caution on deep pericardial sutures for off-pump coronary bypass procedures. *Ann. Thorac. Surg.* 2003;76:339.
[7] Velissaris T, Jonas MM, Ohri SK. Hemodynamic advantage of right heart decompression during off-pump Surgery. *Asian Cardiovasc. Thorac. Ann.* 2010;18:17-21.
[8] George SJ, Amrani M. Mitral annulus distortion during beating heart surgery: a potential cause for hemodynamic disturbance-a three-dimensional echocardiography reconstruction study. *Ann. Thorac. Surg.* 2002;73:1424-30.
[9] Right ventricular support for off-pump coronary artery bypass grafting studied with bi-ventricular pressure±volume loops in sheep. *Eur. J. Cardiothorac. Surg.* 2001;19:179-184.
[10] Gulielmos V, Kappert U, Eller M, et al. Improving Hemodynamics by atrial pacing during off-pump bypass surgery. *Heart Surg. Forum* 2006;6:E179-82.
[11] Hart JC. Maintaining hemodynamic stability and myocardial performance during off-pump coronary bypass surgery. *Ann. Thorac. Surg.* 2003;75:S740-4.
[12] Bergsland J, Salerno TA , Karamanoukian HL, Soltoski PR. "Single suture" for circumflex exposure in off-pump coronary artery bypass grafting. *Ann. Thorac. Surg.* 1999;68:1428-30.
[13] de Carvahlo Lima R, de Escobar MA, Diniz R, et al. How much myocardial revascularization can we do without extracorporeal circulation? *Heart Surg. Forum* 2002;5:163-7.
[14] Ricci M, Karamanoukian HL, D'Ancona G, Bergsland J, Salerno TA. Exposure and mechanical stabilization in off-pump coronary artery bypass grafting via sternotomy. *Ann. Thorac. Surg.* 2000;70:1736-1740.
[15] Fernandez AL, García-Bengochea JB, Alvarez J, et al. Apical suction leads to severe ischemia of the ventricular apex. *Eur. J. Cardiothoracic. Surg.* 2006;29:506-510.
[16] George SJ, Kapetanakis EI, Dhadwal K, et al. A three-dimensional echocardiographic comparison of a deep pericardial stitch versus an apical suction device for heart positioning during beating heart surgery. *Eur. J. Cardiothorac. Surg.* 2007;32:604-610.
[17] Mathison M, Edgerton JR, Horswell JL, Akin JJ, Mack MJ. Analysis of hemodynamic changes during beating heart surgical procedures. *Ann. Thorac. Surg.* 2000;70:1355-60.

[18] Selvanayagam JB, Petersen SE, Francis JM, et al. Effects of off-pump versus on-pump coronary surgery on reversible and irreversible myocardial injury. *Circulation* 2004;109:345-50.
[19] Lemma M, Mangini A, Redaelli A, Acocella F. Do cardiac stabilizers really stabilize? Experimental quantitative analysis of mechanical stabilization. *Interact CardioVasc. Thorac. Surg.* 2005;4:222-226.
[20] Burfeind WR, Duhaylongsod FG, Samuelson D, Leone BJ. The effects of mechanical cardiac stabilization on left ventricular performance. *Eur. J. Cardiothorac. Surg.* 1998;14:285-289.
[21] Oliveira PPM, Braile DM; Vieira RW, et al. Hemodynamic disorders related to beating heart surgery using cardiac stabilizers: experimental study. *Rev. Bras. Cardiovasc.* 2007;22:407-415.
[22] Rousou JA, Engelman RA, Flack III JE, Deaton DW. Fenestrated felt facilitates anastomotic stability and safety in off-pump coronary bypass. *Ann. Thorac. Surg.* 1999;68:272-273.
[23] Rama A, Mohammadi S, Leprince P, Gandjbakhch I. A simple method for heart stabilization during off-pump multi-vessel coronary artery bypass grafting: surgical technique and short term results. *Eur. J. Cardiothorac. Surg.* 2001;19:105-107.

In: Off-Pump Coronary Artery Bypass Grafting
Editors: Shahzad G. Raja and Mohamed Amrani
ISBN: 978-1-62081-549-6
© 2012 Nova Science Publishers, Inc.

*Chapter V*

# Conduits for Coronary Artery Bypass Grafting

*Guo-Wei He*

Professor of Surgery, Nankai University,
Senior Cardiac Surgeon, TEDA International Cardiovascular Hospital
Tianjin, China and Clinical Professor of Surgery, Department of Surgery
Oregon Health and Science University,
Portland, Oregon, US

## Abstract

In comparison with standard saphenous vein grafts, use of the internal mammary artery as a coronary artery bypass graft has resulted in superior long-term results. This is obviously related to the differences in biological characteristics between the venous and arterial grafts.

However, even arterial grafts are not uniform in their biological characteristics. The difference in the perioperative behavior of the grafts and in the long-term patency may be related to different characteristics.

These should be taken into account when selecting arterial grafts, some of which are subjected to more active pharmacological intervention during and after operation, to achieve satisfactory results.

To better understand the biological behavior of the grafts, their common features and the differences, a clinical classification may be useful for a practicing surgeon. Based on experimental studies of vasoreactivity as well as taking into account the anatomical, physiological, and embryological considerations, we proposed a functional classification for arterial grafts that may be useful clinically.

This classification provides explanation for the difference in patency of various conduits. This chapter discusses the biological characteristics of various conduits available for coronary artery bypass grafting, provides an insight into decision making for choice of conduits and describes antispastic protocols and strategies to ensure better patency rates especially for arterial grafts.

# Introduction

Surgical myocardial revascularization is proven to be one of the most effective and long-lasting therapies in the treatment of ischemic heart disease.

The choice of the graft conduit is crucial to the success of coronary artery bypass grafting (CABG) because the patency of a coronary conduit is closely associated with an uneventful postoperative course and better long-term patient survival.

From the beginning of coronary bypass surgery venous conduits particularly the great saphenous vein has been the most frequently used coronary conduit.

However, over the last decade or so, coronary bypass graft surgery with arterial revascularization of all diseased coronaries has shown to be efficient because arterial grafts have better long-term patency, especially internal mammary artery (IMA), compared with venous grafts [1,2].

Early vein graft failure coupled with occlusion is the most important limitation of saphenous vein grafts.

Nevertheless, vein grafting is still an integral part of cardiac surgical practice. The difference in patency rates is obviously related to the differences in biological characteristics between the venous and arterial grafts.

This chapter provides an overview of the differences in characteristics between various conduits and focuses on arterial grafts.

# Differences in Biological Characteristics between the Venous and Arterial Grafts

Back in early days for CABG, the biological characteristics and the differences between the venous and arterial grafts already attracted research interests.

There is a large body of literature including our own work that demonstrated that there are differences between venous and arterial grafts. Those differences may be listed as:

1) veins are more susceptable to vasoactive substances than arteries [3];
2) the venous wall is supplied by the vaso vasorum whereas the arterial wall may be supplied through the lumen in addition to the vaso vasorum [4];
3) the endothelium of arteries may secrete more endothelium-derived relaxing factor (EDRF) [5] and may release more nitric oxide (NO) [6,7] and endothelium-derived relaxing factor (EDRF) [6,7]; and
4) the structure of the vein is more suited to low pressure whereas the artery, to high pressure. After grafting to the aorta-coronary system, in a high pressure system, venous grafts have to adapt to the high pressure.

These differences may account for the difference in the long-term patency rate.

# Arterial Grafts: Biological Characteristics

## Are There Any Differences among Arterial Grafts?

Based on the superior long-term results of the IMA, other arteries have been used in CABG [8-14]. Those arterial conduits are the radial artery (RA) [8], the gastroepiploic artery (GEA) [9], the inferior epigastric artery (IEA) [10,11], the splenic artery [12], the subscapular artery [13], and the inferior mesenteric artery [14], the descending branch of lateral femoral circumflex artery [15], and the ulnar artery [16]. In addition, the intercostal artery [17] has also been suggested to be used as a graft. The long-term patency rates for IMA are well established. The long-term patency for RA [18-23] and GEA [24-27] are also well established now in addition to the early reports [28-30]. It is expected that other arterial conduits will have good long-term results as the IMA does.

This expectation is based on a hypothesis that all arterial conduits have similar biological characteristics such as contractility, relaxing characteristics, endothelial function, and anatomical structure. However, histological studies have revealed that there are major differences among various grafts in terms of structure of smooth muscle such as elastic lamellae [4,31].

These differences reveal that arterial grafts, although are arteries, are not uniform either in anatomy or in function. On the other hand, comparative functional studies [32-36] have demonstrated that there are differences in arterial grafts with regard to contractility and endothelial function. Our previous studies have demonstrated that the endothelium of the IMA releases more NO than the RA at both basal and stimulated levels. Further, the IMA has more hyperpolarizing effect to bradykinin-stimulated release of EDRF than the RA does [37]. In addition, we have recently [38] further demonstrated that the expression and function of endothelial nitric oxide synthase messenger RNA and protein are higher in the internal mammary artery than in radial artery.

These differences are the anatomical and physiological basis of the divergent clinical manifestations of the grafts and may also account for possible differences in the postoperative graft function and long-term patency rates. It is often observed during CABG that the tendency to develop spasm for different arterial grafts during surgical dissection and during perioperative period is different. It has been the observation of many surgeons that GEA has a higher tendency to spasm than IMA [39]. Similarly, during the early days of using RA grafts in the 1970s, spasm of the RA was a serious problem that, together with a low patency rate, led to the abandonment of this arterial graft from the clinical use [27]. Only after the development of a method to overcome spasm of this arterial graft it was re-used again [40,41].

## Biological Characteristics

All arterial grafts for CABG are conductance arteries (in the sense opposite to "resistance" arteries). A common feature of arterial grafts is that removal of these arteries would not usually affect the blood supply to the organ and only under the extreme situation it is a concern. The common physiological role of these conductance arteries is to carry blood flow to perfuse corresponding organs such as the heart (the coronary artery), the stomach or other visceral organs (the GEA, the splenic artery, and the inferior mesenteric artery), the hand (the RA), and the body wall (the IMA, IEA, and the subscapular artery).

However, there may be differences in the function of these arteries owing to the fact that the organs they perfuse have a different physiological role so the flow required or the flow reserve for the organs may be different. The differences among these arteries can be described from the view of anatomy, physiology, pharmacology, and embryology at the organ, tissue, or cellular/molecular level.

## Anatomy

The differences in the gross anatomy among the arterial grafts are obvious since they are at different locations of the body and supply different organs. There is evidence showing that the anatomical structure of the arteries are divergent [4,31]. One of the most obvious differences with regard to the structure is that some arteries contain more smooth muscle cells in their wall and therefore are less elastic such as the GEA, IEA, and RA. In contrast, others may be more elastic, containing more elastic laminae such as the IMA [4]. These differences in structure may account for the difference in physiological and pharmacological reactivity of the conduits.

## Contractility and Incidence of Spasm of Arterial Grafts

The true cause of vasospasm is still vague. However, it is reasonably presumed that vasospasm is the extreme form of vasoconstriction that may be the response of a vessel to many stimuli (spasmogens). These stimuli may be physical (such as mechanical stimulation or temperature changes) or pharmacological (such as nerve stimulation or vasoconstrictor substances).

Important vasoconstrictor substances, which may be spasmogens for blood vessels, are [35,42]: (1) endothelium-derived contracting factors such as endothelin; (2) prostanoids such as thromboxane $A_2$ ($TxA_2$) and prostaglandin $F_{2\alpha}$ ($PGF_{2\alpha}$); (3) circulating sympathomimetic substances ($\alpha$-adrenoceptor agonists) such as norepinephrine and synthetic $\alpha_1$-adrenoceptor agonists (methoxamine or phenylephrine); (4) platelet-derived contracting substances such as 5-hydroxytryptamine (5-HT) and $TxA_2$; (5) substances released from mast cells and basophils such as histamine; (6) muscarinic receptor agonists such as acetylcholine; (7) renin-angiotensin system-related substances such as angiotensin II [43]; (8) neuropeptides such as arginine vasopressin [44] or intestinal peptide [45]; (9) depolarizing agent, potassium ion; and (10) In addition, we have recently demonstrated that human urotensin II may also be a spasmogen for the human IMA and RA [46,47].

The contractility of arterial grafts in response to the above mentioned vasoconstrictors has been extensively studied [32-36,42-57]. We have suggested that there are basically two types of vasoconstrictors that are important spasmogens in arterial grafts [35]. Type I (endothelin, prostanoids ($TxA_2$ and $PGF_{2\alpha}$), $\alpha_1$-adrenoceptor agonists) are the most potent vasoconstrictors and they produce strong contractility of arterial grafts when endothelium is intact. Type II vasoconstrictors (such as 5-HT) only induce a weak vasoconstriction when endothelium is intact. However, those vasoconstrictors probably play an important role in the spasm of arterial grafts if endothelium is lost by surgical handling or by diseases such as diabetes.

The difference among arterial grafts with regard to the response to these vasoconstrictors is the magnitude of the response and the sensitivity to the spasmogen. Although all arterial grafts react to the above vasoconstrictors there is a general trend that some arteries react to vasoconstrictors in a stronger manner than others do. This is best reflected by the fact that the GEA reacts more strongly to vasoconstrictors $K^+$, TXA2, ET-1, and norepinephrine than other arteries [34]. In the comparison between the RA and IMA, the RA has higher response to norepinephrine and 5-HT [33], angiotensin, and endothelin-1 [48]. Clinically, although all arterial grafts may develop vasospasm, it more frequently develops in GEA [39] and RA [41] than in IMA and IEA. Postoperative vasospasm and occlusion is the cause accounting for the early abandonment of the RA [41] and a possible cause for the abandonment of the GEA in some cardiac surgical centers.

However, there are groups of arteries that are similar in their contractility to vasoconstrictors. In fact, we have shown that IMA and IEA are in this group [34,36]. The response of these two arteries to a number of vasoconstrictors, such as endothelin, U46619, or $K^+$, is similar [34,36].

## Comparison of Arterial Grafts and Coronary Arteries

In general, coronary arteries are highly reactive vessels and coronary spasm is a well-known phenomenon. To directly compare the pharmacological reactivity of the human coronary artery and the bypass grafts in vitro is difficult for obvious reason – lack of the human coronary artery. We have tried to do so with the human coronary artery taken from the diseased and explanted heart in transplantation [34]. We can only presume that the reactivity of normal coronary arteries may be equal to or higher than that of arterial grafts, as we demonstrated in the canine vessels [3]. However, when the large coronary artery has atherosclerotic disease it may be less reactive to vasoconstrictors compared to arterial grafts, although the reactivity of the micro-coronary artery may remain high.

## Receptors in Smooth Muscle

Most vasoconstrictors except potassium ion contract arterial grafts by activating a specific receptor. Some receptors on the smooth muscle of the arterial grafts have been characterized. For example, the IMA is an $\alpha 1$-adrenoceptor-dominant artery with little $\alpha 2$- or $\beta$-function [49,58]. In contrast, the RA has both $\alpha 1$- and $\alpha 2$-function although its $\beta$-function is also weak [50].

Other receptors functionally demonstrated in arterial grafts are ETA, ETB [51], 5-HT [52], angiotensin [53], TP (thromboxane-prostanoid) [54], vasopressin V1 receptors [44,55], and vasoactive intestinal peptide [45] receptors in the IMA. There are fewer reports on the receptors in other arterial grafts [34,45,48]. Moreover, we have recently revealed that human urotensin II receptor (hUT receptor) exists in the human IMA [46,47] and RA [46].

## Receptors in Endothelium and Endothelial Function

Receptors are also located in the cellular membrane of the endothelial cell in the arterial grafts. For example, common stimuli for EDRF such as acetylcholine, bradykinin, and substance P are present in the endothelium of arterial grafts [32,36,48]. The vascular endothelial growth factor (VEGF)-induced, endothelium-dependent relaxation, mediated by both NO and prostacyclin in the IMA has been shown mainly through the KDR-receptors, rather than Flt-1 receptors [59]. Most recently, we have shown that corticortropin-releasing factor (CRF) receptors CRF1, CRF2α, and CRF2β are present in the human IMA [60]. The CRF urocortin-induced endothelium-dependent relaxation in the IMA is likely through CRF receptors allocated in the endothelium of the IMA [60].

The above receptors in the endothelium usually mediate endothelium-dependent relaxation but the differences in these receptors among the arterial grafts are to be further studied.

We have been trying to compare the endothelial function among arterial grafts and found that IMA has more endothelium-dependent relaxation than the IEA in response to acetylcholine and calcium ionophore A23187 [36] although it is still uncertain whether this is due the intrinsic physiological differences or due to the higher incidence of atherosclerosis in the IEA [31,36]. In addition, others also found differences regarding the endothelial function among arterial grafts [56,57].

Most importantly, we have previously found that the IMA releases more NO and has more hyperpolarization to endothelium-derived hyperpolarizing factor (EDHF) stimulus bardykinin than the saphenous vein [6] but also than the RA [37]. In fact, NO and EDHF are the two major EDRFs in arteries [61,62]. Our recent study has further demonstrated that the higher NO release from the IMA is probably due to the higher expression of the endothelial NO synthase (eNOS) in the IMA than in the RA [38]. These direct and quantitative studies reveal that the IMA has superior endothelial function as the intrinsic characteristic that is closely related to its excellent long term patency.

## Smooth Muscle Relaxation

Compared to the differences in the endothelium-dependent relaxation, no major differences have been observed among arterial grafts in the endothelium-independent relaxation (such as to nitroglycerine), which is often used as the index for the function of the relaxation properties in the smooth muscle [32,36] although there may be some differences in response to vasodilator substances with regard to the sensitivity [45]. The clinical implications of this need to be determined.

## Embryological Consideration

Commonly used arterial grafts belong to different groups of arteries in various locations of the body and can be divided into somatic arteries and splanchnic arteries [63].

Somatic arteries, supplying the body wall, include the IMA, the IEA, the subscapular artery, and the intercostal artery. In comparison, splanchnic arteries, supplying visceral organs, include the GEA, the splenic artery, and inferior mesenteric artery. From embryology [63], somatic arteries are developed from intersegmental branches to the body wall whereas splanchnic arteries are from segmental branches of primitive dorsal aorta to supply the digestive tube.

Arteries that supply extremities — limb arteries belong to a special type. Upper limb arteries are developed from somatic arteries whereas lower limb arteries, from the dorsal root of the umbilical artery.

## Physiological Consideration

Arterial grafts for coronary surgery are conduit arteries. The physiological function is to carry blood flow to organs. Owing to the fact that the organs they supply have different physiological functions, these arteries are entitled to adapt to the need for blood supply to individual organs. Therefore, the structure and the reactivity of these arteries are different. This explains why some of them are more spastic (more reactive to vasoconstrictors) than others.

## Segmental Difference

The reactivity of the grafts varies along the length of conduit arteries. For example, the main portion (the mid portion, composed more than 60% of the total length of the graft) of the IMA is less reactive compared to the distal portion and the proximal portion [64,65]. The major muscular components are located at the two ends of the artery (muscular regulator) [66]. This may be also true in other arterial grafts such as GEA, IEA, and the radial artery. In particular, the distal end is more efficient as the physiological regulator for the flow because this part contains relatively more smooth muscle cells and is smaller in diameter. Those characteristics are physiologically important in regulating blood flow distribution. However, when such arteries are used as bypass grafts, those characteristics may be detrimental. In terms of preventing vasospasm of the arterial grafts, trimming off the small and highly reactive distal end of the grafts (either IMA, GEA, IEA, or other grafts) may be important and clinically feasible [64].

## Incidence of Atherosclerosis

In general, the incidence of atherosclerosis in the four major arterial grafts is low, compared with the LAD [4]. In fact, atherosclerosis is absent or only mildly present in all four arterial grafts. Early studies already demonstrated that the incidence of atherosclerosis in IMA is low [67] and it is frequently seen from angiograms that a patent IMA exists with a stenotic vetebral artery. In contrast, the incidence of atherosclerosis at the proximal end of the IEA may be high as seen in a small group of patients [31,36] that may be related to the fact that the incidence of atherosclerosis is higher in the lower limb arteries than the upper limb arteries and the IEA is the first branch of the external iliac artery [37]. The atherosclerosis incidence in the GEA is low as recently studied by us [31] and others [68].

The incidence of atherosclerosis is low in the IMA grafts [1,2], even 15 to 21 years later [69]. There is evidence showing that it could be also low in the GEA [68] and RA [70].

## Pharmacology of Vasoactive Substances in Arterial Grafts

Arterial grafts are reactive conductance arteries. Pharmacological reactivity of arterial grafts to vasoactive substances in arterial grafts includes the reactivity to vasoconstrictor substances as well as to spasmolytic vasodilator substances. Since this is a large topic, it is impossible to include it in this chapter. The reader may find reference [71] useful as it reviews this issue. Our original studies on this topic are also recommended for reading [42-44,46-50,53,54,59,71-113].

# Arterial Grafts: Clinical Classification and Scientific Considerations for Clinical Choice

As discussed above, arterial grafts are not uniform in their biological characteristics. The difference in the perioperative behavior of the grafts and in the long-term patency may be related to different characteristics. These should be taken into account in the use of arterial grafts, some of which are subjected to more active pharmacological intervention during and after operation to obtain satisfactory results. To better understand the biological behavior of the grafts, their common features and the differences, a clinical classification may be useful for a practicing surgeon.

## Clinical Classification

Based on experimental studies on the vasoreactivity, taken together with anatomical, physiological, and embryological considerations described above, we proposed a functional classification for arterial grafts that may be useful clinically [34,114].

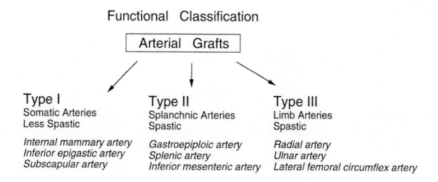

Figure 1. Functional classification of arterial grafts. (Reproduced with permission from He G-W. Arterial grafts for coronary artery bypass grafting: biological characteristics, functional classification, and clinical choice. Ann. Thorac. Surg. 1999;67:277-84 © Society of Thoracic Surgeons).

Our classification suggests that there are three types of arterial grafts as follows.

Type I: somatic arteries;
Type II: splanchnic arteries;
Type III: limb arteries.

From anatomical considerations, somatic arteries (Type I) are located in and supply blood to the body wall. The IMA is a typical example of this type of arteries. In addition, other somatic arteries such as IEA, the subscapular artery, or the intercostal artery belong to this type and their contractility may be similar to the IMA, as already demonstrated for the IEA [4] although there are no data available yet for the others. The IEA although histologically was demonstrated as a muscular artery [4], its pharmacological reactivity [34] as well as embryological origin is similar to the IMA. The wall of the IEA is thinner than the GEA [46]. Therefore, we classified this artery as Type I, together with the IMA.

Splanchnic (visceral) arteries (Type II) supply blood to visceral organs. The GEA is a typical example. Other splanchnic arteries such as the splenic artery and the inferior mesenteric artery belong to this type and their reactivity may be similar to GEA although no data are available yet. Type III arteries are located in the limb. The RA is a typical example. Other limb arteries such as the ulnar artery and the lateral femoral circumflex artery are also classified as Type III.

As already mentioned, the Type II artery GEA and the Type III artery RA have higher pharmacological reactivity to vasoconstrictors. This characteristic may be extended to all Type II and Type III arteries.

Type II arteries are prone to spasm because of the higher contractility of splanchnic arteries. This characteristic of splanchnic arteries has a physiological role as blood flow through splanchnic arteries is subject to tremendous changes under various circumstances to accord with the function of the alimentary tract. The flow increases after meals and decreases under critical situations.

In contrast, Type I arterial grafts (somatic arteries) are less reactive than Type II grafts because they are mainly "less reactive" conduit arteries except at the end of the artery, which is a muscular regulator for blood flow, as demonstrated in the human IMA [64-66].

As to Type III, these arteries are located in limbs, represented by the radial artery, and have higher tendency for spasm compared to somatic arteries (Type I).

It is the common clinical observation that usually arteries at extremities are prone to spasm at either physiological status or under pathological condition (as seen in Raynaud's disease).

The prevalence of vasospasm of arterial grafts is also correlated with their endothelial function. We have recently demonstrated that the Type I artery IMA releases more nitric oxide (NO) and has higher EDHF-mediated relaxation and hyperpolarization than the Type III artery RA [37,38]. In other words, the Type I artery particularly the IMA may prove to have the best endothelial function among arterial grafts and this certainly contributes to the superior patency of this graft.

Importantly, most of the studies comparing the endothelial function among arterial grafts are performed in the vascular segments taken from the coronary artery bypass grafting patients who are old with coronary disease; the superior endothelial function of the IMA may merely reflect the fact that this artery is usually free from atherosclerosis whereas other type

(Type II and III) arteries are usually more involved in atherosclerotic changes that diminish the endothelial function.

Because Type II and III arteries are prone to spasm due to higher contractility, they require more active pharmacological intervention [34,37,48].

Also as aforementioned, our classification is based on pharmacological studies as well as anatomical and embryological considerations.

The reason to classify arterial grafts on contractility rather than relaxation is that although vascular reactivity is composed of contractility and relaxation, the latter depends on the contractility. Relaxation occurs only in an artery that is already contracted and therefore is secondary to existing contraction.

There are clinical implications relating to this classification. First, this clinical classification may have an implication with regard to search for new arterial grafts or to predict the behavior of a graft. As far as vasospasm is concerned, Type I arteries may be less spastic than Type II and Type III, particularly when its most reactive portion — the distal section is trimmed off [64,65,115]. The less spastic characteristics are obviously advantageous perioperatively. In fact, in common clinical practice since 1980s, the IMA has been used as the first choice of arterial grafts and is always used to graft the most important coronary artery – the left anterior descending artery.

With this classification, the surgeon may predict the behavior of the arterial graft and to choose an optimal pharmacological method to overcome vasospasm. For the Type II or III arteries, more active pharmacological intervention is necessary in order to prevent or treat vasospasm in these arteries.

The most important issue of coronary grafting is the long-term patency of the graft including the anastomosis. Apart from technical factors, the long-term patency is related to the endothelial function. Vasospasm is also related to the long-term patency as seen in the early use of the RA that encountered a severe spastic problem and that had reduced patency of the RA graft [40,41]. Even in the largest series from Tatoulis and colleagues who are highly experienced with arterial grafting, the patency for RA was 89% at 4 years, compared to 98% of the patency for the left IMA at 5 years [19]. Although technical factors such as target vessels may be involved in this difference, the aforementioned differences in the endothelial function regarding NO and EDHF between the IMA and RA may play a role.

Further, the arteries in the same type may have different long-term patency due to the prevalence of the atherosclerosis either in the native artery or in the graft, or other factors. The Type I artery IMA has well established and superior long-term patency. On the other hand, the patency of the IEA, another Type I artery, is lower than IMA [116,117]. Several factors may account for this as: (1) the IEA is used as a free graft; (2) the IEA is very small at the distal end that increases the technical difficulties [118]; (3) the size of the proximal IEA is less than 2 mm that makes it technically challenging to construct aortic anastomosis [118]; and (4) the IEA, at least at the proximal part, has higher incidence of atherosclerosis that may influence the patency [4]. The new technique to use the IEA is, therefore, to trim off the very small part of the distal end and the atherosclerotic proximal end to be used as a part of composite graft [118]. In this way, use of the IEA may reach a similar patency rate comparable to the IMA. The patency rate of Type II and III arteries is not as well established as that of the IMA. Suma [119] reported that the cumulative patency rate estimated by the Kaplan-Meier method was 96.6% at 1 month, 91.4% at 1 year, 80.5% at 5 years, and 62.5% at 10 years. Causes of late occlusion were primary anastomotic stenosis and anastomosis to a less critically stenosed coronary artery. Voutilainers and associates [120] reported 82.1% (23/26) of the GEA grafts were patent at 5 years. From these studies, the patency of the GEA, as a Type II artery, is acceptable but not as superior as the IMA that was 95% at 10 years and 88% at 15 years [19]. The patency rate of the RA is more dramatic. There was a disappointing 35% incidence of narrowing or occlusion of the RA [121].

With modified technique, avoiding skeletonization and using calcium antagonists, the early patency increased to 93.5% at 9 months [41], 83% at 5 years [122] for Acar's group and 93.1% to 95.7% in other groups [123,124] at 3-21 months in the early stage of the use of RA. In addition, Tatoulis and associates reported that the radial artery patency at 1 year was 96% and at 4 years it was 89% [19].

These results may suggest that Type II and III arteries may have inferior patency to that of the IMA. However, if the vasospasm and the technical problem can be overcome and the endothelial function is well preserved, the patency of the Type II and III arteries may significantly improve. In summary, arterial grafts are biologically divergent conductance arteries. They can be functionally and clinically classified as three types.

Type II (such as GEA) and Type III (such as RA) are more spastic than Type I (such as IMA). In order to obtain the best results, antispastic therapy, preservation of endothelial function, and other technical modifications are essential particularly in Type II and III arteries.

## Antispastic Protocols for Conduits

There are a few antispastic protocols available in different units around the world. We present the following protocols used in our practice. These protocols are also adopted by other cardiac surgeons in various countries.

## The GW HE Protocol (Modified UHK Protocol) for Use in Arterial Grafting [77,78]

Based on the above pharmacological studies, we have developed an antispastic protocol - The GW HE Protocol (modified UHK Protocol) - for use in arterial grafting.

The solution (VG solution) was originally developed for IMA and saphenous vein harvesting and later was expanded to a protocol for RA grafting. As a protocol for RA grafting, it includes pre-, intra-, and post- operative management.

### 1. Preoperative for RA Grafting (Not Necessary for Other Grafts)

1) Allen test for both arms;
2) Doppler flow examination for the ulnar artery during Allen test and for the RA flow to demonstrate its patency.

## 2. Intraoperative

1) Use verapamil plus nitroglycerin (VG) solution (see below) topically during harvesting;

The components of the VG solution [75-78] are as follows:

| | |
|---|---|
| verapamil hydrochloride | 5 mg |
| nitroglycerine (NTG) | 2.5 mg |
| heparin | 500 Unit |
| 8.4% NaHCO3 | 0.2 mL |
| Ringer's solution | 300 ml |

This solution gives the concentration of about 30 μMol/L of verapamil or NTG in an isotonic solution of pH 7.4.

2) The RA is removed as soon as dissected from the arm and stored in the VG solution at room temperature;
3) Once the harvesting of the RA is started, low dose nicardipine (0.5 mg per hour; 5 mg in 100 ml D5W, IV at the rate of 10 ml per hour) is given systematically.

## 3. Postoperative

1) Nicardipine IV at the same dose until the patient is able to take oral calcium antagonists.
2) Oral intake of low dose of one of the calcium antagonists for at least 6-12 months. This can be nicardipine 20 mg twice a day; or verapamil 120-240 mg per day (A test dose 120 mg is recommended); or diltiazem at appropriate low dose. The choice of the calcium antagonist (nicardipine/diltiazem/verapamil) is based on the availability, the patient condition particularly the heart rate, and the preference of the cardiologist

Use of beta-blockers should be cautious when some of the calcium antagonists are given.
During harvesting of the IMA, this solution is used to spray on the pedicle as well as injected into the lumen.

# The GW HE Antispastic Solution No. 2 (NG Solution) for use in Arterial Grafting

## Design of the NG Cocktail

Since verapamil is not available in all places and its bradycardia effect may prevent the simultaneous use of β-blocker, also due to the fact that new generations of calcium antagonists have been developed, we designed a new cocktail that is composed of a second generation of dihydropyridin calcium antagonist – nicardipine and NTG. We tested this cocktail and reported the excellent effect of this solution on both human IMA and RA [125].

We tested the effect of nicardipine and NTG at the concentration of 30 µMol/L (-4.5 log M) on the human IMA and RA segments in the organ chamber. From previous studies [42,53,71,74-78,81,84,91-93,96,110] this concentration was expected to have maximal or nearly maximal effect.

The components of the clinical (NG) cocktail are as follows:

Nicardipine hydrochloride    5 mg
NTG                          5 mg
8.4% NaHCO3                  0.3 mL*
Normosol-R solution          300 ml
(Heparin 500 Unit could be added).

This cocktail gives concentration of about 30 µMol/L (-4.5 log M) of nicardipine or 60 µMol/L (-4.3 log M) NTG in an isotonic solution of pH 7.1.

*The pH of NG (Nicardipine hydrochloride 5 mg and NTG 5 mg) in Normosol-R solution (300 mL) without adding $NaHCO_3$ is 6.6. When the amount of 8.4% $NaHCO_3$ added is more than 0.3 ml, the solution becomes gradually turbid until pH = 7.4 with 8.4% $NaHCO_3$ 0.5 mL added.

This however, does not affect the antispastic effect as seen in the results of the present study because the effect of NG solution at the concentration of 30 µMol/L (-4.5 log M) was tested in the organ bath with PH =7.4 and a slight turbid look.

We presented here these two solutions for choice as antispastic protocol during arterial grafting. Our experimental studies [75-78,125] have demonstrated that these solutions are effective vasodilator cocktails that release vasoconstriction caused by all mechanisms including depolarizing and receptor mechanisms, unlike some other solutions such as α-adrenoceptor antagonists that are only effective to reverse adrenoceptor-mediated spasm and calcium antagonists alone that are only effective to reverse depolarizing agent ($K^+$)-mediated spasm. Our clinical trials have demonstrated that these are excellent vasodilators to reverse or prevent spasm [75,76,110].

## Conclusion

Coronary artery bypass grafting is one of the most outstanding surgical achievements of the 20th century. Over its 50-year history patient outcomes have become excellent owing to technical refinements, myocardial protection, the use of antiplatelet and anticholesterol drugs, and the continued search for better conduits. The performance of conduits used for bypass remains the most important prognostic factor.

Over the past 50 years a number of conduits have been employed and some extensively studied in an attempt to identify the conduit capable of providing best long-term patency in the native coronary arterial system, with the left internal mammary artery being the conduit of choice due to its excellent patency rates. The quest for second best, however, continues. Arterial conduits appear to be superior when grafted to tight stenosis but improving results with the saphenous vein mean that veins remain popular with surgeons. More supportive evidence is required to guide practice.

# References

[1] Loop FD, Lytle BW, Cosgrove DM, et al. Influence of the internal- mammary-artery graft on 10-year survival and other cardiac events. *N. Engl. J. Med.* 1986;314:1-6.
[2] Barner HB, Standeven JW, Reese J. Twelve-year experience with internal mammary artery for coronary artery bypass. *J. Thorac. Cardiovasc. Surg.* 1985;90:668.
[3] He G-W, Angus JA, Rosenfeldt FL. Reactivity of the canine isolated internal mammary artery, saphenous vein, and coronary artery to constrictor and dilator substances: Relevance to coronary bypass graft surgery. *J. Cardiovasc. Pharmacol.* 1988;12:12-22.
[4] Van Son JAM, Smedts F, Vincent JG, Van Lier HJ, Kubat K. Comparative anatomic studies of various arterial conduits for myocardial revascularization. *J. Thorac. Cardiovasc. Surg.* 1990;99:703-7.
[5] Lüscher TF, Diederich D, Siebenmann R, et al. Difference between endothlium-dependent relaxation in arterial and in venous coronary bypass grafts. *N. Engl. J. Med.* 1988;319:462-7.
[6] Liu ZG, Ge ZD, He GW. Difference in endothelium-derived hyperpolarizing factor-mediated hyperpolarization and nitric oxide release between human internal mammary artery and saphenous vein. *Circulation* 2000;102[suppl III]: III-296-III-301.
[7] Zhang RZ, Yang Q, Yim AP, Huang Y, He GW. Different role of nitric oxide and endothelium-derived hyperpolarizing factor in endothelium-dependent hyperpolarization and relaxation in porcine coronary arterial and venous ystem. *J. Cardiovasc. Pharmacol.* 2004;43:839-850.
[8] Carpentier A, Guermonprez JZ, Deloche A, Frechette C, Dubost C. The aorta-to-coronary radial artery bypass graft: a technique avoiding pathological changes in grafts. *Ann. Thorac. Surg.* 1973;16:111-21.
[9] Pym J, Brown PM, Charrette EJP, Parker JO, West RO. Gastroepiploic-coronary anastomosis: a viable alternative bypass graft. *J. Thorac. Cardiovasc. Surg.* 1987;94:256-9.
[10] Puig LB, Ciongolli W, Cividanes GV, et al. Inferior epigastric artery as a free graft for myocardial revascularization. *J. Thorac. Cardiovasc. Surg.* 1990;99:251-5.
[11] Buche M, Schoevaerdts JC, Louagie Y, et al. Use of the inferior epigastric artery for coronary bypass. *J. Thorac. Cardiovasc. Surg.* 1992;103:665-70.
[12] Edwards WS, Lewis CE, Blakeley WR, Napolitano L. Coronary artery bypass with internal mammary and splenic artery grafts. *Ann. Thorac. Surg.* 1973;15:35-9.
[13] Mills NL, Dupin CL, Everson CT, Leger CL. The subscapular artery: An alternative conduit for coronary bypass. *J. Card. Surg.* 1993;8:66-71.
[14] Shatapathy P, Aggarwal BK, Punnen J. Inferior mesenteric artery as a free arterial conduit for myocardial revascularization. *J. Thorac. Cardiovasc. Surg.* 1997113:210-1.
[15] Tatsumi TO, Tanaka Y, Kondoh K, et al. Descending branch of lateral femoral circumflex artery as a free graft for myocardial revascularization: a case report. *J. Thorac. Cardiovasc. Surg.* 1996;112:546-7.

[16] Buxton BF, Chan AT, Dixit AS, et al. Ulnar artery as a coronary bypass graft. *Ann. Thorac. Surg.* 1998;65:1020-4.

[17] Van Son JAM, Smedts F, Korving J, Guyt A, de Kok LB. Intercostal artery: histomorphometric study to assess its suitability as a coronary bypass graft. *Ann. Thorac. Surg.* 1993;56:1078-81.

[18] Tatoulis J, Buxton BF, Fuller JA, et al. Long-term patency of 1108 radial arterial-coronary angiograms over 10 years. *Ann. Thorac. Surg.* 2009;88:23-9.

[19] Tatoulis J, Buxton BF, Fuller JA. Patencies of 2127 arterial to coronary conduits over 15 years. *Ann. Thorac. Surg.* 2004;77:93-101.

[20] Schwann TA, Zacharias A, Riordan CJ, et al. Sequential radial artery grafts for multivessel coronary artery bypass graft surgery: 10-year survival and angiography results. *Ann. Thorac. Surg.* 2009 ;88:31-9.

[21] Hayward PA, Hare DL, Gordon I, Buxton BF. Effect of radial artery or saphenous vein conduit for the second graft on 6-year clinical outcome after coronary artery bypass grafting. Results of a randomised trial. *Eur. J. Cardiothorac. Surg.* 2008;34:113-7.

[22] Schwann TA, Zacharias A, Riordan CJ, et al. Does radial use as a second arterial conduit for coronary artery bypass grafting improve long-term outcomes in diabetics? *Eur. J. Cardiothorac. Surg.* 2008;33:914-23.

[23] Nezić DG, Knezević AM, Milojević PS, et al. The fate of the radial artery conduit in coronary artery bypass grafting surgery. *Eur. J. Cardiothorac. Surg.* 2006;30:341-6.

[24] Eda T, Matsuura A, Miyahara K, et al. Transplantation of the free gastroepiploic artery graft for myocardial revascularization: long-term clinical and angiographic results. *Ann. Thorac. Surg.* 2008;85:880-4.

[25] Hirose H, Amano A, Takanashi S, Takahashi A. Coronary artery bypass grafting using the gastroepiploic artery in 1,000 patients. *Ann. Thorac. Surg.* 2002;73:1371-9.

[26] Suma H, Wanibuchi Y, Furuta S, et al. Comparative study between the gastroepiploic and the internal thoracic artery as a coronary bypass graft. Size, flow, patency, histology. *Eur. J. Cardiothorac. Surg.* 1991;5:244-7.

[27] Suma H, Tanabe H, Yamada J, Mikuriya A, Horii T, Isomura T. Midterm results for use of the skeletonized gastroepiploic artery graft in coronary artery bypass. *Circ. J.* 2007 ;71:1503-5.

[28] Lytle BW, Cosgrove DM, Ratliff NB, Loop FD. Coronary artery bypass grafting with the right gastroepiploic artery. *J. Thorac. Cardiovasc. Surg.* 1989;97:826-31.

[29] Suma H, Wanibuchi Y, Terada Y, Fukuda S, Takayama T, Furuta S. The right gastroepiploic artery graft: clinical and angiographic midterm results in 200 patients. *J. Thorac. Cardiovasc. Surg.* 1993;105:615-23.

[30] Grandjean JG, Boonstra PW, Heyer P, Ebels T. Arterial revascularization with the right gastroepiploic artery and internal mammary arteries in 300 patients. *J. Thorac. Cardiovasc. Surg.* 1994;107:1309-16.

[31] van Son JAM, Smedts FM, Yang CQ, He GW. Morphometric study of the right gastroepiploic and inferior epigastric artery. *Ann. Thorac. Surg.* 1997;63:709-15.

[32] Dignan RJ, Yeh T Jr, Dyke CM, et al. Reactivity of gastroepiploic and internal mammary arteries: relevance to coronary artery bypass grafting. *J. Thorac. Cardiovasc. Surg.* 1992;103:116-22.

[33] Chardigny C, Jebara VA, Acar C, et al. Vasoreactivity of the radial artery. Comparison with the internal mammary artery and gastroepipoic arteries with implications for coronary artery surgery. *Circulation* 1993;88[part II]:115-27.

[34] He G-W, Yang C-Q: Comparison among arterial grafts and coronary artery. An attempt at functional classification. *J. Thorac. Cardiovasc. Surg.* 1995;109:707-15.

[35] He G-W, Yang C-Q, Starr A: An overview of the nature of vasoconstriction in arterial grafts for coronary surgery. *Ann. Thorac. Surg.* 1995;59:676-683.

[36] He G-W, Acuff TE, Yang C-Q, Ryan WH, Mack MJ. Functional comparison between the human inferior epigastric artery and internal mammary artery: Similarities and differences. *J. Thorac. Cardiovasc. Surg.* 1995;109:13-20.

[37] He GW, Liu ZG. Comparison of nitric oxide release and endothelium-derived hyperpolarizing factor-mediated hyperpolarization between human radial and internal mammary arteries. *Circulation* 2001;104 [suppl I]: I-344-I-349.

[38] He GW, Fan L, Grove KL, Furnary A, Yang Q. Expression and function of endothelial nitric oxide synthase messenger RNA and protein are higher in internal mammary than in radial arteries. *Ann. Thorac. Surg.* 2011;92:845-50.

[39] Suma H. Spasm of the gastroepiploic artery graft. *Ann. Thorac. Surg.* 1990;49:168-9.

[40] Fisk RL, Bruoks CH, Callaghan JC, Dvorkin J. Experience with the radial artery graft for coronary bypass. *Ann. Thorac. Surg.* 1976;21:513-8.

[41] Acar C, Jebara VA, Portoghese M, et al. Revival of the radial artery for coronary bypass grafting. *Ann. Thorac. Surg.* 1992;54:652-60.

[42] He G-W, Buxton B, Rosenfeldt F, Angus JA. Reactivity of human isolated internal mammary artery to constrictor and dilator agents. Implications for treatment of internal mammary artery spasm. *Circulation* 1989; 80(Suppl):I-141-I-150.

[43] Liu MH, Floten HS, Furnary A, He GW. Inhibition of vasoconstriction by angiotensin receptor antagonist GR117289C in arteries grafts. *Ann. Thorac. Surg.* 2000;70:2064-9.

[44] Wei W, Floten HS, He GW. Interaction between vasodilators and vasopressin in internal mammary artery and clinical significance. *Ann. Thorac. Surg.* 2002;73:516-22.

[45] Luu TN, Dashwood MR, Chester AH, Tadjkarimi S, Yacoub MH. Action of vasoactive intestinal peptide and distribution of its binding sites in vessels used for coronary artery bypass grafts. *Am. J. Cardiol.* 1993;71:1278-82.

[46] Chen ZW, Yang Q, Huang Y, Fan L, Li XW, He GW. Human urotensin II in internal mammary and radial arteries of patients undergoing coronary surgery. *Vascul. Pharmacol.* 2010 ;52:70-6.

[47] Bai XY, Liu XC, Yang Q, Tang XD, He GW. The interaction between human urotensin II and vasodilator agents in human internal mammary artery with possible clinical implications. *Ann. Thorac. Surg.* 2011;92:610-6.

[48] He GW, Yang CQ. Radial artery has higher receptor-selective contractility but similar endothelium function compared to mammary artery. *Ann. Thorac. Surg.* 1997;63:1346-52.

[49] He GW, Shaw J, Hughes CF, Yang CQ, et al. Predominant $\alpha_1$-adrenoceptor mediated contraction in the human internal mammary artery. *J. Cardiovasc. Pharmacol.* 1993;21:256-63.

[50] He GW, Yang CQ. Characteristics of adrenoceptors in the human radial artery: clinical implications. *J. Thorac. Cardiovasc. Surg.* 1998;115:1136-41.

[51] Seo B, Oemar BS, Siebenmann R, et al. Both ETA and ETB receptors mediate contraction to endothelin-1 in human blood vessels. *Circulation* 1994;89:1203-8.

[52] Yildiz O, Cicek S, Ay I, Tatar H, Tuncer M. 5-HT1-like receptor-mediated contraction in the human internal mammary artery. *J. Cardiovasc. Pharmacol.* 1996;28:6-10.

[53] He GW, Yang CQ. Comparison of nitroprusside and nitroglycerin in inhibition of angiotensin II and other vasoconstrictor-mediated contraction in human coronary bypass conduits. *Br. J. Clin. Pharmacol.* 1997;44:361-367.

[54] He GW, Yang CQ. Effects of thromboxane $A_2$ antagonist GR32191B on prostanoid and nonprostanoid receptors in the human internal mammary artery. *J. Cardiovasc. Pharmacol.* 1995;26:13-19.

[55] Liu JJ, Phillips PA, Burrell LM, Buxton BB, Johnston CI. Human internal mammary artery responses to non-peptide vasopressin antagonists. *Clin. Exp. Pharmacol. Physiol.* 1994;21:121-4.

[56] Ochiai M, Ohno M, Taguchi J, et al. Responses of human gastroepiploic arteries to vasoactive substances: comparison with responses of internal mammary artery and saphenous veins. *J. Thorac. Cardiovasc. Surg.* 1992;104:453-8.

[57] Mugge A, Barton MR, Cremer J, et al. Different vascular reactivity of human internal mammary artery and inferior epigastric arteries in vitro. *Ann. Thorac. Surg.* 1993;56:1085-9.

[58] He G-W, Buxton BF, Rosenfeldt BF, et al. Weak β-adrenoceptor mediated relaxation in human internal mammary artery. *J. Thorac. Cardiovasc. Surg.* 1989;97: 259-66.

[59] Wei W, Jin H, Chen ZW, et al. Vascular endothelial growth factor-induced nitric oxide- and PGI2-dependent relaxation in human internal mammary arteries: a comparative study with KDR and Flt-1 selective mutants. *J. Cardiovasc. Pharmacol.* 2004;44:615-21.

[60] Chen ZW, Huang Y, Yang Q, et al. Urocortin-induced relaxation in the human internal mammary artery. *Cardiovasc. Res.* 2005;65:913- 20.

[61] He G-W, Yang C-Q, Graier WF, Yang JA. Hyperkalemia alters EDHF-mediated hyperpolarization and relaxation in coronary arteries. *Am. J. Physiol.* 1996;271 (*Heart Circ. Physiol.* 40):H760-H767.

[62] Ge ZD, Zhang XH, Fung PC, He GW. Endothelium-dependent hyperpolarization and relaxation resistance to N(G)-nitro-L-arginine and indomethacin in coronary circulation. *Cardiovasc. Res.* 2000;46:547-56.

[63] Williams PL, Warwick R, Dyson M, Bannister LH, ed. Gray's anatomy. New York: Churchill Livingstone, 1989:213-9.

[64] He G-W. Contractility of the human internal mammary artery at the distal section increases toward the end. Emphasis on not using the end of the IMA for grafting. *J. Thorac. Cardiovasc. Surg.* 1993;106:406-11.

[65] He G-W, Acuff TE, Yang C-Q, Ryan WH, Mack MJ. The mid and the proximal sections of the human internal mammary artery are not "passive conduit". *J. Thorac. Cardiovasc. Surg.* 1994;108:741-6.

[66] He G-W, Yang C-Q. Vascular reactivity of gastroepiploic artery. *J. Thorac. Cardiovasc. Surg.* 1995;110:1569-70.

[67] Sims FH. A comparison of coronary and internal mammary arteries and implications of the results in the etiology of arteriosclerosis. *Am. Heart J.* 1983;105:560-566.

[68] Suma H. Gastroepiploic artery graft: coronary artery bypass graft in patients with diseased ascending aorta - using an aortic no-touch technique. *Operative Techniques in Cardiac and Thoracic Surgery* 1996;1:185-195.

[69] Barner HB, Barnett MG. Fifteen- to twenty-one-year angiopraphic assessment of internal thoracic artery as a bypass conduit. *Ann. Thorac. Surg.* 1994;57:1526-8.

[70] Desai ND, Cohen EA, Naylor CD, Fremes SE; Radial Artery Patency Study Investigators. A randomized comparison of radial-artery and saphenous-vein coronary bypass grafts. *N. Engl. J. Med.* 2004;351:2262-4.

[71] He GW, Yang CQ. Pharmacological studies and guidelines for the use of vasodilators for arterial grafts. In: He GW, editor. Arterial grafting for coronary artery bypass surgery. Berlin: Springer, 2$^{nd}$ Ed. 2006:39-44.

[72] Cooper GJ, Locke TJ. The *in vitro* response of human internal mammary artery to vasodilators. *J. Thorac. Cadiovasc. Surg.* 1994;107:1155-6.

[73] Jett GK, Guyton RA, Hatcher CR, Abel PW. Inhibition of human internal mammary artery contractions. An *in vitro* study of vasodilators. *J. Thorac. Cardiovasc. Surg.* 1992;104:977-82.

[74] He GW, Yang CQ, Mack MJ, et al. Interaction between endothelin and vasodilators in the human internal mammary artery. *Br. J. Clin. Pharmacol.* 1994;38:505-12.

[75] He GW, Rosenfeldt F, Angus JA. Pharmacological relaxation of the saphenous vein during harvesting for coronary artery bypass grafting. *Ann. Thorac. Surg.* 1993;55:1210-7.

[76] He GW, Rosenfeldt FL, Angus JA, Buxton BF. Pharmacological dilatation of internal mammary artery during surgery. *J. Thorac. Cardiovasc. Surg.* 1994;107:1440-4.

[77] He GW, Yang CQ. Use of verapamil and nitroglycerin solution in preparation of radial artery for coronary grafting. *Ann. Thorac. Surg.* 1996;61:610-4.

[78] He GW. Verapamil plus nitroglycerin solution maximally preserves endothelial function of the radial artery. comparison to papaverine solution. *J. Thorac. Cardiovasc. Surg.* 1998;115:1321-7.

[79] Cunningham JN. Papaverine hydrochloride preservation of vein grafts. *J. Thorac. Cardiovasc. Surg.* 1982; 84:933-4.

[80] Chavanon O, Cracowski JL, Hacini R, et al. Effect of topical vasodilators on gastroepiploic artery graft. *Ann. Thorac. Surg.* 1999;67:1295-8.

[81] He GW, Shaw J, Yang CQ, et al. Inhibitory effects of glyceryl trinitrate on α-adrenoceptor mediated contraction in the internal mammary artery. *Br. J. Clin. Pharmacol.* 1992;34:236-43.

[82] Cooper GJ, Wilkinson GAL, Angelini GD. Overcoming perioperative spasm of the internal mammary artery: which is the best vasodilator? *J. Thorac. Cardiovasc. Surg.* 1992;104:465-8.

[83] He GW, Yang CO, Gately H, et al. Potential greater than additive vasorelaxant actions of milrinone and nitroglycerin on human conduit arteries. *Br. J. Clin. Pharmacol.* 1996;41:101-7.

[84] He GW, Yang CQ. Comparison of vasorelaxant effect of nitroprusside and nitroglycerin in the human radial artery. *Br. J. Clin. Pharmacol.* 1999;48:99-104.

[85] Zabeeda D, Medalion B, Jackobshvilli S, et al. Comparison of systemic vasodilators: effects on flow in internal mammary and radial arteries. *Ann. Thorac. Surg.* 2001;71:138-41.

[86] Shapira OM, Xu A, Vita JA, et al. Nitroglycerin is superior to diltiazem as a coronary bypass conduit vasodilator. *J. Thorac. Cardiovasc. Surg.* 1999;117:906-11.

[87] Cable DG, Caccitolo JA, Pearson PJ, et al. New approaches to prevention and treatment of radial artery graft vasospasm. *Circulation* 1998; 10;98(19 Suppl):II15-21.

[88] Lobato EB, Janelle GM, Urdaneta F, Martin TD. Comparison of milrinone versus nitroglycerin, alone and in combination, on grafted internal mammary artery flow after cardiopulmonary bypass: effects of alpha-adrenergic stimulation. *J. Cardiothorac. Vasc. Anesth* 2001;15:723-7.

[89] He G-W, Acuff TE, Ryan WH, et al. Inhibitory effects of calcium antagonists on α-adrenoceptor mediated contraction in the internal mammary artery. *Br. J. Clin. Pharmac.* 1994;37:173-9.

[90] Rosenfeldt FL, He GW, Buxton BF, Angus JA. Pharmacology of coronary artery bypass grafts. *Ann. Thorac. Surg.* 1999;67:878-88.

[91] He GW, Yang CQ. Comparative study on calcium channel antagonists in the human radial artery: clinical implications. *J. Thorac. Cardiovasc. Surg.* 2000;119:94-100.

[92] Wei Wei, H. Storm Floten, He GW. Interaction between vasodilators and vasopressin in internal mammary artery and clinical significance. *Ann. Thorac. Surg.* 2002;73:516-22.

[93] He GW and Yang CQ. Inhibition of vasoconstriction by phosphodiesterase III inhibitor milrinone in human conduit arteries used as coronary bypass grafts. *J. Cardiovasc. Pharmacol.* 1996;28:208-14.

[94] Liu JJ, Doolan LA, Xie B, Chen JR, Buxton BF. Direct vasodilator effect of milrinone, an inotropic dgug, on arterial coronary bypass grafts. *J. Thorac. Cardiovasc. Surg.* 1997;113:3108-13.

[95] He GW. Effect of milrinone on coronary artery bypass grafts (letter to the editor). *J. Thorac. Cardiovasc. Surg.* 1997;114:302-4.

[96] He GW, Yang CQ. Vasorelaxant effect of phosphodiesterase-inhibitor milrinone in the human radial artery used as coronary bypass graft. *J. Thorac. Cardiovasc. Surg.* 2000;119:1039-45.

[97] Wei W, Yang CQ, Furnary A, He GW. Greater vasopressin-induced vasoconstriction and inferior effects of nitrovasodilators and milrinone in the radial artery than in the internal thoracic artery. *J. Thorac. Cardiovasc. Surg.* 2005;129:33-40.

[98] Cracowski JL, Stanke-Labesque F, Chavanon O, et al. Vasorelaxant actions of enoximone, dobutamine, and the combination on human arterial coronary bypass grafts. *J. Cardiovasc. Pharmacol.* 1999;34:741-8.

[99] He GW, Yang CQ. Inhibition of vasoconstriction by thromboxane A2 antagonist GR32191B in the human radial artery. *Br. J. Clin. Pharmacol.* 1999;48:207-15.

[100] He GW and Yang CQ. Inhibition of vasoconstriction by potassium channel opener aprikalim in human conduit arteries. *Br. J. Clin. Pharmacol.* 1997;44:353-9.

[101] Liu MH, Floten HS, Furnary A, Yim APC, He GW. Effect of potassium channel opener (KCO) aprikalim on the receptor-mediated vasoconstriction in the human internal mammary artery (IMA). *Ann. Thorac. Surg.* 2001;71:636-41.

[102] Ren Z, Floten HS, Furnary A, et al. Effects of potassium channel opener KRN4884 on human conduit arteries used as coronary bypass grafts. *Br. J. Clin. Pharmacol.* 2000;50:154-60.

[103] Mussa S, Guzik TJ, Black E, et al. Comparative efficacies and durations of action of phenoxybenzamine, verapamil/nitroglycerin solution, and papaverine as topical

antispasmodics for radial artery coronary bypass grafting. *J. Thorac. Cardiovasc. Surg.* 2003;126:1798-805.

[104] Corvera JS, Morris CD, Budde JM, et al. Pretreatment with phenoxybenzamine attenuates the radial artery's vasoconstrictor response to alpha-adrenergic stimuli. *J. Thorac. Cardiovasc. Surg.* 2003;126:1549-54.

[105] Conant AR, Shackcloth MJ, Oo AY, et al. Phenoxybenzamine treatment is insufficient to prevent spasm in the radial artery: the effect of other vasodilators. *J. Thorac. Cardiovasc. Surg.* 2003;126:448-54.

[106] Liu MH, Floten HS, Yang Q, He GW. Inhibition of vasoconstriction by AJ-2615, a novel calcium antagonist with $\alpha_1$-adrenergic receptor blocking activity in human conduit arteries used as bypass grafts. *Br. J. Clin. Pharmacol.* 2001;52:279-87.

[107] Liu MH, Floten HS, Furnary A, He GW. Inhibition of vasoconstriction by angiotensin receptor antagonist GR117289C in arteries grafts. *Ann. Thorac. Surg.* 2000;70:2064-9.

[108] Liu JJ, Johnston CI, Buxton BF. Synergistic effect of nisoldipine and nitroglycerin on human internal mammary artery. *J. Pharmacol. Exp. Therap.* 1994;268:434-40.

[109] Chanda J, Brichkov I, Canver CC. Prevention of radial artery graft vasospasm after coronary bypass. *Ann. Thorac. Surg.* 2000;70:2070-4.

[110] He GW, Fan KY, Chiu SW, Chow WH. Injection of vasodilators into arterial grafts through cardiac catheter to relieve spasm. *Ann. Thorac. Surg.* 2000;69:625-8.

[111] Kiemeneij F, Vajifdar BU, Eccleshall SC, et al. Evaluation of a spasmolytic cocktail to prevent radial artery spasm during coronary procedures. *Catheter Cardiovasc. Interv.* 2003;58:281-4.

[112] Koike R, Suma H, Kondo K, Oku T, Satoh H, Fukuda S, Takeuchi A. Pharmacological response of internal mammary artery and gastroepiploic artery. *Ann. Thorac. Surg.* 1990;50:384-6.

[113] Liu ZG, Liu XC, Yim APC, He GW. Direct measurement of nitric oxide release from saphenous vein: abolishment by surgical preparation. *Ann. Thorac. Surg.* 2001;71:133-7.

[114] He GW. Arterial grafts for coronary artery bypass grafting: biological characteristics, functional classification, and clinical choice. *Ann. Thorac. Surg.* 1999;67:277-84.

[115] He GW. Spasm of internal mammary artery: is it a secret? *J. Thorac. Cardiovasc. Surg. 1993;106:381-2.*

[116] Cremer J, Mügge A, Schulze M, et al. The inferior epigastric artery for coronary bypass grafting: functional assessment and clinical result. *Eur. J. Cardiothorac. Surg.* 1993;7:243-247.

[117] Perrault LP, Carrier M, Hebert Y, et al. Early experience with the inferior epigastric artery in coronary artery bypass grafting. *J. Thorac. Cardiovasc. Surg.* 1993;106:928-930.

[118] Calafiore AM. Use of the inferior epigastric artery for coronary revascularization. *Operative Techniques in Cardiac and Thoracic Surgery* 1996;1:147-159.

[119] Suma H, Isomura T, Horii T, Sato T. Late angiographic result of using the right gastroepiploic artery as a graft. *J. Thorac. Cardiovasc. Surg.* 2000;120:496-8.

[120] Voutilainers S, Verkkala K, Jarvinen A, Keto P. Angiographic 5-year follow-up study of right gastroepiploic artery grafts. *Ann. Thorac. Surg.* 1996;62:501-505.

[121] Carpentier A. Discussion of: Geha AS, Krone RJ, McCormick JR, Baue AE. Selection of coronary bypass: Anatomic, physiological, and angiographic considerations of vein and mammary artery grafts. *J. Thorac. Cardiovasc. Surg.* 1975;70:429-430.

[122] Acar C, Ramsheyi A, Pagny JY, et al. The radial artery for coronary artery bypass grafting: clinical and angiographic results at five years. *J. Thorac. Cardiovasc. Surg.* 1998;116:981-9.

[123] Calafiore AM, Di Giammarco G, Teodori G, et al. Radial artery and inferior epigastric artery in composite grafts: Improved midterm angiographic results. *Ann. Thorac. Surg.* 1995;60:517-524.

[124] Brodman RF, Frame R, Camacho M, et al. Routine use of unilateral and bilateral radial arteries for coronary artery bypass graft surgery. *J. Am. Coll. Cardiol.* 1996;28:959-963.

[125] He GW, Fan L, Furnary A, Yang Q. A new antispastic solution for arterial grafting: nicardipine and nitroglycerin cocktail in preparation of internal thoracic and radial arteries for coronary surgery. *J. Thorac. Cardiovasc. Surg.* 2008;136:673-80.

In: Off-Pump Coronary Artery Bypass Grafting
Editors: Shahzad G. Raja and Mohamed Amrani

ISBN: 978-1- 62081-549-6
© 2012 Nova Science Publishers, Inc.

*Chapter VI*

# Techniques of Conduit Harvesting for Coronary Artery Bypass Grafting

*David O. Moore, Lonnie J. Ginn and Michael J. Mack*

Heart Hospital Baylor Plano, Plano, Texas
and Medical City Dallas Hospital, Cardiopulmonary Research Science
and Technology Institute, Dallas, Texas, US

## Abstract

Coronary artery bypass grafting (CABG) continues to be an effective and frequently performed procedure for multi-vessel coronary disease. The choice and meticulous acquisition of conduits is critical to the success of these operations. The goal of accomplishing complete revascularization often requires multiple conduits. The challenge with each patient is to obtain the optimal conduits for the best target vessels in that particular individual. The focus of this chapter will be the review of harvesting techniques as well as complications associated with the harvest of the most commonly used conduits today. These will include saphenous vein, internal thoracic arteries and the radial artery. General overview of each conduit with respect to target vessel destination and patency will also be discussed. Particular attention will be directed towards the evolution of endoscopic vein harvest and the optimal treatment of the harvested conduit. The issue of patency in endoscopically harvested veins when compared to veins harvested in the standard open manner will also be addressed. The choice of conduit is often greatly influenced by the desire to minimize operative and anesthetic time and to perform the operation efficiently. The surgeon often relies upon physician assistants and other surgical assistants involved in the procedure to procure much of the needed graft material. In keeping with this fact, the technical aspects of endoscopic vein harvest will be detailed by one of the authors (LG), an experienced physician assistant. The quality of the conduit obtained is key to the ultimate short- and long-term success of the operation. Patience and persistence, sometimes at the expense of speed, is required to obtain the best conduits available. A technically superb operation can be foiled by the use of poor conduits or conduits that have been damaged by poor harvesting technique.

# Introduction

The STS (Society of Thoracic Surgeons) database provides insight into present patterns in cardiovascular practice. In 2010, 78% of the patients undergoing first time isolated coronary bypass surgery had 3 or more distal anastamoses, confirming the need for multiple conduits especially saphenous veins. The left internal thoracic artery (LITA) graft is used in 90.6% of patients, bilateral internal thoracic artery grafts were used in only 3.9%, radial artery (RA) in 5.3%, and isolated right internal thoracic artery (RITA) in 0.4%. SV was harvested endoscopically in 77.3% of the cases. It is therefore important to continue to improve vein harvest technology and techniques while encouraging increased use of the arterial conduits which clearly are beneficial to patients.

# Saphenous Vein

Many patients would attest that the greatest advance in cardiothoracic surgery has been the advent of endoscopic vein harvest. The long and often painful leg incisions, the hallmark of the earlier era of CABG are not frequently seen today. Questions remain however if the endoscopic vein harvest (EVH) technique compromises graft patency by causing damage to the vein that may occur with this minimally invasive approach. This issue came to the forefront in a post hoc analysis of the PREVENT IV study [1]. This study evaluated a large patient population undergoing coronary bypass surgery in multiple well-established medical centers in the U.S. 3000 patients were evaluated, 1753 having EVH and 1247 undergoing standard open vein removal. The method of vein harvest was determined by the surgeon and therefore was not randomized. 2000 of these patients were in an angiography cohort of which 75% had an angiogram for review. The median time for angiographic follow-up was 12.6 months. The total number of vein grafts in this group for evaluation was 4290. Clinical outcomes including death, myocardial infarction, and the need for repeat revascularization were also analyzed in the entire group over a 3 year follow-up period. The baseline characteristics were similar between patients who underwent endoscopic harvesting and those who had open conduit harvest. Patients who underwent endoscopic harvesting had higher rates of vein graft failure at 12 and 18 months when compared to the open harvest group. At 3 years endoscopic harvesting was also associated with higher death rates, myocardial infarction, or repeat revascularization. The conclusion was that endoscopic vein harvesting was independently associated with vein graft failure and adverse clinical outcomes. These findings have prompted reevaluation of the harvest techniques and the general handling of venous conduits. The industry leaders have responded with improved technology and ongoing research. It must however be highlighted that graft patency is a complex multifactorial issue with many variables including surgical technique, quality of recipient vessels, degree of stenosis, competitive flow, and quality of the conduit all being important. These variables exist and influence graft patency regardless of the harvest technique. There is also the patient's metabolic and innate coagulation milieu to consider. Factors such as diabetes control, lipid management and platelet inhibition must all be significant factors. Despite the complexity of the graft patency issue it is incumbent upon the cardiovascular surgical community to continue to explore all of these facets including vein harvest technology in order to achieve better outcomes.

## **Historical Perspective and Evolving Techniques**

Interest in vein harvest and preservation has existed for many years. As early as 1980, studies focused on endothelial preservation of vein grafts [2]. Electron microscopy was used to evaluate the effects of various solutions and distention pressures on the venous conduit. Cold blood solution and avoidance of high distention pressures was found to result in the best preservation of endothelium. The open, "no touch" technique was considered important with minimal instrumentation of the vein and careful ligation of venous tributaries well away from the vein itself. Bridging methods of harvest were developed which avoided the long, continuous incision but did require more traumatic manipulation of the vein. In the early days of endoscopic vein harvest the focus was more on the minimally invasive approach and not necessarily on the issue of conduit preservation. There has been an evolution over recent years, which addresses the issue of vein trauma, thermal damage and clot formation in the harvested veins. Lower energy and heat producing systems have been developed. Larger tunnels are now created to decrease the risk of thermal injury and heparin is now generally administered at the onset of vein harvest in order to reduce the risk of clot formation within the vein. Sophisticated methods of vein graft analysis have evolved including optical coherence tomography (OCT) [3]. OCT is an imaging modality that utilizes near-infrared light analogous to B-mode ultrasound to create cross-sectional and three-dimensional images of blood vessels [4]. It was originally designed for use in transparent tissues such as those present in the eye. Over time it has increasingly been utilized in the evaluation of atherosclerotic plaque in coronary vessels as well as cerebrovascular disease. It is possible to identify vulnerable, lipid laden plaques that are considered unstable. These images are in real time and have had good in-vitro histological confirmation studies done. One of the challenges with this imaging modality is the interference that blood in the imaged vessel creates. Presently balloon occlusion with frequent saline flushes provides the clear conditions for optimal image quality. Use of this modality is readily adaptable to vein harvest and conduit assessment. Recently a number of studies have used this imaging system to evaluate veins as well as radial arteries harvested for coronary bypass procedures. These images allow for the identification of damaged segments of vein and clots within the vein that otherwise would not have been appreciated. One such study explored the experience of the vein harvesting physician assistant. [3] It also compared some open technique veins to those harvested endoscopically. It was clear that experience was a factor in endoscopic vein harvest and those veins taken in an open manner were less likely to have damage demonstrated by OCT. Veins harvested by a less experienced individual had more intimal disruptions, adventitial injury and branch point tears. CT angiography imaging was done on the fifth postoperative day to evaluate graft patency. The rate of graft attrition was similar between the two groups (6.45% vs. 4.34%). However those veins having at least 4 intimal or medial disruptions showed significantly worse patency (67% vs. 96%). This was an underpowered study (85 EVH cases and 10 open cases) but does shed light on the types of injuries seen in EVH harvested veins that otherwise would have gone unnoticed.

There have been a number of studies over the past decade that have clearly supported the benefits of EVH. A prospective, randomized evaluation of 144 patients from the University of Western Ontario was published in 2001 [5]. The incidence of leg wound infection was significantly reduced in the EVH group and double blinded histological assessment of harvested vein showed no significant damage in either group. The majority of infections occurred after discharge as expected. Post operative leg pain, mobilization, and overall patient satisfaction was significantly improved in the endoscopic group.

A larger, more recent study was published by the Northern New England Cardiovascular Study Group [6]. In this retrospective study 8542 patients underwent isolated CAB during the 2001 to 2004 time period. The use of endoscopic vein harvest increased from 34% to 75 % during that time frame. 52.5 % of the study cohort had EVH. The main outcomes of the study evaluated were the incidence of death and repeat revascularization within 4 years of the index admission. Wound complications and postoperative bleeding were also reported. Leg wound infections were significantly less in the patients undergoing EVH however the bleeding complications slightly increased in this group. Mortality was reduced in the EVH group to a significant degree and the incidence of repeat revascularization was increased in the EVH group but to an insignificant degree. The study concludes that EVH is not associated with harm when compared to open techniques of vein harvest. This study did not address the issue of vein patency or quality of the conduit. The clinical outcomes evaluated in the retrospective review however supported the expected benefits of EVR with no significant increase in mortality or need for repeat revascularization.

A number of other studies have appeared in the literature over the past ten years which are favorable for equivalent clinical outcomes comparing open vein harvest and EVH. A Canadian study published in 2009 retrospectively reviewed 5825 patients operated between the years 1998 to 2007 [7]. 32% of these patients had EVH. Median follow-up was 2.6 years. EVH was associated with fewer leg wound infections and had no association with adverse in–hospital or midterm adverse outcomes.

In 2005 Aziz and colleagues published a meta-analysis evaluating the current literature regarding EVH vs. open vein harvest [8]. Clinical outcomes analyzed included leg wound issues as well as postoperative myocardial infarction. The macroscopic quality of the conduit, the veins requiring repair and the number of repairs required were evaluated. Finally some data was available on graft patency studies but the small sample size, varying follow-up period, and mode of assessment of patency made these data unsuitable for meta-analysis. The results revealed that the number of veins requiring repair were similar in the two groups however the EVH group that required repair had a significantly higher number of repairs than the open group. No difference in the incidence of myocardial infarction was observed.

In summary, the review of the literature is complex with many variables making clear conclusions problematic. The ideal study would entail a large, randomized, prospective population of patients with macroscopic as well as microscopic evaluation of the veins for damage. Clear documentation of the target vessel quality would have to be provided and short and long term patency assessment would need to be obtained. Such a study would be very difficult to conduct for multiple reasons, the most problematic being randomization to open harvest when patient satisfaction with EVH is so well established. The literature has provided both physicians and industry with information that has enhanced the focus on less traumatic techniques in vein harvest. Optimal handling of the tissue and vein preparation is evolving.

# Evolution of Endoscopic Vein Harvesting (EVH)

Endoscopic vessel harvesting (EVH) was first introduced in the 1990s with the use of a lighted laryngoscope and first described by Lumsden and Eaves-"Laryngoscope Harvest of the Saphenous Vein"[9]. This procedure incorporated the "bridging technique" with the laryngoscope in order to get better visualization of the vein (Figure 1). This technique gained acceptance and was later modified and augmented using a hooded dissector on a rigid scope to guide longer instrumentation. A commercial disposable product was developed, Handheld Lighted Retractor and Dissector (Ethicon, Inc, Cincinnatti, OH) for saphenous vein harvest that included a tool port and endoscopic clips and scissor devices to ligate and divide branch tributaries.

Several other manufacturers followed with self-retaining lighted retractor systems that facilitated vein harvesting through multiple short incisions. Others incorporated inflated balloon blunt dissection in an attempt to create a working space around the vein. However these techniques could not demonstrate widely accepted functionality because of poor visualiztion and cumbersome instrumentation. The balloon dissection mechanisim could not always reliably be positioned with the vein trunk within dissected tunnel.

EndoSaph™ produced by General Surgical Innovations used an elongated balloon inflated with fluid to create a working space. In the mid to late 1990s Albert K. Chin M.D., who is now referred to as the "Father of EVH", introduced the Vasoview™ device [10]. Vasoview™ is a system and technique that incorporated two concepts which modernized EVH. Vasoview™ revolutionized EVH by first improving visualization and secondly, creating an optimum working space around the vessel during the harvest. Vasoview™ was originally introduced by CTS Origin and CTS Origin was subsequently purchased by Guidant Corporation and Vasoview™ underwent several iterations of improvement and continued research and development by Guidant Corporation. Guidant subsequently merged with Boston Scientific Corporation in 2006 and the Guidant cardiovascular surgery products which included Vasoview™ were sold to Maquet, a cardiovascular innovation company in Europe. Vasoview™ revolutionized EVH by optimizing visualization and workspace. A transparent conical tip was attached directly to the end of the endoscope permitting visualization through the conical tip.

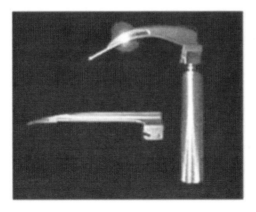

Figure 1. Standard lighted laryngoscope with Mac and Miller blades. (Photo courtesy Albert K. Chin M.D).

The transparent conical tip is used for blunt dissection. Dr. Chin's optically transparent 2mm conical tip allowed for blunt dissection of the perivascular tissues away from the vein trunk and branches without damaging or piercing the adventitia. The transparent conical blunt dissecting tip markedly improved visualization during dissection by preventing the tissues and fluids from coming in direct contact and blurring the endoscope (Figures 2, 3, 4 and 5).

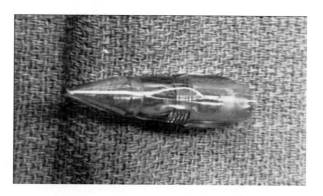

Figure 2. Transparent conical blunt dissection tip. (Photo by Lonnie J. Ginn PA-C).

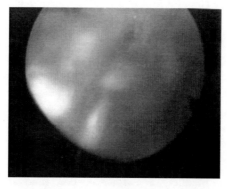

Figure 3. Compromised visualization with a bare scope during initial dissection. (Photo courtesy Albert K. Chin M.D).

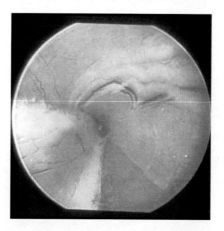

Figure 4. Improved visualization through the transparent conical tip during initial dissection. (Photo courtesy Albert K. Chin M.D).

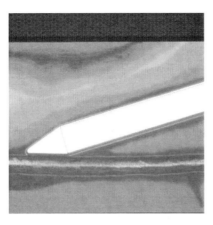

Figure 5. Tapered conical tip concept. (Photo courtesy Albert K. Chin M.D).

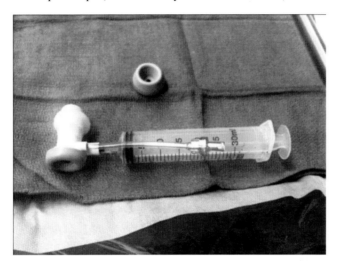

Figure 6. Blunt tip trocar port has an inflatable balloon to form a seal around the incision. (Photo by Lonnie J. Ginn PA-C).

The design and length of the conical dissection tip also proved to be a key feature by allowing appreciation of anatomical features through its transparency and easily allowing dissection with the 2mm hemi-spherical distal tip. It was also in the 1990s that technology was developed around laparoscopic procedures using balloon dissectors in the peritoneal and retroperitoneal spaces for dissection. These laparoscopic procedures used $CO_2$ gas as means of insufflating and maintaining a separation of the dissected tissue planes thus creating optimal visualization within the peritoneal cavity. Dr. Chin recognized $CO_2$ insufflation as a means of improving visualization within an EVH tunnel. He incorporated the use of a sealed trocar port to introduce the scope into a closed working area and used CO2 insufflation to improve visualization by preventing the working space tunnel from collapsing around the dissection (Figure 6). With the above noted advancements it became possible to visualize and perform blunt dissection around the main trunk of the vein. The mobilization of the small branch tributaries out of the connecting tissues while creating an improved workspace around the vein trunk could be achieved (Figure 7).

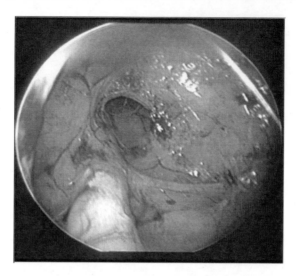

Figure 7. Superior visualization and dissection maintained by $CO_2$ insufflation created an ideal workspace to ligate and divide branch tributaries. (Photo courtesy Albert K. Chin M.D).

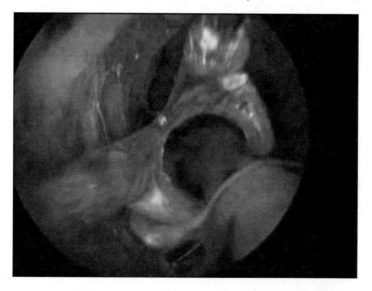

Figure 8. Open ringed retractor for manipulating the vein. (Photo by Lonnie J. Ginn PA-C).

The second stage of Dr. Chin's EVH device focused on ligating and dividing branch tributaries after all blunt dissection using the transparent conical dissection tip was completed. A device containing three items was developed that incorporated a lighted endoscope, a cautery/cutting instrument used for ligation and division of branches and an open ringed retractor for manipulating the vein (Figures 8, 9 and 10).

The tool port endoscopic device was introduced into the $CO_2$ insufflated working space through the same trocar port used for blunt tip dissection. Early usage of multiple ports for separate instrumentation demonstrated a lack of coordination and impeded a natural work flow. Using a long instrument in a tunnel with a long endoscope commonly created a competition for position often referred to as a "sword fighting" effect.

# Techniques of Conduit Harvesting for Coronary Artery Bypass Grafting

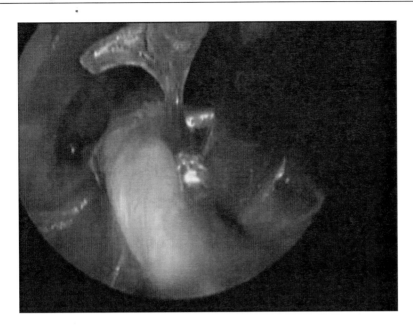

Figure 9. Cautery/cutting instrument used for ligation and division of branches. (Photo by Lonnie J. Ginn PA-C).

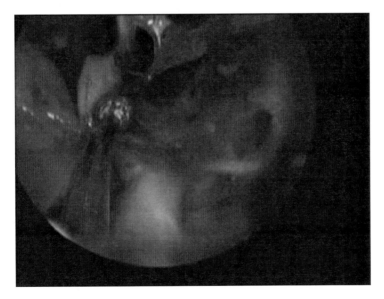

Figure 10. Retracted side branch. (Photo by Lonnie J. Ginn PA-C).

Dr. Chin substantially improved this functionality by incorporating all three items inline and fixed within the same working cannula thereby eliminating the clumsy "sword fighting". EVH now had a platform for stable instrumentation within an adequate workspace with optimum visualization.

Tributary branch ligation and division has been accomplished by several endoscopic instruments. Bipolar cautery arced electrical current between two poles and placed across the tributaries has shown to be an acceptable means of desiccating the branches.

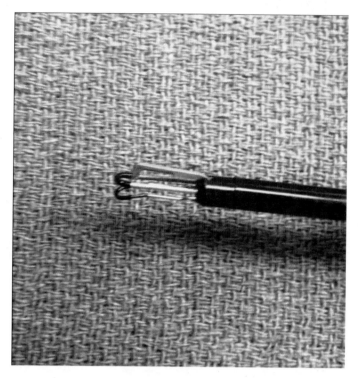

Figure 11. Bisector device with retractable knife blade. (Photo by Lonnie J. Ginn PA-C).

The use of curved endoscopic scissor or a bisector bipolar device consisting of two elongated wire loops placed on each side of the branch to apply bipolar cautery ultimately divided by a retractable guillotine blade has been shown as an effective strategy to divide branches (Figure 11).

Most recently, The HemoPro II™, a third generation device has been developed that applies pressure and heat through a small set of curved jaws that simultaneously ligate and divide branch tributaries.

This newest device of pressure and heat is gaining a wide user preference because of its superior sealing of branches minimizing oozing of blood in the tunnel and its overall best protection from thermal injury by containing the heating element completely within the confines of the jaws of the instrument along with an electronic circuitry cutoff mechanism that prevents the jaws from overheating (Figures 12 and 13).

Over the past 10 years, endoscopic vein harvesting (EVH) has become the preferred technique of vein harvesting for patients undergoing CABG in the United States. Open vein harvest (OVH) technique uses long incisions made along the medial aspect of the leg. This technique along with short incision, or skip incision "skin bridging" harvest technique has been associated with significant wound complications including dehiscence, hematoma, wound infection, cellulitis, edema, and pain. Postoperative wound complications can increase cost and length of stay in the hospital.

EVH has been shown to reduce wound complications and increase patient mobility and overall satisfaction with reduced leg pain. [5, 6].

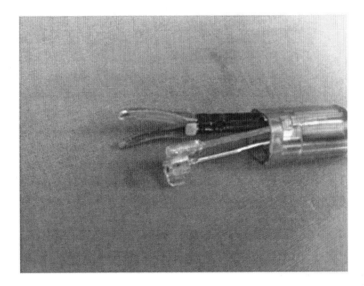

Figure 12. Maquet HemoPro II™ with open ringed retractor. (Photo by Lonnie J. Ginn).

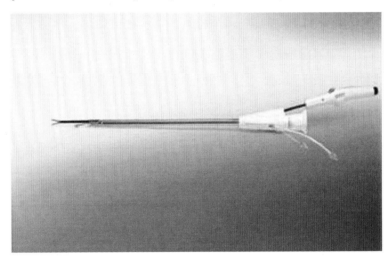

Figure 13. Maquet HemoPro II™ (Maquet Website Photo).

Graft failure related to EVH has been attributed to vein damage associated with the harvest process. Injuries resulting from excessive manipulation, avulsion of tributaries, and thermal spread from cautery devices are well described. Clot formation in the vein thought to be related to blood stasis has also been observed. Bleeding, hematomas, wound infections, and saphenous nerve injury leading to numbness and pain do occasionally occur. Rarely $CO_2$ embolism has been reported usually associated with disruption of a major venous tributary [11]. More detail regarding these complications and their avoidance will be provided in the following discussion of the EVH procedure.

Harvester experience, technique and a time constraints all play a major role in the quality of the conduit ultimately obtained.

# Technique of EVH

## Pre-Operative Assessment

Pre-operative preparation including history and physical examination for previous injury, vein stripping or leg swelling can all be good indicators for underlying vein quality. Co-morbid conditions including, diabetes, peripheral vascular disease, congestive heart failure, lymphedema and history of deep venous thrombosis can impact wound healing and the quality of the vein available. Vein mapping with ultrasound can be beneficial for locating and evaluating vein quality in obese or excessively swollen lower extremities. Ultrasound is also beneficial in identifying venous abnormalities such as duplicate systems and varicosities.

## Positioning

Supine frog-leg position with a small roll of surgical towels under the knee or a special frog-leg designed pillow allow for best positioning for EVH procedures.

## Incision

An incision above or below the knee is based on user preference. . Longitudinal, transverse and oblique incisions are all acceptable each offering advantages and disadvantages. Incisions that follow skin tension lines can enhance wound healing and cosmesis. Transverse incisions may allow easier locating of the vein where a longitudinal incision allow for easier mobilization of the vein around the port site where endoscopic harvesting is impaired by the port itself. All offer small advantages and equally small disadvantages and become the users preference and discretion and are driven by the individual patient size and tissue qualities. Another consideration is to make incisions along the corresponding tension lines of the skin. Manipulating the scope across the knee, especially on bony arthritic knees in elderly patients can be difficult. Incisions above the knee do allow for an easier vein harvest of the thigh. The need for additional lengths of vein from the lower leg can make traversing the knee from an incision in the thigh (above the knee) difficult .Harvesting the vein from the lower leg where there is typically a tighter, less compliant space can be challenging with the endoscopic approach. It is also important to keep the skin incision to a minimum. In locating, and identifying the vein, the use of retractors can create a stretching out of the incision. In closed systems using a $CO_2$ insufflation, a large incision can create a CO2 leak around the port site and impair visualization in a collapsing tunnel.

## $CO_2$ Insufflation

$CO_2$ is frequently used to improve visibility and control of the tissues. $CO_2$ is used in a closed system to create an endoscopic tunnel or in an open system used as blower used to clear blood, fluid or tissue debris from the working area. $CO_2$ insufflation can however create the potential for $CO_2$ embolization. Attention to vein and tissue fragility is important in the prevention of tears or fenestrations that could potentially allow for an embolism to occur. It is important to be familiar with and correctly set the pressures and $CO_2$ flow within the manufacturer's recommendations. Attention to the patient's central venous pressure (CVP) and limiting the insufflation to a pressure setting below the CVP can also reduce the risk of embolization. Positive end expiratory pressure (PEEP) can also be adjusted to decrease the CVP/tunnel pressure gradient. A sudden rise in end tidal $CO_2$ accompanied by a drop in systemic pressure is an early indicator of a $CO_2$ embolism. Intra-operative transesophageal echocardiogram monitoring is also valuable for revealing evidence of micro-embolization of $CO_2$.

## Intra-Luminal Clots and Fibrin Strands

Intra-luminal clots and fibrin strands can develop within the vein during the harvest process. This is most likely due to the stasis that occurs within the vein during the manipulation of harvesting as well as thermal or mechanical injury. The use of a vein with small clots within can lead to coronary embolization or intimal hyperplasia causing early or acute graft closure. Intra-luminal clots and fibrin strands can be potentially minimized and eliminated by pre-heparinizing the patient immediately prior to vein manipulations and increased external pressures from $CO_2$. A low dose of 3000 to 5000 units of Heparin intravenously is considered sufficient to reduce the incidence of intra-luminal clot and fibrin strand formations during endoscopic vein harvesting.

## Thermal Injury

Thermal injury is another means of vein injury that can lead to early graft failure. Thermal injury can also be occult and not readily visible with microscopic or other tissue viability assessment. Prevention of thermal injury is best performed by allowing adequate margins between the cautery and main vein trunk. Ensure that tributary branches are thoroughly dissected to allow a length of tissue shrinkage when branches desiccate from the heat of the cautery. Short bursts of a low cautery setting rather a prolonged cautery application also allow the user to visualize tissue desiccation, transference of heat and tissue margins as branches are sealed and divided.

## Dissecting the Conduit and Exposing Tributary Branches

A systematic approach allows harvesters to develop confidence and skills and ultimately become efficient. The "ABCD" of endoscopic vein harvest is useful in organizing and teaching the technique. Create a dissection plane (A)bove the vein followed by a similar plane (B)elow. After both above and below blunt dissection planes are completed, a sharp dissector with cautery is used to dissect all (C)ircumferential branches. Ultimately the vein trunk is (D)ivided using an endo-loop or skin puncture technique. Recommended sequence of approach is to locate and identify the vein, and mobilize tributary branches in the proximity of the port site under direct vision by using a suitable retractor. After white balancing and focusing the scope, the dissection tip is applied to vein and the superficial plane is advanced to the length of the working scope using "blunt" dissection by a plowing motion. It is important to use short plowing motions to prevent branch avulsions or fenestration in the main vein trunk.

In a closed system, it is best to advance the scope a short 1-2 cm motion, then pull the scope back and allow the $CO_2$ to penetrate and lift the dissected plane as the scope is advanced.

The short motion appears to "tease" the tissue planes apart. Keep the dissection plane as near to vein as possible to prevent bleeding in the tunnel. Adipose (fat) tissue surrounding the vein is commonly vascular and disruption can create unnecessary bleeding in the workspace. After, the superficial plane is developed; a plane directly below is similarly created. A sharp dissecting device with cautery or tissue sealing technology is used next to ligate and divide branches.

Divided branches should be long enough to adequately apply silk suture ties and or ligature clips in preparing the conduit for grafting use. Larger branches will need more length to accommodate silk ties and ligature clips. Larger branches also desiccate and shrink more than smaller ones. To create more space and allow for a safe length in branch ligation and division, harvesters may use a "window" technique. The "window" technique involves creating fenestrations or "windows" in the fascia surrounding tributary branches. Releasing the surrounding fascia allows the branch to be retracted further away from the surrounding tissue for application of the cautery and sharp dissector.

## Vessel Removal and Preparation

It is important to be sure all tributary branches are ligated and divided along the length of the vein before ligating the proximal or distal end for removal. Any missed branches or connective tissue is more difficult to ligate and divide endoscopically after the ends have been divided. Generally it is recommended to create a small incision over the concerned area and ligate and divide the branch using direct vision rather expose the vein trunk to potential injury.

Several appropriate techniques are used for ligation, division and removal of the vein from the leg. Most commonly used is a skin puncture with a #11 blade followed by blunt puncture of the fascia with a hemostat or like instrument. When making the puncture the "stab" in the skin is superficial and not near the larger deep neurovascular structures. The vein is grasped by the clamp and gently pulled back through the skin. Slow, gentle traction is used to pull the vein through the skin.

Careful attention is directed in the area of the saphenous-femoral junction especially with patients with fragile tissues. The vein is then clamped, divided and ligated with silk ties. It is important to realize that when the vein retracts back into the leg that as it pulls through the skin it does not pull off the ligating suture tie.

A double tie or a suture ligature is best to prevent disruption of the ligation and significant bleeding inside the tunnel.

# Radial Artery

In the 1970s, the radial artery was introduced as an arterial conduit for coronary bypass operations [12]. Initial enthusiasm for the conduit was tempered by the radial artery's propensity to spasm as well as concerns regarding hand ischemia. Uncertainty associated with patency and reliability of radial grafts resulted in very limited use of this conduit until a resurgence of interest occurred in the early 1990s [13]. Methods used to overcome spasm as well as the introduction of calcium-channel blockers revived interest in the radial artery. The advantage of arterial conduits regarding resistance to atherosclerotic disease was becoming more apparent and a number of encouraging publications regarding patency appeared in the literature. Over time the radial artery has been established as a very good arterial conduit option when handled properly. Minimally invasive harvest techniques have been developed. However, the time required as well as the potential for trauma and spasm in the artery have limited their utilization. Radial graft patency studies have demonstrated failure in three general ways [14]. Complete occlusion, string sign, and short, focal areas of narrowing. No evidence of atherosclerotic deterioration has been observed. The radial artery is very vasoreactive and therefore is very sensitive to competitive flow. Placement of these conduits to large coronary arteries with only moderate degrees of stenosis may well lead to occlusion or string sign and therefore should be placed only to totally occluded vessels or those with a high degree of stenosis.

Good clinical preoperative assessment of the patient provides much useful information regarding the potential use of the radial artery as a conduit. The non-dominant arm is usually chosen however in situations of limited conduit options both arms can be considered. Palpable radial and ulnar pulses, along with a clearly negative Allen test are the initial assessment. In questionable situations Doppler assessment confirms the integrity of the palmar arch and the adequacy of ulnar collateral circulation. Some reports in the literature recommend the routine use of Doppler evaluation which is certainly a reasonable approach [15]. The presence of a pulse in the distal radial artery with temporary proximal occlusion at the time of harvest confirms good collateral flow. Excellent, detailed anatomic description and harvest technique references have been described [16,17]. The radial artery is generally harvested using low cautery and taken as a pedicle graft. The harmonic scalpel has also been used to limit the potential of thermal injury [18]. Care must be taken to avoid the lateral antebrachial cutaneous nerve which results in some numbness in the arm if injured. Most of the multiple, small radial artery branches are cauterized and the larger ones clipped. The artery is treated topically with dilute papaverine or other antispasmodic solutions. One technique that works well is cannulation of the distal radial artery with a small angiocath after division and gently injecting the antispasmodic solution. This is done while the proximal portion is intact resulting in gentle dilation of the conduit. Complications of radial artery harvest are infrequent and usually limited to some paresthesias of the hand, limited areas of arm numbness, hematomas and occasionally infection. The use of calcium channel blockers during the postoperative period has been advocated to block the radial artery propensity for spasm. The use of long term oral calcium channel blockers is sometimes done empirically as well [17].

## Internal Thoracic Arteries

The use of the left internal thoracic artery (LITA) to the left anterior descending (LAD) artery has become a measure of quality in cardiac surgery programs. This of course is due to the wealth of data that demonstrates the superiority of this conduit for long term patency, especially when used as an in-situ graft to the LAD [19]. The STS Database confirms that the LITA is used in over 95% of first time coronary bypass procedures. The internal thoracic artery (ITA) is almost always free of any atherosclerosis and remains free from atherosclerotic degeneration when used as a coronary graft. Despite this fact the right internal thoracic artery (RITA) continues to have limited use [20].

Concerns for sternal wound infection, extra time required for harvest, and the uncertainty of where and how to use the graft contribute to the infrequent use of the RITA. It is more difficult to use the RITA as an in-situ graft because of inadequate length. It has also been shown to have less than optimal patency when used with the Right Coronary Artery, probably due to competitive flow. Additional length can be obtained by skeletonizing the artery at the time of harvest. The RITA can be passed through the transverse sinus to reach an intermediate or high obtuse marginal branch of the circumflex.

The RITA is also used as a free graft with the proximal anastamotic site on the LITA or a vein hood on the aorta. The RITA and LITA are most frequently harvested as a pedicle but some advocate the skeletonization technique in order to obtain better length and possibly reduce the degree of devascularization of the sternum [21].

Bipolar low cautery is often utilized in this technique. Complications of ITA harvest include sternal devascularization and subsequent wound infection, phrenic nerve injury, and rarely chylothorax secondary to lymphatic disruption [22,23].

## Conduit Preparation

The optimal treatment of conduits after harvest in preparation for grafting has been extensively studied. It is clear from all studies that over distention of vein grafts will lead to endothelial disruption. Various solutions have been developed to assist in the reduction of conduit spasm. An excellent review of this topic was published in The Annals of Thoracic Surgery in 1999 [24].

Rosenfeldt and associates discuss the causes of venous and arterial conduit spasm and the solutions effective in managing this problem. Papaverine is one of the more frequently used vasodilators. It has a low pH and could potentially damage endothelium unless buffered with albumin or blood. Topical use is effective and less likely to cause damage to the conduit. Glyceryl trinitrate-verapamil combination is effective in both saphenous vein and arterial conduits.

It is safe to use intraluminally and has a rapid onset and prolonged action. Gentle hydrostatic dilation of veins treated with antispasmodic solution results in less damage to endothelium. Special syringes have been developed which limit the degree of pressure distention.

# Conclusion

The choice of the graft conduit is crucial to the success of CABG because the patency of a coronary conduit is closely associated with an uneventful postoperative course and better long-term patient survival.

From the beginning of coronary bypass surgery venous conduits particularly the greater saphenous vein has been the most frequently used coronary conduit.

However, over the last decade or so, coronary bypass graft surgery with arterial revascularization of all diseased coronaries has shown to be efficient because arterial grafts have better long-term patency, especially LITA, compared with venous grafts. In addition to the inherent characteristics of the various conduits, quality of the conduit obtained is key to the ultimate short- and long-term success of the operation.

Patience and persistence, sometimes at the expense of speed, is required to obtain the best conduits available. A technically superb operation can be foiled by the use of poor conduits or conduits that have been damaged by poor harvesting technique.

Table 1. Intraoperative vasodilator agents for use with vascular grafts

| Agent | Optimal Concentration | Advantages | Disadvantages | Comment |
|---|---|---|---|---|
| Papaverine in electrolyte solution | 1.6 mmol/L (0.6 mg/mL) | Powerful dilator regardless of the cause of the spasm | Acid pH could damage endothelium | Improves early patency. Suitable for topical use. |
| Papaverine in blood or albumin | 2.7 mmol/L (1.0 mg/mL) | Blood or protein to buffer acidity | When blood-based solution used topically it obscures operative field | Suitable for topical and intraluminal use. |
| Glyceryl trinitrate-verapamil combination | GTN: 37 µmol/L (8.3 µg/mL) V: 34 µmol/L (16.7 µg/mL) | Rapid onset, prolonged action, suitable for all vessels | Multi-ingredient | Has been validated in ITA, saphenous vein, and radial artery. |
| Sodium nitroprusside | 1.7 mmol/L (0.5 mg/mL) | Effective on ITA | Systemic hypotension if it enters circulation, weak dilation in saphenous vein | More effective in arterial than in venous grafts. |

GTN= glyceryl trinitrate; ITA=internal thoracic artery; V=verapamil.

# Acknowledgments

The authors wish to acknowledge the kindness of Albert K. Chin M.D. in providing his permission to use his figures.

# References

[1] Lopes RD, Hafley GE, Allen KB, et al. Endoscopic versus open vein-graft harvesting in coronary-artery bypass surgery. *N. Engl. J. Med.* 2009;361:235-44.

[2] Gundry SR, Jones M, Ishihara T, Ferrans VJ. Optimal preparation techniques for human saphenous vein grafts. *Surgery* 1980;88:785-94.

[3] Desai P, Kiani S, Thiruvanthan N, et al. Impact of the learning curve for endoscopic vein harvest on conduit quality and early graft patency. *Ann. Thorac. Surg.* 2011;91:1385-91.

[4] Farooq MU, Khasnis A, Majid A, Kassab MY. The role of optical coherence tomography in vascular medicine. *Vasc Med* 2009;14:63-71.

[5] Kiaii B, Moon BC, Massel D, et al. A prospective randomized trial of endoscopic versus conventional harvesting of the saphenous vein in coronary artery bypass surgery. *J. Thorac. Cardiovasc. Surg.* 2002;123:204-12. Erratum in: *J. Thorac. Cardiovasc. Surg.* 2002;123:1224.

[6] Dacey LJ, Braxton JH Jr, Kramer RS, et al; Northern New England Cardiovascular Disease Study Group. Long-term outcomes of endoscopic vein harvesting after coronary artery bypass grafting. *Circulation* 2011;123:147-53.

[7] Ouzounian M, Hassan A, Buth KJ, et al. Impact of endoscopic versus open saphenous vein harvest techniques on outcomes after coronary artery bypass grafting. *Ann. Thorac. Surg.* 2010;89:403-8.

[8] Aziz O, Athanasiou T, Panesar SS, et al. Does minimally invasive vein harvesting technique affect the quality of the conduit for coronary revascularization? *Ann. Thorac. Surg.* 2005;80:2407-14.

[9] Lumsden AB, Eaves FF. Endoscopic vein harvest. In: Bostwick J, Eaves FF, Nahai F, eds. Endoscopic plastic surgery. St. Louis: Quality Medical Publishing; 1995:535–47.

[10] Chin A. Endoscopic Techniques and Technology in Cardiac Surgery. Vol 1, Number 1, March 2010. 66 -76.

[11] Tamim M, Omrani M, Tash A, El Watidy A. Carbon dioxide embolism during endoscopic vein harvesting. *Ann. Thorac. Surg.* 2010;89:661-70.

[12] Carpentier A, Guermonprez JL, Deloche A, Frechette C, DuBost C. The aorta-to-coronary radial artery bypass graft. A technique avoiding pathological changes in grafts. *Ann. Thorac. Surg.* 1973;16:111-21.

[13] Acar C, Jebara VA, Portoghese M, et al. Revival of the radial artery for coronary artery bypass grafting. *Ann. Thorac. Surg.* 1992;54:652-9.

[14] Tatoulis J, Buxton BF, Fuller JA, et al. Long-term patency of 1108 radial arterial-coronary angiograms over 10 years. *Ann. Thorac. Surg.* 2009;88:23-9.

[15] Jarvis MA, Jarvis CL, Jones PR, Spyt TJ. Reliability of Allen's test in selection of patients for radial artery harvest. *Ann. Thorac. Surg.* 2000;70:1362-5.

[16] Reyes AT, Frame R, Brodman RF. Technique for harvesting the radial artery as a coronary artery bypass graft. *Ann. Thorac. Surg.* 1995;59:118-26.

[17] Sajja LR, Mannam G, Pantula NR, Sompalli S. Role of radial artery graft in coronary artery bypass grafting. *Ann. Thorac. Surg.* 2005;79:2180-8.

[18] Brazio PS, Laird PC, Xu C, et al. Harmonic scalpel versus electrocautery for harvest of radial artery conduits: reduced risk of spasm and intimal injury on optical coherence tomography. *J. Thorac. Cardiovasc. Surg.* 2008;136:1302-8.

[19] Loop FD, Lytle BW, Cosgrove DM, et al. Influence of the internal-mammary-artery graft on 10-year survival and other cardiac events. *N. Engl. J. Med.* 1986;314:1-6.

[20] Tatoulis J, Buxton BF, Fuller JA. The right internal thoracic artery: the forgotten conduit--5,766 patients and 991 angiograms. *Ann. Thorac. Surg.* 2011;92:9-15.

[21] Saso S, James D, Vecht JA, et al. Effect of skeletonization of the internal thoracic artery for coronary revascularization on the incidence of sternal wound infection. *Ann. Thorac. Surg.* 2010;89:661-70.

[22] Deng Y, Byth K, Paterson HS. Phrenic nerve injury associated with high free right internal mammary artery harvesting. *Ann. Thorac. Surg. 2003;76:459-63.*

[23] Choong CK, Martinez C, Barner HB. Chylothorax after internal thoracic artery harvest. *Ann. Thorac. Surg.* 2006;81:1507-9.

[24] Rosenfeldt FL, He GW, Buxton BF, Angus JA. Pharmacology of coronary artery bypass grafts. *Ann. Thorac. Surg.* 1999;67:878–888.

In: Off-Pump Coronary Artery Bypass Grafting
Editors: Shahzad G. Raja and Mohamed Amrani

ISBN: 978-1- 62081-549-6
© 2012 Nova Science Publishers, Inc.

*Chapter VII*

# Technique of Off-Pump Multivessel Coronary Artery Bypass Grafting through Median Sternotomy

*Bryon J. Boulton[1] and John D. Puskas[2]*
[1]Emory University, The Emory Clinic
Atlanta, Georgia, US
[2]Emory University, Emory Healthcare
Emory University Hospital Midtown
Atlanta, Georgia, US

## Abstract

Off-pump coronary artery bypass (OPCAB) grafting continues to be a useful technique for coronary revascularization. Current literature comparing off-pump vs. on-pump coronary artery bypass has failed to demonstrate the superiority of one technique over the other. Small prospective randomized controlled trials continue to show equivalent in-hospital outcomes and continue to raise concerns about vein graft patency and completeness of revascularization. Larger observational analyses are better powered to statistically compare in-hospital outcomes in both low and high-risk patients and in general have shown more favorable in-hospital outcomes and equivalent long-term outcomes with off-pump compared with on-pump coronary artery bypass. The benefits of off-pump techniques may be more apparent for patients at high risk for complications associated with cardiopulmonary bypass and aortic manipulation. This chapter takes an in-depth look into all aspects of OPCAB to give the surgeon just adopting the technique a firm foundation upon which to incorporate OPCAB into his/her practice as well as to providing the experienced OPCAB surgeon a few new tricks to address the many challenges with the procedure. Highlights of the preoperative evaluation are reviewed followed by a detailed examination of the surgical and anesthetic preoperative considerations. The major focus of this chapter addresses the technical considerations and caveats of OPCAB and is designed to provide a thorough understanding of the procedure laid out in a logical step-wise fashion as one would perform the procedure in the operating room.

# Introduction

Over the last 15 years there has been increasing interest in performing coronary artery bypass grafting (CABG) without the use of cardiopulmonary bypass. This growth in off-pump coronary artery bypass (OPCAB) grafting has been largely driven by increasing recognition of the deleterious effects of cardiopulmonary bypass and the desire to avoid the diffuse inflammatory response, multi-organ dysfunction, and neurocognitive complications that may follow. Increasing clinical experience with OPCAB has allowed analysis of outcomes following the procedure and demonstrated improved clinical outcomes in both prospective randomized trials and large, risk-adjusted, retrospective comparisons among various patient populations [1-7]. This chapter takes an in-depth look into all aspects of OPCAB to give both the surgeon just adapting the technique a firm foundation upon which to incorporate OPCAB into his/her practice, to providing the experienced OPCAB surgeon a few new tricks to address the many challenges with the procedure. Highlights of the preoperative evaluation are reviewed followed by a detailed examination of the surgical and anesthetic preoperative considerations. The major focus of this chapter addresses the technical considerations and caveats of OPCAB and is designed to provide a thorough understanding of the procedure laid out in a logical step-wise fashion as one would perform the procedure in the operating room (OR).

# Preoperative Considerations

### Evaluation

The preoperative evaluation of the patient begins with a complete history and physical examination. If a radial artery harvest is considered, patients with an inconclusive Allen's test should undergo radial and ulnar artery duplex examinations. Criteria for preoperative carotid duplex evaluation include left main disease, peripheral vascular disease, carotid bruits, history of cerebrovascular accident, history of heavy tobacco use, and age > 65. If significant carotid disease is detected, further workup is pursued, and typically staged carotid endarterectomy followed by coronary revascularization are performed. Absolute contraindications to OPCAB include cardiogenic shock, ischemic arrhythmias and anatomic factors preventing rotation of the heart, such as previous left pneumonectomy and severe pectus excavatum. Relative contraindications include significantly intramyocardial coronary arteries, and small or calcified coronary arteries. Such coronary arteries can only be bypassed safely with the benefit of considerable experience with OPCAB techniques. Patients with significant left main disease and recent myocardial infarction can be safely revascularized with OPCAB, and should be generally considered good candidates for this approach.

# Surgeon Considerations

Surgeon interest in and commitment to OPCAB is usually tied to a conviction that the technical challenges inherent to the procedure are worth overcoming so that the patient may benefit from avoidance of cardiopulmonary bypass. Despite the spectrum of attitudes and commitment to OPCAB, there is increasing recognition that there are certain subgroups of patients, such as those with severe atherosclerosis of the ascending aorta, for whom OPCAB is strongly advised.

Individual surgeon experience in OPCAB is an important determinant in patient selection for OPCAB. The unique technical challenges of OPCAB grafting and its relative unfamiliarity have raised concern that adoption of OPCAB may lead to poorer outcomes during each surgeon's learning curve. However, with careful patient selection, OPCAB surgery can be gradually assimilated into clinical practice while preserving and ultimately improving clinical outcomes. Very early in a surgeon's experience, it is recommended that patients with depressed left ventricular function, left main disease, and three-vessel disease be excluded from selection for OPCAB. As the surgeon's experience grows, more complex and higher-risk cases can be performed safely off pump. Over time, OPCAB can be applied to a broad spectrum of clinical settings, including patients with advanced age, multivessel disease, depressed left ventricular function, left main disease, and performance of complete arterial revascularization. Gradual assimilation of OPCAB thereby develops surgeon familiarity and comfort with the technique, allowing its broader application to an increasing pool of patients who derive benefit from avoiding cardiopulmonary bypass.

## Anesthesia Considerations

After the appropriate pre-operative preparation and work up is done, the patient is brought to the pre-operative holding area where a radial arterial line and a pulmonary artery catheter are placed. A pulmonary artery catheter is helpful in OPCAB to have an objective measure of pulmonary pressures, volume status and cardiac function during the case; these parameters are frequently utilized by the surgeon in the intra-operative decision making process. The patient's hair is also clipped in the pre-operative holding area from the neck to the feet. Efforts to maintain normothermia should begin in the pre-operative area by placing warm blankets on the patient. The operating room should be prepared accordingly for the patient by refraining from over cooling and placing a Bair Hugger (Bair Hugger; Arizant Healthcare, Eden Prairie, MN) on the operating table that will remain under the patient. All the IV fluids and blood products should be warmed either in preparation for the patient or by actively utilizing a Hotline Blood and Fluid Warming System (Level1; Smiths Medical, Dublin OH).

Much of the anesthetic management of patients during OPCAB surgery is common to the management of patients having conventional CABG surgery on cardiopulmonary bypass. However, because of the challenge to maintain hemodynamic stability during cardiac lifting, positioning, and retracting, the anesthesia team is much more engaged and interactive with the surgeon during the anastomotic portion of the procedure. Familiarity with the OPCAB procedure in general and the unique steps to each operation as dictated by the surgeon are important for successful outcomes. Communication between the anesthesia team and the surgeon before and during the operation is important, particularly when changes in the surgeon's operative plan occur. In understanding the operative steps, the anesthesia team must anticipate and prepare for what is approaching in the operation. For example, before anastomosis of the lateral wall vessels, if the patient is on higher than average pharmacological support, the anesthesia team can administer intravascular volume to obviate the need for increased pharmacological support that might be necessary during cardiac displacement for the lateral wall anastomoses.

The principle challenge in the intraoperative anesthetic management of patients undergoing OPCAB is maintenance of hemodynamic stability during the lifting and retracting of the heart necessary to obtain exposure to coronary targets. Significant alterations in blood pressure and cardiac output occur, particularly with rightward retraction of the heart for lateral wall exposure. Acutely, this is typically related to decreases in preload and left ventricular filling because the vena cavae, right ventricular outflow tract, and pulmonary veins may be partially kinked with this maneuver. An effective first-line response is the administration of IV fluids. An assessment of the patient's intravascular volume status is made before manipulation of the heart and preload is optimized in this way. To compensate for the acute changes in preload that occur during heart manipulation, placement of the patient in steep Trendelenburg position can rapidly increase preload to support ventricular filling during cardiac displacement. Aggressive use of table tilt in the operating room is particularly useful when moment-to-moment changes in blood pressure are desired. For example, when rightward displacement of the heart is anticipated Trendelenburg position is helpful. When moderate hypotension is desired before placement of a partial occluding vascular clamp on the ascending aorta, brief use of reverse Trendelenburg position is preferable to administration of pharmacological vasodilators, since the fluid shift that occur with table tilt are more readily reversible. In general, steep Trendelenburg position mimics sudden intravenous administration of a large volume of fluid, but is much more readily reversible and does not lead to long-term volume overload.

## **Operative Approach**

The surgeon should enter OR with a detailed plan delineating the overall strategy as well as contingency plans should there be any issues that arise during the case. OPCAB regularly requires several intraoperative decisions that are determined by factors discovered or issues that have developed during the operation. The following describes a typical operative course for a patient undergoing multivessel OPCAB.

The patient is taken to OR where she/he is intubated in the usual fashion. After this, a 1000mg aspirin rectal suppository and a temperature recording urinary catheter are placed. The pre-operative aspirin is placed because of the concern for maintaining graft patency in the early post-operative period as OPCAB patients do not benefit from cardiopulmonary bypass-related coagulopathy. It is for this reason also that plavix is administered in the immediate post operative period. Some studies have suggested that OPCAB patients may exhibit a relative hypercoagulable state in the peri-operative period, as has been demonstrated in general and orthopedic surgical patients[8].

The patient is then prepped and draped in the standard fashion for cardiac surgery. An unprimed cardiopulmonary bypass machine is always in the room with the lines set up on the pump, but not passed off to the sterile field. Cell saver, external defibrillator paddles, and a pacing cable are set up and handed off the sterile field.

The chest is opened in the usual fashion utilizing a median sternotomy to approach the mediastinum. The left and/or right internal mammary artery (LIMA/RIMA) is harvested utilizing the Rultract (Rultract; Cleveland OH) or Couetil (Vitalcor; Westmont IL) retractor. During this process the left and/or right pleural spaces are opened widely, but the right pleural space is not routinely opened if only the LIMA is harvested. 5000 units of IV heparin are administered at the time of vein harvest to minimize fibrin strand formation during the harvesting procedure. Radial artery and/or greater saphenous vein endoscopic harvesting is performed simultaneously while the internal mammary artery is harvested. Simultaneous conduit harvesting after IV heparin administration has not been associated with increased blood loss during the procedure. Once the internal mammary artery(ies) has been successfully dissected from the chest wall, 1.5 mg/kg (180 units/kg) of IV heparin is administered to achieve a targeted activated clotting time (ACT) of >350 seconds. The ACT is rechecked and heparin redosed every 30 minutes to maintain this level of anticoagulation. This redosing typically requires 3000 units of heparin to maintain ACT > 350 seconds, since normothermic OPCAB patients metabolize heparin more quickly than hypothermic patients do during cardiopulmonary bypass.

After administration of heparin, the mammary pedicle is divided, intraluminal papaverine is administered into the mammary artery, and then the distal branches of the artery are clipped to allow for it to distend until it is anastomosed to the left anterior descending (LAD) coronary artery. A sternal retractor (OctoBase; Medtronic Inc., Minneapolis MN or Maquet Sternal Retractor Blades; Maquet Inc., Wayne NJ) that is designed to act as a platform base for OPCAB stabilizers and positioners (ACROBAT and XPOSE product lines, Maquet Inc., Wayne NJ or Octopus and Starfish product line, Medtronic Inc., Minneapolis MN) is used. A generous inverted-T shaped pericardiotomy is performed dividing the pericardium along the diaphragm to its anterior limits to allow for cardiac displacement during the operation, while paying attention to the location of the phrenic nerves. Frequently the right and left pericardiophrenic artery and vein are encountered and clipped to prevent postoperative hemorrhage. The diaphragmatic attachments to the sternum are divided as are the right and left pericardial fat pads to allow further room for cardiac displacement. Two rolled towels can be placed under the right corner of the sternal retractor to elevate the retractor to prevent cardiac compression against the retractor or right sternal edge during rightward cardiac displacement.

Pericardial traction sutures are placed below the cut edge of the pericardium on the left side to allow for rightward cardiac rotation on the vena caval axis, thus facilitating exposure of the lateral wall of the left ventricle. The aortopulmonary window may be dissected to allow for placement of a partial-occlusion vascular clamp to perform proximal anastomoses.

Epiaortic ultrasound is performed on all patients before manipulating the aorta, and is the most sensitive method of identifying atherosclerotic lesions of the ascending aorta and aortic arch. Most importantly it allows the surgeon to selectively place either partially occluding vascular clamps or clampless proximal anastomotic devices (Heartstring III; Maquet Inc., Wayne NJ) to minimize the risk of atheroembolism. A grade III, IV or V lesion in the ascending aorta should preclude the placement of a vascular clamp on the ascending aorta. In this scenario, the epiaortic ultrasound can guide the placement of a clampless proximal anastomosis in an uninvolved area of the ascending aorta. In rare cases when there is no free area of the ascending aorta, the innominate artery, or either RIMA or LIMA pedicle can be used as a proximal bypass inflow source.

A deep pericardial traction suture is then placed roughly two-thirds of the distance between the inferior vena cava and the left pulmonary vein at the point where the pericardium reflects behind the left atrium. Care is taken to avoid the underlying esophagus, left lung, descending aorta, and pulmonary veins. This suture is then placed in a soft rubber catheter to prevent cardiac damage. This stitch is used to elevate the heart out of the pericardial well to facilitate exposure of the coronary targets. Placing a moist laparotomy pad lateral to the suture may aid in this exposure and may dampen cardiac motion. Moving this stitch towards the left shoulder causes the heart to elevate and rotate towards the patient's right, exposing the LAD and diagonal coronary artery branches.

## Sequence of Coronary Grafting

In OPCAB, the selected sequence of grafting is important in maintaining hemodynamic stability and avoiding myocardial ischemia. As a general principle, hemodynamic stability is best preserved by grafting any *collateralized* vessel(s) first and then constructing the proximal anastomosis(es) for these grafts. *Collateralizing* vessels are grafted last. This strategy prevents interruption of vital blood flow from the collateralizing vessel during its grafting. If the LIMA-LAD is performed first, a long pedicle may be necessary to avoid undue tension placed on the anastomosis during cardiac positioning while performing the other required anastomoses.

A preferred sequence of grafting is as follows:

1. Perform the anastomosis to the completely occluded, collateralized vessel(s) first. The collateralizing vessel may then be safely grafted. This strategy will minimize myocardial ischemia.
2. The LIMA-LAD anastomosis should be performed first especially if the LAD is collateralized or in cases of tight left main stenosis. The anastomosis is performed last when the LAD is the collateralizing vessel.
3. The proximal anastomosis can be performed first or early after the distal anastomosis if the target is a critical, collateralized vessel. This allows simultaneous perfusion during the occlusion of the collateralizing vessel and minimizes overall myocardial ischemia.
4. Beware of the large, moderately stenosed right coronary artery. The right coronary artery, particularly if large and dominant, can cause problems when occluded during OPCAB. Acute occlusion of a moderately stenotic right coronary artery may lead to severe hemodynamic compromise due to bradycardia, secondary to AV node ischemia. The surgeon must be prepared to use an intracoronary shunt or epicardial pacing to correct bradyarrhythmias promptly.
5. Beware of mitral regurgitation in OPCAB. Prolonged cardiac displacement combined with mitral regurgitation may contribute to a downward hemodynamic spiral. Progressive elevation of pulmonary pressures and increasing regurgitation on TEE may signal impending heart failure. Ischemic mitral regurgitation should be addressed early in the procedure. This is accomplished by grafting and perfusing the culprit vessel responsible for papillary muscle dysfunction.

6. If none of these above principles dictate otherwise, the lateral wall targets are grafted last as these tend to require cardiac positioning that can compromise venous return more significantly than the anterior or inferior wall targets positions require.
7. Importantly, graft sequence should be individualized for each patient, depending on anatomic patterns of coronary occlusion and collateralization, myocardial contractility, atherosclerosis of the ascending aorta, conduit availability, and graft geometry.

## Cardiac Displacement and Presentation of Coronary Targets

It is important to understand that the cardiac displacement techniques for exposure of the inferior and lateral wall coronary arteries are different. For the lateral wall vessels, such as the obtuse marginals and ramus intermedius, the right pericardial traction sutures are released first and the left pericardial traction sutures are pulled taut on the sternal retractor to begin displacing the heart. The right limb of the sternal retractor is routinely elevated on two rolled towels, creating space for rightward cardiac displacement. Occasionally the right pleural space is opened or a relaxing incision is made on the diaphragmatic pericardium to allow the apex of the heart to be elevated and rolled under the sternum on the vena caval axis without compressing the caval vessels or the apex of the heart against the sternum. The patient is placed in steep Trendelenburg position to facilitate venous return and the table is rotated to the patient's right. The deep stitch is pulled taut towards the patient's left and secured to the sternal retractor. The cardiac positioner and stabilizer (ACROBAT and XPOSE product lines, Maquet Inc., Wayne NJ or Octopus and Starfish product line, Medtronic Inc., Minneapolis MN) are mounted on the right side of the sternal retractor platform (OctoBase; Medtronic Inc., Minneapolis MN or Maquet Sternal Retractor Blades; Maquet Inc., Wayne NJ). The positioner is often best placed on the left ventricular lateral wall rather than on the apex to facilitate optimal exposure of circumflex marginal coronary artery targets.

For the inferior wall vessels, such as the posterior descending artery, left ventricular branch of the right coronary artery, or posterolateral obtuse marginal branch, the deep stitch is pulled towards the patient's left hip or feet and secured to the retractor or drapes. It is very important that tension on the right sided pericardial sutures is released. The coronary stabilizer is mounted to the left limb of the sternal retractor. The patient is placed in Trendelenburg position and rotated to the patient's right. The base of the heart is elevated so the apex is oriented towards the ceiling with the cardiac positioner, which is placed on the right limb of the sternal retractor.

In contrast to the lateral and inferior wall vessels, the anterior wall vessels (LAD and diagonals) are exposed with very little manipulation of the heart. The deep stitch is secured to the patient's left lateral side and the coronary stabilizer is placed over the anterior wall from the caudal or left side of the sternal retractor. An apical positioner is not routinely necessary for grafting of the anterior wall. Care is taken to divide the pericardium to allow the LIMA pedicle to fall posteriorly into the left chest, medial and posterior to the apex of the left lung.

## Coronary Stabilization and Grafting

The current stabilization devices on the market (XPOSE product lines, Maquet Inc., Wayne NJ or Octopus product lines, Medtronic Inc., Minneapolis MN) utilize suction rather than compression to maintain epicardial capture. This allows for coronary stabilization at the mechanical median of the cardiac cycle, and thus minimal interference with ventricular function. Once the device is applied, a few cardiac cycles may be needed for the heart to recover. If hemodynamics are compromised, as evidenced by decreased systolic blood pressure or elevated pulmonary artery pressures, the degree of compression or cardiac position should be adjusted to find the median point in the cardiac cycle. This can be done by adjusting the stabilizer arm's tension while still maintaining suction. The malleable arms of both devices can be spread apart after epicardial capture to improve visualization. They also can be independently bent up, down, or curved to maximize epicardial tissue "capture" and coronary visualization. Epicardial fat retractors are thus infrequently needed, but can be helpful in patients with intramyocardial coronary arteries or when the coronary arteries are buried in excessive epicardial fat.

After optimal exposure is obtained, a soft silastic vessel loop with a blunt-tip needle (Quest Medial, Allen TX) is looped around the target vessel for occlusion. The loop is placed proximal to the planned anastomosis – never distally-- to avoid trauma to the coronary outflow of the bypass graft. This silastic loop should be placed widely around the coronary artery target vessel, encompassing a generous amount of epicardial tissue, to avoid arterial injury. Care should be taken during placement to avoid entering the ventricle or damaging epicardial veins. When this occurs, a superficial epicardial suture generally stops the bleeding. The vessel loop should be directed out of the surgeon's field of view, and this may be aided with a loose pericardial suture acting like a pulley.

If the target vessel is poorly collateralized, an interval test occlusion of 2-5 minutes can be used to determine how well the regional ischemia will be tolerated. This also induces ischemic preconditioning. Moreover, if the test occlusion is not well tolerated, an intracoronary shunt (Clearview Intracoronary shunt, Medtronic Inc., Minneapolis MN) can then be placed prior to beginning suturing the anastomosis. This also gives the surgeon some measure of assurance before committing to the anastomosis by creating an arteriotomy. Once the distal anastomosis is underway, it is critical for the anesthesia team to be communicating continuously with the surgeon, and quickly addressing any changes in hemodynamics. Bradyarrhythmias, most frequently encountered during right coronary grafting, can be promptly treated with epicardial pacing, or placement of an intracoronary shunt.

The target vessel is occluded by applying the minimal necessary tension to the silastic vessel loop. This tension will allow for the vessel to be lifted slightly above the plane of the epicardial fat and improve visualization. The target vessel is opened with a coronary knife and the arteriotomy is extended with coronary scissors. The field is kept free of blood by dispersing the retrograde bleeding with a humidified $CO_2$ blower (Clearview Blower/Mister, Medtronic Inc., Minneapolis MN). Occasionally, when a vessel is completely occluded proximally, an intracoronary shunt is required because the mister/blower is unable to create satisfactory visualization in the presence of significant retrograde bleeding. To minimize vessel trauma, it is important for the surgeon's assistant to blow on the target only when the surgeon is placing the needle through the tissue of the conduit or target vessel. Excellent visualization is critical for a precise anastomosis, with the intima visualized for each stitch on the conduit and target vessel. Magnification with a 3.5x loups, headlight, and Castro needle holders are used for all anastomoses. An 8-0 monofilament suture is used to optimize precision, unless severe calcification mandates the use of a heavier 7-0 monofilament suture needle. As with all coronary artery anastomoses, the needle should be rotated through the coronary vessel without any torquing to avoid trauma to the vessel. With practice and fastidious technique a precise coronary anastomosis can be reliably achieved despite the minimal movement of the vessel during OPCAB.

## Myocardial Protection Strategies

A number of myocardial protection strategies were developed early in the experience of OPCAB and remain in use. The importance of maintaining good systemic blood pressure by optimizing preload conditions and the use of vasopressors as part of conscientious anesthetic management cannot be overemphasized. Even delaying initiation of the anastomotic process to allow for resuscitation of a hypovolemic patient may be necessary to allow for hemodynamic stability and thus good myocardial protection. Optimal placement of coronary stabilizers and cardiac positioners to allow for adequate exposure of the target vessel without excessively compressing the cardiac chambers or inhibiting venous return is a vital part of myocardial protection during OPCAB. Another strategy of myocardial protection is the sequence of anastomoses during the OPCAB procedure. Selecting an occluded, collateralized vessel first in the sequence of anastomoses allows for this territory to be reperfused and then secondarily perfuse other territories via reversed flow across the collateral bed during the anastomosis of their respective arteries.

Early proximal anastomosis before distal anastomosis can allow for immediate reperfusion of the ischemic territory after distal anastomosis. The common rationale of anastomosing the LIMA-LAD first is that this graft requires little cardiac displacement and its reperfusion benefits hemodynamic stability during subsequent lifting of the heart to graft other vessels of the heart. If a large territory of myocardium is perfused by a target vessel, and lifting is necessary for adequate exposure, the operative sequence might be to first perform the proximal anastomosis for that target vessel, then perform the LIMA-LAD, to allow for added hemodynamic stability during lifting and exposure for the distal anastomosis of the target vessel.

An intracoronary shunt (ClearView Intracoronary Shunts; Medtronic, Inc. Minneapolis, MN) may be placed if significant ischemia or hemodynamic compromise occurs after target vessel occlusion. Commercially available shunts range in size from 1.0mm to 3.0mm in 0.25mm increments. While these are used infrequently, they are kept available in the operating room for all cases. Intracoronary shunts may be particularly helpful with a large, dominant right coronary artery which can cause bradyarrhythmias when occluded; intramyocardial vessels, and with critical anatomy. The shunt is removed after completion of the anastomosis prior to tying the suture. Air is allowed to be expelled from the anastomosis prior to tying the suture. The conduit should be occluded with an atraumatic bulldog clamp until the proximal anastomosis is performed in order to prevent retrograde bleeding and loss of coronary perfusion pressure.

At times, to maintain hemodynamic stability, especially in a patient with a low ejection fraction, an intra-aortic balloon pump (IABP) may be placed. It is best for this to be placed at the beginning of the operation in anticipation of potential problems rather than in response to the development of hemodynamic issues during the operation. Frequently, the IABP reduces or eliminates the need for inotropic support during the exposure and occlusion of target vessels during OPCAB. This can also allow patients with severe proximal multivessel coronary artery disease, recent myocardial infarction, and severe ventricular dysfunction to have adequate hemodynamics and myocardial protection during OPCAB. With experience and gradual application of the principles described above, virtually all coronary vessels can be safely exposed, stabilized, and grafted by off-pump techniques.

## Proximal Anastomoses

Proximal anastomoses to the aorta are commonly performed with an aortic partial occlusion clamp. The systolic pressure is brought down to roughly 90-95 mmHg prior to application of the clamp. This can be frequently achieved with simple placement of the patient in reverse Trendelenburg positioning, and decreasing any pharmacological support the patient may be on, without having to pharmacologically decrease the systolic blood pressure. Once the side-biting, partial clamp is applied, aortotomies are created with a 4.0mm aortic punch. Vein graft anastomoses are performed with 5-0 or 6-0 monofilament suture and arterial anastomoses are performed with 6-0 or 7-0 monofilament suture. Any graft that is taken as a 'T' graft off the LIMA is anastomosed with an 8-0 monofilament. Air emboli are prevented by placing an atraumatic bulldog clamp on the conduit before beginning the anastomoses. The aorta is de-aired by removing the partial-occluding clamp after completion of the final proximal anastomosis before tying down the suture, and the vein grafts are de-aired by puncturing with a 25-gauge needle and then removing the atraumatic bulldog clamps after the air has been expelled. Arterial grafts are not punctured, but allowed to back bleed prior to the removal of the clamp.

As mentioned previously, prior to the placement of the partial-occluding, side-biting clamp, the aorta is always scanned with an epiaortic ultrasound. Clamping is not performed in patients with diffuse grade III, grade IV, or grade V atherosclerotic disease. In these scenarios, the epiaortic ultrasound is used to identify an uninvolved segment of the aorta. A clampless proximal aortotomy system (Heartstring III, Maquet, Inc., Wayne NJ) is utilized creating a beveled, hand-sewn proximal anastomosis. This is done with a monofilament suture on a RB-2 needle sized according to the conduit being used. If no suitable location can be identified on the aorta, a 'T' graft is created off the LIMA or RIMA. Alternatively, the RIMA may also be harvested and used as an inflow source.

After completion and reperfusion of all grafts, protamine is administered (0.75 to 1.0 mg/kg) to partially correct the ACT to around 150 seconds or roughly near baseline, depending on surgeon preference. As hemostasis is being achieved, a chest tube is placed into each opened pleural space and the mediastinum. Temporary epicardial pacing wires are only placed if they have been needed during the procedure. The chest is closed in the standard fashion with sternal wires and running absorbable sutures in the fascia, subcutaneous, and subcuticular layers. Morbidly obese diabetic patients may benefit from use of retention sutures rather than a subcuticular closure to reduce risk of sternal wound infection.

## Robotic and Hybrid Coronary Revascularization

Off-pump coronary revascularization has evolved to include several minimally invasive options, including robotic LIMA harvest and LIMA-LAD anastomosis via a 3-4cm left anterior micro-thoracotomy ("robotic EndoACAB"). The many technical considerations of this operation are beyond the scope of this chapter, but it is a very useful technique for highly selected patients who require a single LIMA-LAD graft. Application of this technique has been combined with percutaneous revascularization in 'hybrid' procedures. This procedure is performed for patients with multi-vessel coronary artery disease, especially for those with LAD disease and a single other diseased vessel. In this procedure the LIMA is harvested thorascopically or with robotic assistance and is anastomosed to the LAD through a small anterior left micro-thoractomy, and the remainder of the lesions are treated with percutaneous coronary intervention. Future advancements in miniaturization and the application of robotics to cardiac surgery may expand our ability to revascularize more complex coronary anatomy and apply these advanced techniques more broadly.

## Conclusion

As with adopting other new techniques, there is a learning curve associated with OPCAB. With persistence and careful attention to detail, this technique can be mastered and performed reliably in most patients. Complete revascularization can be achieved in all patients and OPCAB has been shown to provide superior outcomes compared with conventional on-pump coronary artery bypass grafting in multiple high-risk patient subgroups, including women, and in patients with aortic atherosclerosis, prior stroke, severe pulmonary disease and decreased renal function. [7,9] It is an essential part of the modern cardiac surgeon's armamentarium.

## References

[1] Ascione R, Lloyd CT, Underwood MJ, Gomes WJ, Angelini GD. On-pump versus off-pump coronary revascularization: evaluation of myocardial function in a prospective randomized study. *Eur. J. Cardiothorac. Surg.* 1999;15:685-90.

[2] Angelini GD, Taylor FC, Reeves BC, Ascione R. Early and midterm outcome after off-pump and on-pump surgery in beating heart against cardioplegic arrest studies (BHACAS 1 and 2): a pooled analysis of two randomized controlled trials. *Lancet* 2002;359:1194-9.

[3] Cleveland JC Jr, Shroyer AL, Chen AY, Peterson E, Grover FL. Off-pump coronary artery bypass grafting decreases risk-adjusted mortality and morbidity. *Ann. Thorac. Surg.* 2001;71:165-9.

[4] Khan NE, De Souza A, Mister R, Flather M, Claque J, Davies S, Collins P, Wang D, Sigwart U, Pepper J. A randomized comparison of off-pump and on-pump multi-vessel coronary-artery bypass surgery. *N. Eng. J. Med.* 2004;350:21-8.

[5] Plomondon ME, Cleveland JC Jr, Ludwig ST, Grunwald GK, Kiefe CI, Grover FL, Shroyer AL. Off-pump coronary artery bypass is associated with improved risk-adjusted outcomes. *Ann. Thorac. Surg.* 2001;72:114-9.

[6] Puskas JD, Williams WH, Duke PG, et al. Off-pump coronary artery bypass grafting provides complete revascularization with reduced myocardial injury, transfusion requirements, and length of stay: a prospective randomized comparison of two hundred unselected patients undergoing off-pump versus conventional coronary artery bypass grafting. *J. Thorac. Cardiovasc. Surg.* 2003;125:797-808.

[7] Puskas JD, Kilgo PD, Lattouf OM, et al. Off-pump coronary bypass provides reduced mortality and morbidity and equivalent 10-year survival. *Ann. Thorac. Surg.* 2008;86:1139-46.

[8] Geerts WH, Berggvist D, Pineo GF, Heit JA, Samama CM, Lassen MR, Colwell CW. Prevention of venous thromboembolism: American College of Chest Physicians evidence-based clinical practice guidelines, 8th edition. *Chest* 2008;133(6 Suppl):381S-453S.

[9] Puskas JD, Edwards FH, Pappas PA, et al. Off-pump techniques benefits men and women and narrow the disparity in mortality after coronary bypass grafting. *Ann. Thorac. Surg.* 2007;84:1447-56.

In: Off-Pump Coronary Artery Bypass Grafting
Editors: Shahzad G. Raja and Mohamed Amrani

ISBN: 978-1- 62081-549-6
© 2012 Nova Science Publishers, Inc.

*Chapter VIII*

# Technique of Minimally Invasive Direct Coronary Artery Bypass (MIDCAB) Grafting

*Piroze M. Davierwala, David M. Holzhey and Friedrich W. Mohr*
Department of Cardiac Surgery, Heart Center
University of Leipzig, Leipzig, Germany

## Abstract

Minimally invasive direct coronary artery bypass (MIDCAB) surgery usually involves revascularization of the anterior wall using the left internal mammary artery (LIMA) as the bypass graft. Performance of this operation is quite demanding and has a steep learning curve.

Despite that, it has become a procedure associated with low postoperative mortality and morbidity, especially in high-volume centers having surgeons performing this operation on a regular basis.

It can be combined with percutaneous coronary intervention (PCI) to other coronary vessels in a hybrid procedure. It is most commonly performed for single-vessel isolated LAD disease, in which PCI is not advisable (proximal or complex lesions), not successful, or not possible (occluded LAD). It also includes patients who have undergone PCI and stenting of the LAD previously and have presented again with recurrence of symptoms due to development of in-stent restenosis. Similarly, patients with double vessel disease who have already undergone primary angioplasty and stenting of a non-LAD culprit vessel can subsequently undergo LAD revascularization by a MIDCAB operation.

MIDCAB surgery is a very attractive operation for the patient due to excellent cosmesis and an early and quick recovery. It can be performed very elegantly and effectively by highly experienced surgeons, with not only good short and mid-term results but also excellent long-term outcomes. This chapter focuses on the historical aspects, indications, contraindications, technique and results of MIDCAB and provides an overview of the authors' experience with this strategy for revascularizing isolated proximal LAD stenosis.

## Introduction

The proximal left anterior descending artery (LAD), defined as the part of the LAD from its origin at the bifurcation of the left main coronary artery to the first major septal branch, can supply up to 50% of the left ventricle. As a result, a large area of the myocardium is at risk, when this segment of the LAD has a high grade stenosis [1]. Minimally invasive direct coronary artery bypass (MIDCAB) surgery using the left internal mammary artery (LIMA) as the bypass graft is one of the established treatment options for isolated proximal LAD lesions and has gained widespread acceptance. It is now the preferred method of surgical revascularization for isolated coronary artery disease of the anterior wall at some centers. The major pros in favour of MIDCAB surgery are the minimal access and the LIMA graft to the LAD, which has stood the test of time. Although, performing the operation is quite demanding and has a steep learning curve, it has become a procedure associated with low postoperative mortality and morbidity, especially in high-volume centers having surgeons performing this operation on a regular basis [2].

The alternative procedures available for the treatment of anterior wall coronary disease are conventional on- or off-pump coronary artery bypass grafting (CABG) or percutaneous coronary intervention (PCI). For the last four to five decades, on-pump CABG has enabled cardiac surgeons all over the world to achieve excellent results, despite the ever-increasing risk profile of the patients. However, majority of the complications occurring after on-pump CABG can be attributed to cardiopulmonary bypass (CPB) and myocardial protection. This is especially true in high-risk patients currently undergoing CABG.

Off-pump CABG for single-vessel LAD disease eliminates all the risks involved in on-pump CABG, except one and that is the potential risk of superficial and deep sternal wound infection. MIDCAB surgery avoids CPB and a sternotomy and their related complications.

Improvement of symptoms in patients with single-vessel LAD disease has been achieved by both, percutaneous transluminal coronary angioplasty (PTCA) and CABG [3]. However, several studies published in literature have consistently proven that the incidence of medium-term adverse events and repeat revascularization of the target lesion were higher after PTCA than conventional CABG in these patients [4,5]. Although the rate of restenosis reduced drastically after the advent of stents [6], randomized trials comparing stenting and MIDCAB revealed a significantly higher reintervention rate after stenting and similar results for mortality and reinfarction at mid- to long-term follow-up [7,8]. Diegler and colleagues reported that the rate of repeated revascularization of the target vessel for restenosis after stenting was 29% versus 8% after MIDCAB (p=0.003). 79% patients were free from angina after six months, as compared to 62% in the stenting group (p=0.03) [9]. The application of drug-eluting stents (DES) did reduce the risk of in-stent restenosis [10], however in a randomized comparison of MIDCAB surgery versus sirolimus-eluting stenting in isolated proximal LAD stenosis, Thiele et al. reported a repeat revascularization rate of 0% in patients who underwent MIDCAB as compared to 6.2% in those who underwent stenting. Although perioperative complications occurred more often after surgery, they did not influence quality of life at 12-month follow-up and the overall rate of major adverse cardiovascular events

(MACE) [11]. This chapter discusses the historical aspects, indications, operative technique and results of MIDCAB surgery.

## Historical Aspects

The initial attempts to revascularize the myocardium date back to the 6$^{th}$ decade of the 20$^{th}$ century, a long time before the utilization of CPB for CABG. In 1952, Arthur Vineburg described his technique of myocardial revascularization by rerouting internal mammary artery into heart muscle, allowing side branches to bleed into, and nourish, heart muscle [12].

However it was not until the early 1960s that direct coronary artery grafting was established as the norm in coronary surgery due to the foresight and perseverance of a few surgeons. In 1961, Goetz and coworkers reported their experience with nonsutured internal mammary artery (IMA) anastomoses. They connected the right IMA (RIMA) to the right coronary artery (RCA) on the beating heart by means of a tantalum ring [13]. The main group that should be credited with the development of minimally invasive coronary surgery was the clinic in St. Petersburg, directed by Vasilii I. Kolesov, the pioneer and founder of coronary revascularization, as described by Olearchyk [14]. He introduced direct suturing anastomosis between the IMAs and coronary ateries and performed the first operation in February 1964, and until May 1967, his clinic was the only site where coronary revascularization was systematically performed [15].

In 1973, Garrett and colleagues reported a case of saphenous vein graft performed on beating heart 9 years earlier in 1964 [16]. Trapp and Bisarya [17], in Canada and Ankeney [18], in the United States tried to propagate off-pump CABG against the popular trend of performing CABG with CPB on an arrested heart in a bloodless, motionless surgical field. This trend continues for the next 2 decades, when it gradually came to light that many of the complications occurring after on-pump CABG were attributed to CPB. It was not until the early 1990s that the perception regarding off-pump CABG began to change. The revival of the concept of performing CABG in a minimally invasive manner was to perform the operation without CPB and though a small incision. This concept was proposed in 1995 by Benetti [19] and further propagated by several investigators like Calafiore and colleagues [20] and Subramanian and coworkers [21]. This innovative approach, which combined the off-pump technique with the minimally invasive approach, came to be known as MIDCAB or the left anterior small thoracotomy (LAST) operation. It is now widely used by some centers for revascularization of the anterior wall myocardium.

## Indications

The commonest pathology for which patients undergo a MIDCAB operation, is single-vessel isolated LAD disease, in which PTCA is not advisable (proximal or complex lesions), not successful, or not possible (occluded LAD). It also includes patients who have undergone PCI and stenting of the LAD previously and have presented again with recurrence of symptoms due to development of in-stent restenosis. Similarly, patients with double vessel disease who have already undergone primary angioplasty and stenting of a non-LAD culprit vessel can subsequently undergo LAD revascularization by a MIDCAB operation. Performance of this operation in an emergency situation like iatrogenic dissection of the LAD in the catheterization laboratory is controversial. One can argue in favour of a MIDCAB operation in such situations when the patient is hemodynamically stable, without overt signs of ongoing ischemia and the operation is to be performed by an experienced surgeon, who can expedite the procedure efficiently. However, such situations could be considered as relative contraindications for MIDCAB surgery.

The indications of MIDCAB surgery can be further extended to patients with double vessel with LAD disease, in whom a second vessel (right coronary or circumflex arteries) is occluded and recanalized or with a mild stenosis or stenosis that could be dilated and stented later; patients with LAD disease and disease of two other vessels with a combination of the situations previously described. The latter constellation is called the "hybrid" MIDCAB procedure.

Patients suffering from multiple comorbidities like chronic obstructive pulmonary disease, chronic renal insufficiency, diffuse cerebrovascular and peripheral vascular disease, malignancy and those with advanced age are at an extremely high risk for CPB. In addition, patients with severe uncontrolled insulin-dependent diabetes mellitus, obesity, renal failure or immune deficiency have a higher predilection for deep sternal wound infections. Such patients would be better served by a MIDCAB procedure followed by PCI of the other vessels if required. Patients with multivessel disease with poor left ventricular function, ischemic cardiomyopathy and congestive heart failure, who are not transplant candidates, have a very high predicted mortality for conventional CABG. Jacobs et al. reported an actuarial 4-year survival of 85.6% and the event-free survival including freedom from angina, MACE, and reintervention of 81.5% in this patient group. They showed that MIDCAB carries a lower incidence of in-hospital death, neurological events, and perioperative myocardial infarction with comparable midterm result, when compared to conventional CABG in high-risk patients [22]. MIDCAB surgery is also a good option for patients, who require redo CABG. LIMA to LAD grafts can be performed for failed saphenous vein grafts to the LAD.

There are certain anatomical considerations that should be minutely scrutinized in every patient, so as to assess the feasibility of performing the operation comfortably and safely. A mid-distal (2-4 cm distal to the second diagonal branch) noncalcified LAD greater than 1.75 mm in diameter, total occlusion of the LAD with good collaterals to the distal segment, a thin tubular vertically positioned heart and a slim patient are ideal candidates for a MIDCAB operation.

## Contraindications

There are probably only two absolute contraindications to MIDCAB surgery; (a) an occluded left subclavian artery and (b) a patient in cardiogenic shock with LAD as the culprit vessel requiring emergent revascularization. In the second situation, the sole aim is to execute the operation as quickly and safely as possible. In MIDCAB surgery, longer time is required to harvest the LIMA and perform the anastomosis.

The other contraindications for MIDCAB can be regarded as relative, and are dependent on the experience and expertise of the operating surgeon. Intramyocardial LADs, calcified

LADs and LADs with a diameter less than 1.5 mm pose a real challenge for the operating surgeon. The threshold to convert to a sternotomy should be low in such patients.

Extreme obesity increases the difficulty of the operation at every stage; LIMA harvest becomes a grinding task because it is difficult to visualize it, not only due to the difficult exposure through the thick chest wall, but also due to the fact that it is enveloped in a thick layer of fat, especially in its proximal part. The heart is also very fatty and exposure of a deeply seated LAD can be technically demanding through a small incision. Finally, performing the LIMA-LAD anastomosis is also more challenging than usual as it has to be performed deep in the chest through the restricted access.

# Operative Procedure

## Preoperative Assessment

Preoperative assessment of the patient is extremely important prior to MIDCAB surgery in order to justify the indication for surgery. Patients requiring emergent revascularization and those with severe COPD may not be ideally suited to MIDCAB surgery. The importance of physical examination of the patient cannot be undermined. Obesity, chest contour (better visualization of the LIMA with increasing curvature of the chest wall) and length of the thorax (proximal LIMA access becomes more difficult with increasing length of the chest) should be carefully assessed. The chest radiograph not only helps to confirm the physical findings, but also give the surgeon an approximate idea about the position of the heart (horizontal or vertical), its size and the width of the intercostal spaces. The preoperative coronary angiogram is the most important investigation, which enables the surgeon to decide about the feasibility of the patient to undergo MIDCAB surgery. The course (whether it reaches the apex or falls significantly short of it or is it intramyocardial) and the size of the LAD, the quality of its wall (diffuse disease or calcification), the degree of stenosis (the higher the grade of stenosis, the better is the tolerance to occlusion), accompanying arteries (a large diagonal running parallel to the LAD may be mistaken to be the LAD and grafted) and the position of stents if the artery has been previously stented.

## *Patient Positioning and Monitoring*

The patient is placed in a supine position with the left chest elevated by about 30 degrees from the horizontal plane by placing a bolster under it. The arms of the patient lie at the sides. This affords access to the left chest for the LIMA harvest. The left groin of the patient is always available for emergent institution of CPB if required. A perfusionist and a heart-lung machine are always on standby. A catheter is usually inserted into the left femoral artery in very obese patients to facilitate quick incorporation of CPB in an emergency situation. External pacing and defibrillator pads are also attached. Monitoring is performed with arterial and central venous catheters. The pulmonary artery catheter is placed only in patients with a left ventricular ejection fraction less that 30%. Changes in ST segment are monitored using a on-line 5-channel electrocardiogram. The urinary bladder is catheterized. Transesophageal echocardiography is used in patients with poor left ventricular function or when a patient unexpectedly becomes hemodynamically unstable during the operative procedure. A warming blanket is always used and the room temperature is maintained at 22°C.

## Surgical Technique

The incision is a 5-6 cm anterolateral muscle-sparing minithoracotomy, located 2-3 cm inferior to the nipple. The left hemithorax is entered through the 4$^{th}$ or 5$^{th}$ left intercostal space after the patient is connected to single lung ventilation. A specially designed IMA access retractor is used for IMA harvesting under direct vision. The technique of LIMA harvest, whether pedicled or skeletonized, is at the discretion of the operating surgeon. The proximal three quarters of the LIMA can usually be harvested with this retractor. For harvest of the lower quarter of the LIMA, rib retraction and immobilization of the myocardial surface a second device is used. In obese patients, the large amount of pericardial fat sometimes obscures the vision of the LIMA especially in its proximal third. This can be overcome either by removal of this fat or by retraction of the fat inferiorly and laterally with a retraction suture. The whole length of the LIMA is harvested in most cases; however in some patients with a long chest it may be possible to take it down only up to the 2$^{nd}$ rib. Calafiore and colleagues have shown that 76.9% of the LADs needed a LIMA length of 9 cm or less to be grafted. Hence, the whole length of the LIMA is not necessary to reach the LAD in a MIDCAB procedure. Harvesting the distal LIMA segment is more important for its mobility to reach the LAD. The concern, that partial harvest of the LIMA may give rise to the possibility of competitive flow with the LAD, has also been put to rest by Luise and colleagues who showed that the flow reserve in the LIMA remained unchanged, even when it was partially harvested [23]. The patient is then heparinised with 100-150 IU/kg of heparin. The activated clotting time is maintained at a level above 300 seconds throughout the operation. The pericardium is then opened longitudinally and the LAD is identified. The position of the LAD and its accompanying diagonal branches must be correlated with that on the angiography film. The distal end of the LIMA is transected only after the target vessel identified, is confirmed to be the LAD. Two 6.0 polypropelene sutures are used to hold the LIMA against the upper edge of the chest incision, following which, the distal end of the LIMA is prepared for anastomosis. A reusable pressure stabilizer without suction, which can be attached to the rib retractor, is used to stabilize the LAD. This can be attached to the superior or inferior blade of the rib spreader depending on the location of the thoracotomy incision in relation to the site of anastomosis on the LAD. It is then secured at the site of the potential anastomosis. Two 6.0 polypropylene sutures are used retract the epicardial fat, if the LAD is deeply embedded in it. A 4.0 polypropylene pledgeted tourniquet is passed around the LAD proximal to the site of anastomosis (Figure 1). No ischemic preconditioning is used. The LAD is opened and the tourniquet is snared just enough to stop the forward flow in the LAD. Shunting of the LAD can be used alternatively and can be recommended when ischemic changes are seen in ECG tracings on the monitor, excessive retrograde flow of blood from the distal LAD or in patients with a large LAD with a lower grade stenosis (60-70%) or in whom the anastomosis is performed more proximally. Such patients have a higher chance of developing ischemia upon proximal occlusion of the LAD. Distal occlusion should be always avoided. The anastomosis is performed using one running 8-0 or 7-0 polypropylene suture, starting at the heel of the anastomosis (Figure 2).

If the LIMA is pedicled, both sides of the pedicle are fixed to the epicardium. Following this, the flows in the LIMA are checked with the commercially available Doppler flow probes.

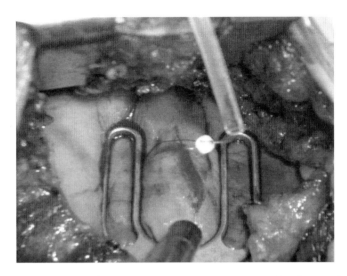

Figure 1. Stabilization of the LAD with a pressure stabilizer and preparation for proximal occlusion of the LAD.

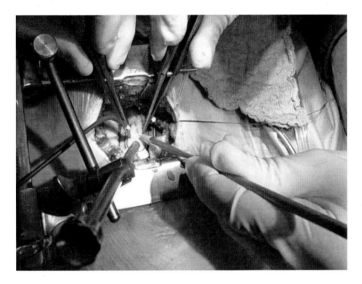

Figure 2. Operative field immediately before incision of the LAD.

The anastomosis is checked for hemostasis. The pericardium is usually closed around the apex. The rest of the defect is closed by approximating the pericardial fat with the medial edge of the pericardium, so as to cover the distal segment of the LIMA. This protects the LIMA from being pushed anteriorly by the left lung upon inflation. Once hemostasis is checked, a single chest drain is inserted into the left pleural cavity. The anesthetist is then asked to inflate the left lung. At this stage, it is extremely important to prevent the lung from pushing the LIMA anteriorly, in order to prevent an avulsion. The LIMA should lie medial to the lung after it is completely inflated. An intercostal nerve block is then administered and the spread ribs are approximated. The thoracotomy is then closed in layers. Patients, who become extremely unstable during the course of the operation and develop low output syndrome refractory to medical management, are immediately connected to CPB by cannulation of the left femoral vessels. Patients, in whom LIMA is injured or is too short, or the LAD is not visible along its entire length or is heavily calcified or anastomotic problems or right ventricle injuries occur are patients who require conversion to a sternotomy. Some patients do not tolerate single-lung ventilation and need conversion.

*Postoperative Management*

Postoperative management does not differ from that for other off-pump CABG patients. MIDCAB patients are usually good candidates for the fast-track recovery concept. The patient can be extubated in the operating room itself or shortly thereafter in the cardiovascular intensive care unit (CVICU). The utilization of precisely the right quantity of anaesthetic and sedative medications is crucial to avoid postoperative atelectasis of the left lung, especially in the first few postoperative days. Some studies published in literature have shown that the degree of pain encountered by patients with an anterolateral minithoracotomy is higher as compared to sternotomy, especially during the first three days after surgery [24].

# Results

The MIDCAB procedure is generally acknowledged as a challenging operation with a substantial learning curve (Figure 3) [2]. However, almost all published series report excellent results. This is probably due to the fact that most publications in literature are from centers harboring surgeons with a lot of experience in MIDCAB surgery. The following sections give a brief overview of the results of MIDCAB surgery as well as long-term outcomes in a series of 1768 consecutive patients, who underwent MIDCAB surgery at our institution (Table 1).

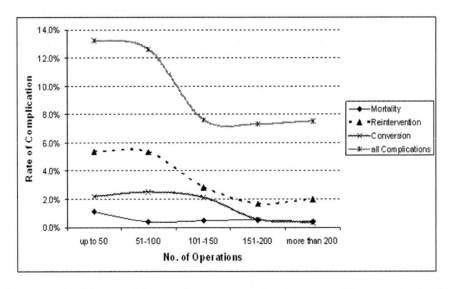

Figure 3. Average development of the most important complications rates with surgeon's experience.

## Table 1. Preoperative patient characteristics and risk factors of the study population

| Preoperative variable | Number | Percentage |
|---|---|---|
| Total number of patients | 1768 | |
| Mean age (Mean ± SD) | 63.4 ± 10.8 | |
| Male (n, %) | 1273 | 72% |
| Mean Body Mass Index (Mean ± SD) | 27.3 ± 3,9 | |
| Long-term smokers (n, %) | 573 | 32.4% |
| Arterial hypertension (n, %) | 1416 | 80.1% |
| Diabetes (n, %) | | |
| Type I | 9 | 0.5% |
| Type II without insulin | 307 | 17.4% |
| Type II with insulin | 171 | 9.7% |
| Hyperlipoproteinemia (n, %) | 1154 | 65.3% |
| COPD (n, %) | 130 | 7.4% |
| PVD (n, %) | 258 | 14.6% |
| Neurological disorders (n, %) | 65 | 3.7% |
| Renal failure (n, %) | 44 | 2.4% |
| Critical preoperative state (n, %) | 28 | 1.6% |
| Unstable angina pectoris (n, %) | 146 | 8.3% |
| Pulmonary hypertension (n, %) | 14 | 0.8% |
| Implanted pacemaker (n, %) | 52 | 2.9% |
| Implanted ICD (n, %) | 8 | 0.5% |
| Previous cardiac operation (n, %) | 57 | 3.2% |
| Previous stent implantation in target vessel (n, %) | 322 | 18.2% |
| Chronic total occlusion of target vessel (n, %) | 407 | 23.0% |
| Previous stent implantation in other vessels (n, %) | 232 | 13.1% |
| Mean logistic EuroSCORE (Mean ± SD) | 3.8 ± 6.2 | |

COPD: Chronic obstructive pulmonary disease; PVD: Peripheral vascular disease; ICD: Intracardiac defibrillator.

## Procedural Success

Being a challenging operation, one can well imagine that in some patients, one might have to alter plans and convert to a median sternotomy, implement CPB, or use an interposition vein graft between the LIMA and LAD (short LIMA) and in some patients abort the operation right from the outset due to intolerance of the patient to single-lung ventilation. Many a times, these problems can be avoided by careful selection of patients with anatomically favourable conditions for MIDCAB operations. In our series, a "conversion rate" of 2.3% was observed. Median sternotomy and CPB became necessary in 31 (1.75%) and 17 patients (0.96%) respectively. The commonest reasons were an injured LIMA or an intramural LAD. This is consistent with the results of a meta-analysis by Kettering et al. who reported a conversion rate of 1.8% [25].

## Clinical Outcomes

Kettering et al. reported an early mortality of 1.3%[25]. Other single center analyses have reported an early mortality rate between 0% and 2.5% strongly depending on sample size and patient selection [11, 26, 27]. In our series, the combined 30-day and in-hospital mortality was 0.8%.

Postoperative stroke is uncommon in patients undergoing MIDCAB surgery and usually occurs only as a consequence of other complications (need for cardiopulmonary bypass, resuscitation, postoperative ECMO support) or in the presence of other risk factors such as atrial fibrillation. Thus, the reported stroke rates after MIDCAB surgery varied between 0% and 1.5% in the early publications [28-30]. In our series, 7 patients (0.4%) suffered a stroke and one patient (0.06%) developed intracerebral hemorrhage.

Perioperative myocardial infarction is commonly associated with graft occlusion, which is diagnosed by postoperative coronary angiography and more often than not, requires reintervention (see below). 0.8% patients developed myocardial infarction in our series and its range varies between 0% and 3.1% in literature [25].

Other typical complications observed after conventional CABG are rarely seen after MIDCAB surgery. In our series, 3% needed re-exploration for bleeding, 8.2% developed pleural effusion and 8.2% developed transient new atrial fibrillation. A (superficial) wound infection was seen in 1.5% patients.

## Angiographic Follow-Up and Reintervention

A good quality-assessment criterion is postoperative coronary angiography to evaluate the LIMA to LAD graft. Diegeler and colleagues published the largest series of patients, who underwent routine postoperative coronary angiography after MIDCAB surgery.

The postoperative patency rate in more than 700 patients was 95.6% and follow-up at 6 months angiogram of more than 300 patients showed a 94% patency rate [31].

The need for immediate or short term reintervention (surgical revision or percutaneous coronary intervention, PCI), reported in literature, ranges between of 0.4% to 8.9% [11,25,27,32] depicting different levels of experience with this procedure. In our series, a total of 59 patients (3.3%) needed short term reintervention on the target vessel.

In most cases, due to stenosis of the anastomosis, stenosis of the LAD distal to the anastomosis or narrowing or kinking of the LIMA. These problems were managed by PCI/stent-implantation (11 patients) or re-operation (48 patients).

## Long Term Outcomes

The main advantage of the LIMA-to-LAD bypass and therefore, also of MIDCAB operation is the excellent long term outcomes.

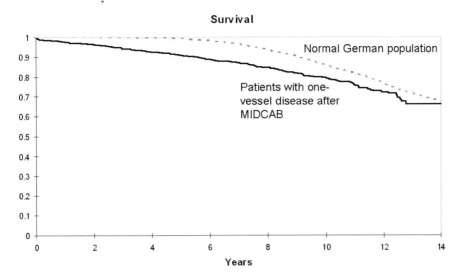

Figure 4. Comparison of survival curves for patients after MIDCAB and an age and gender matched population.

Five year survival ranges between 80% and 95% in different publications including high risk and elderly patients [32-35]. The survival of our patients after MIDCAB compares favourably to an age and gender matched population (Figure 4). In our patient population the actuarial freedom from major adverse cardiovascular and cerebrovascular complications (MACCE) at ten years was 70.9%. This is comparable with other studies [32,33], although the long term data is still sparse.

## Conclusion

MIDCAB surgery is a very attractive operation for the patient due to excellent cosmesis and an early and quick recovery. Although, it is a challenging operation for surgeons, especially for those who are in their learning curve, it can be performed very elegantly and effectively by highly experienced surgeons, with not only good short and mid-term results but also excellent long-term outcomes. It can also be used in combination with PCI as a hybrid procedure.

## References

[1] Varnauskas E. Twelve-year follow-up of survival in the randomized European Coronary Surgery Study. *N. Engl. J. Med.* 1988;319:332-7.

[2] Holzhey DM, Jacobs S, Walther T, Mochalski M, Mohr FW, Falk V. Cumulative sum failure analysis for eight surgeons performing minimally invasive direct coronary artery bypass. *J. Thorac. Cardiovasc. Surg.* 2007;134:663-9.

[3] Hueb WA, Bellotti G, de Oliveira SA, et al. The Medicine, Angioplasty or Surgery Study (MASS): a prospective, randomized trial of medical therapy, balloon angioplasty

or bypass surgery for single proximal left anterior descending artery stenoses. *J. Am. Coll. Cardiol.* 1995;26:1600-5.

[4] Goy JJ, Eeckhout E, Burnand B, et al. Coronary angioplasty versus left internal mammary artery grafting for isolated proximal left anterior descending artery stenosis. *Lancet* 1994;343:1449-53.

[5] Goy JJ, Eeckhout E, Moret C, et al. Five-year outcome in patients with isolated proximal left anterior descending coronary artery stenosis treated by angioplasty or left internal mammary artery grafting. A prospective trial. *Circulation* 1999; 99:3255-9.

[6] Versaci F, Gaspardone A, Tomai F, Crea F, Chiariello L, Gioffrè PA. A comparison of coronary-artery stenting with angioplasty for isolated stenosis of the proximal left anterior descending coronary artery. *N. Engl. J. Med.* 1997; 336:817-22.

[7] Jaffery Z, Kowalski M, Weaver WD, Khanal S. A meta-analysis of randomized control trials comparing minimally invasive direct coronary bypass grafting versus percutaneous coronary intervention for stenosis of the proximal left anterior descending artery. *Eur. J. Cardiothorac. Surg.* 2007;31:691-7.

[8] Thiele H, Oettel S, Jacobs S, et al. Comparison of bare-metal stenting with minimally invasive bypass surgery for stenosis of the left anterior descending coronary artery: a 5-year follow-up. *Circulation* 2005;112:3445-50.

[9] Diegeler A, Thiele H, Falk V, et al. Comparison of stenting with minimally invasive bypass surgery for stenosis of the left anterior descending coronary artery. *N. Engl. J. Med.* 2002;347:561-6.

[10] Moses JW, Leon MB, Popma JJ, et al; SIRIUS Investigators. Sirolimus-eluting stents versus standard stents in patients with stenosis in a native coronary artery. *N. Engl. J. Med.* 2003;349:1315-23.

[11] Thiele H, Neumann-Schniedewind P, Jacobs S, et al. Randomized comparison of minimally invasive direct coronary artery bypass surgery versus sirolimus-eluting stenting in isolated proximal left anterior descending coronary artery stenosis. *J. Am. Coll. Cardiol.* 2009;53:2324-31.

[12] Vineburg A. The treatment of angina pectoris by internal mammary artery implantation supplemented by pericardial fat wrap; covering four years clinical and eight years experimental experience. *Conn. State Med. J.* 1955;19:281-302.

[13] Goetz RH, Rohman M, Haller JD, Dee R, Rosenak SS. Internal mammary-coronary artery anastomosis. A nonsuture method employing tantalum rings. *J. Thorac. Cardiovasc. Surg.* 1961;41:378-86.

[14] Olearchyk AS. Vasilii I. Kolesov. A pioneer of coronary revascularization by internal mammary-coronary artery grafting. *J. Thorac. Cardiovasc. Surg.* 1988;96:13-8.

[15] Kolesov VI. [Initial experience in the treatment of stenocardia by the formation of coronary-systemic vascular anastomoses]. *Kardiologiia* 1967;7:20-5.

[16] Garrett HE, Dennis EW, DeBakey ME. Aortocoronary bypass with saphenous vein graft. Seven-year follow-up. *JAMA* 1973;223:792-4.

[17] Trapp WG, Bisarya R. Placement of coronary artery bypass graft without pump oxygenator. *Ann. Thorac. Surg.* 1975;19:1-9.

[18] Ankeney JL. Off-pump bypass surgery: the early experience, 1969-1985. *Tex. Heart Inst. J.* 2004;31:210-3.

[19] Benetti FJ, Ballester C, Sani G, Doonstra P, Grandjean J. Video assisted coronary bypass surgery. *J. Card. Surg.* 1995;10:620-5.

[20] Calafiore AM, Giammarco GD, Teodori G, et al. Left anterior descending coronary artery grafting via left anterior small thoracotomy without cardiopulmonary bypass. *Ann. Thorac. Surg.* 1996;61:1658-63.

[21] Subramanian VA. Less invasive arterial CABG on a beating heart. *Ann. Thorac. Surg.* 1997;63(6 Suppl):S68-71.

[22] Jacobs S, Holzhey D, Falk V, Garbade J, Walther T, Mohr FW. High-risk patients with multivessel disease--is there a role for incomplete myocardial revascularization via minimally invasive direct coronary artery bypass grafting? *Heart Surg. Forum* 2007;10:E459-62.

[23] Luise R, Teodori G, Di Giammarco G, et al. Persistence of mammary artery branches and blood supply to the left anterior descending artery. *Ann. Thorac. Surg.* 1997;63:1759-64.

[24] Diegeler A, Walther T, Metz S, Falk V, Krakor R, Autschbach R, Mohr FW. Comparison of MIDCAP versus conventional CABG surgery regarding pain and quality of life. *Heart Surg. Forum* 1999;2:290-5.

[25] Kettering K, Dapunt O, Baer FM. Minimally invasive direct coronary artery bypass grafting: a systematic review. *J. Cardiovasc. Surg.* (Torino) 2004;45:255-64.

[26] Mehran R, Dangas G, Stamou SC, et al. One-year clinical outcome after minimally invasive direct coronary artery bypass. *Circulation* 2000;102:2799-802.

[27] Karpuzoglu OE, Ozay B, Sener T, et al. Comparison of minimally invasive direct coronary artery bypass and off-pump coronary artery bypass in single-vessel disease. *Heart Surg. Forum* 2009;12:E39-43.

[28] Jegaden O, Wautot F, Sassard T, etal . Is there an optimal minimally invasive technique for left anterior descending coronary artery bypass? *J. Cardiothorac. Surg.* 2011;6:37.

[29] Boodhwani M, Ruel M, Mesana TG, Rubens FD. Minimally invasive direct coronary artery bypass for the treatment of isolated disease of the left anterior descending coronary artery. *Can. J. Surg.* 2005;48:307-10.

[30] Bucerius J, Gummert JF, Borger MA, et al. Stroke after cardiac surgery: a risk factor analysis of 16,184 consecutive adult patients. *Ann. Thorac. Surg.* 2003;75:472-8.

[31] Diegeler A. Left internal mammary artery grafting to left anterior descending coronary artery by minimally invasive direct coronary artery bypass approach. *Curr. Cardiol. Rep.* 1999;1:323-30.

[32] Holzhey DM, Jacobs S, Mochalski M, et al. Seven-year follow-up after minimally invasive direct coronary artery bypass: experience with more than 1300 patients. *Ann. Thorac. Surg.* 2007;83:108-14.

[33] Sorm Z, Harrer J, Vobornik M,Cermáková E, Vojácek J. Early and long-term results of minimally invasive coronary artery bypass grafting in elderly patients. *Kardiol. Pol.* 2011;69:213-8.

[34] Pompilio G, Alamanni F, Tartara PM, et al. Determinants of late outcome after minimally invasive direct coronary artery bypass. *J. Cardiovasc. Surg.* (Torino) 2007;48:207-14.

[35] Okawa Y, Baba H, Hashimoto M, et al. Comparison of standard coronary artery bypass grafting and minimary invasive direct coronary artery bypass grafting. Early and mid-term result. *Jpn J. Thorac. Cardiovasc. Surg.* 2000;48:725-9.

In: Off-Pump Coronary Artery Bypass Grafting
Editors: Shahzad G. Raja and Mohamed Amrani

ISBN: 978-1- 62081-549-6
© 2012 Nova Science Publishers, Inc.

*Chapter IX*

# Technique of Totally Endoscopic Robot-Assisted Off-Pump Coronary Artery Bypass Grafting

*Eric J. Lehr[1], W. Randolph Chitwood Jr.[2] and Johannes Bonatti[3]*

[1]Swedish Heart and Vascular Institute, Swedish Medical Center
Seattle, WA, US
[2]East Carolina Heart Institute, East Carolina University
Greenville, NC, US
[3]Division of Cardiac Surgery
University of Maryland School of Medicine
Baltimore, MD, US

## Abstract

Robotically assisted beating heart totally endoscopic coronary artery bypass grafting (BHTECAB) is the most advanced form of less invasive surgical coronary revascularization. Single and double vessel procedures have been standardized and are reproducible, while technological advancement and procedural development has lead to triple and even quadruple bypass being performed at a few centers of excellence. BHTECAB can be an elegant surgical component to hybrid revascularization strategies, extending the minimally invasive approach to a wider patient population. A hybrid approach requires consideration of revascularization strategy, and anticoagulant and antiplatelet regimes. With experience, a wide range of surgical revascularization options isd available, including multiarterial grafting with sequential, Y- and T-grafts to all major territories of the myocardium. Larger studies reporting short- to mid-term outcomes are available from several centers around the world. In the major published series totaling 668 cases, in hospital mortality was 0.6%. Conversion to a larger incision is high (14.2%) and operative times are prolonged, but these series represent the learning curves of multiple teams and improve with experience. Mid-term freedom from major adverse cardiac and cerebral events is in line with the results of major studies assessing conventional coronary artery bypass grafting. Patient benefits from BHTECAB may include shorter hospital stays and earlier return to full activity.

Stepwise progression of robotic technology and procedure development will continue to make robotic operations simpler and more efficient, which will encourage more surgeons to take up this technology and extend the benefits of robotic surgery to a larger patient population. As BHTECAB continues to evolve, long-term studies are required to confirm that the outcomes of BHTECAB match those of traditional approaches. This chapter provides an overview of the technique, technology, outcomes, concerns, controversies and future developments associated with BHTECAB.

## Introduction

Surgical pioneers have sought more effective methods of revascularizing the ischemic heart since Carrel sutured a carotid artery graft from the descending thoracic aorta to a coronary artery in a dog in 1910. In the early to mid 1900s, surgical pioneers including Beck, Vineberg, Goetz, Longmire, Demikhov, Favalaro and others developed the foundation supporting Johnson's report of 301 patients undergoing coronary artery bypass grafting (CABG) forming the basis for today's revascularization procedures [1].

With the development of cardiopulmonary bypass, cardioplegic techniques and myocardial protection were introduced and on-pump arrested heart CABG quickly became the gold standard for myocardial revascularization, allowing anastomoses to be performed on a still heart in a bloodless field.

On-pump arrested heart CABG via sternotomy, now one of the most commonly performed surgical procedures, can be performed with outstanding, long-term reproducible results. Further procedural development dictated reducing collateral surgical trauma while maintaining excellent long-lasting outcomes.

Minimally invasive techniques were introduced to cardiac surgery in the mid-1990s [2,3] and off-pump beating heart totally endoscopic coronary artery bypass grafting (BHTECAB) was heralded as the "Holy Grail" of surgical coronary revascularization. Modified cardiopulmonary bypass methods and limited incisions with long shafted instruments under direct vision facilitated minimally invasive valve surgery, but CABG using endoscopic techniques without robotic assistance is technically demanding and has been performed only sporadically [4,5].

Robotic surgery using the da Vinci® surgical system (Intuitive Surgical, Inc., Sunnyvale, CA) with articulating wrist instrumentation has overcome many of the limitations of long-shafted instruments by providing seven degrees of freedom and incorporating three dimensional (3D) visualization, making delicate intracorporeal surgery possible within confined spaces. Loulmet was the first to report a successfully completed totally endoscopic coronary artery bypass grafting TECAB using femoral cannulation and cardioplegic arrest [6].

Further work set the stage for a multicenter study of arrested heart TECAB that lead to approval of the da Vinci® surgical system by the United States Food and Drug Administration in July 2004 [7]. The first generation system however, had only 3 arms (left, right and camera). BHTECAB therefore required the use of external static epicardial stabilizers that generally attached to the operative table and were challenging to apply. This limitation rendered BHTECAB technically quite difficult.

Consequently, conversion was common in early series [8] and some surgeons limited their robotic practice to internal mammary artery (IMA) harvesting and completed the procedure through an anterior thoracotomy, performing a direct hand sutured anastomosis on the beating heart [5]. With the addition of a fourth arm, a dynamic, robotically controlled endoscopic epicardial stabilizer could be applied.

This robotic stabilizer added the capability of making fine adjustments in positioning and myocardial stabilization and provided exposure of lateral wall target vessels, making BHTECAB much more feasible [9].

The scope of robot-assisted coronary operations ranges from IMA harvest with a hand-sewn anastomosis, performed on-pump through a median sternotomy, to multivessel BHTECAB which can include combinations of single, sequential, T or Y grafts, generally based off of one or both IMAs, using radial artery or saphenous vein to construct composite grafts.

Because of the difficulty in constructing robotic proximal aortocoronary graft anastomoses from the left and to increase the range of potential target vessels, we introduced axillary-coronary bypass using saphenous vein [10].

The success of robotic IMA grafting has lead to its inclusion in hybrid (single IMA to LAD and PCI of one or two additional target vessels) and advanced hybrid (double IMA grafting with PCI of one or more additional target vessels) procedures [11,12,13]. As multivessel robotic TECAB is technically demanding and the benefits of off-pump CABG (OPCAB) have been recently questioned, our preferred approach to robotic TECAB is on-pump arrested heart. However, there are number of clinical settings that preclude the use of CPB in TECAB patients or the use of endoaortic occlusion and there are patient subsets that likely truly benefit from avoidance of cardiopulmonary bypass. In addition, some surgeons as well as some patients prefer an off-pump approach. Consequently, BHTECAB is an important tool in the armamentarium of the robotic cardiac surgeon and some surgical groups use BHTECAB as their predominant method.

## The Robot

Although a number of devices were previously available, and others are under development, the only commercially available surgical robot suitable for cardiac surgery at the time of writing is Surgical Intuitive's telemanipulator. The latest iteration, the da Vinci® Si™, consists of 3 primary components: a visioning cart, the 4-arm patient-side cart and the surgeon console (Figure 1).

A dual console system with push-button instrument exchange is also available and facilitates assistance and teaching by providing 3D visioning in 1080i high definition to both surgeon and assistant, allowing them to work together as "pilot and copilot" [14].

Working at the console, the surgeon's movements of the masters, or joysticks are translated and scaled up to 5:1 by the visioning cart into real-time movements of the surgical instruments by the patient cart. A variety of wristed instruments with 7 degrees of freedom are available for 8 mm and 5 mm ports.

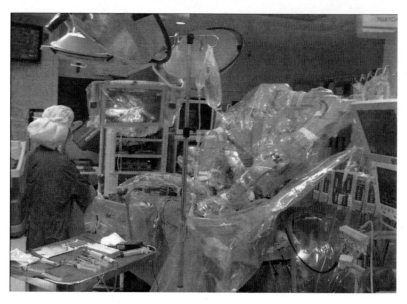

Figure 1. The da Vinci® Si™ telemanipulator consists of a visioning cart, the 4-arm patient-side cart and one or two surgeon consoles. For robotically assisted beating heart totally endoscopic coronary artery bypass grafting, the camera port is positioned in the 5$^{th}$ left intercostal space. Additional ports are placed in the 7$^{th}$ and 3$^{rd}$ intercostal spaces for the left and right arms respectively, and the dynamic stabilizer is positioned through a left subcostal port.

## Patient Selection

Careful patient selection is one of the most important factors to ensure successful outcomes in minimally invasive cardiac surgery. Preoperative assessment should include a history and physical examination, basic laboratory examination and echocardiogram as for a standard open procedure. In addition, pulmonary function testing is required to determine suitability for single lung ventilation and a gated coronary computed tomographic (CT) scan with assessment of the aorta, axillary and femoral arteries assists in assessing a patient's suitability for BHTECAB. This radiological examination provides data regarding heart size, its rotation and position in the mediastinum, and the location and course, whether intramyocardial, of the coronary arteries in relation to the internal mammary arteries. Although there is minimal data in the literature predicting the degree of technical difficulty from preoperative imaging, we have anecdotally found that patients with enlarged hearts, minimal distance between the heart and the thorax wall, and increased distance between the IMA and the target vessel can be more challenging. Vascular assessment aids in determining sites for possible remote cannulation if required either prophylactically or urgently during the procedure [15].

## Indications

Patients should meet the established indications for CABG and be fit to undergo an open CABG procedure. We consider a totally endoscopic approach in all patients meeting the standard guidelines for CABG. Either the surgeon or patient may have a preference for an off-pump approach, or the patient may have contraindications to femoral cannulation or intra-aortic balloon occlusion (femoral arteries < 8mm, moderate or severe aortic or iliac atherosclerosis, ascending aortic > 38 mm, aortic dissection or moderate to severe aortic valve insufficiency). Patients who may be particularly well suited for BHTECAB are those who have single or double vessel disease in large anterior or anterolateral target vessels. Multivessel disease may be treated with endoscopic techniques, in the context of a hybrid treatment regime, or by surgical teams with significant experience.

## Contraindications

Target vessel suitability is among the most important factors for BHTECAB. There are reports in the literature describing multivessel BHTECAB of posterior and inferior wall vessels, but such cases can be difficult even for experts in the field. Small, heavily calcified and intramyocardial vessels also pose significant challenges. Other contraindications to BHTECAB generally include high risk patients (poor left ventricular function [ejection fraction less than 30%], emergency surgery, pulmonary edema, acute myocardial infarction and hemodynamic insufficiency), conditions precluding single lung ventilation (asthma, chronic obstructive pulmonary disease, pulmonary fibrosis), major chest wall deformities limiting intrathoracic space (scoliosis, kyphosis), and high suspicion of intrathoracic adhesions on the operative side (prior thoracic surgery, chest tube insertion or severe thoracic trauma, pleuritis or other inflammatory disease, adhesions on CT scan, empyema, loculated pleural effusion). The requirement for concomitant procedures is generally a contraindication for a BHTECAB. Relative contraindications include prior chest radiation, and morbid obesity, which may limit intrathoracic space in the off-pump setting [15,16]. Peripheral arterial disease is not inherently a contraindication for BHTECAB, and may in fact be an indication for an off-pump rather than an on-pump approach. However, peripheral arterial disease may also be a marker for more advanced coronary arterial disease and could complicate conversion to an on-pump procedure if required. Consideration should be given to the team's level of experience prior to performing complex BHTECAB procedures or offering BHTECAB to patients with multiple comorbidities. However, with sufficient experience even challenging anatomy and higher risk patients can successfully undergo BHTECAB. Although experienced surgeons have successfully managed complex anatomy on the beating heart, vessels that are intramyocardial target, heavily diseased, or require endarterectomy [17] or pose similar challenges are probably better grafted on an arrested heart or through a sternotomy. The indications and contraindications for BHTECAB are still evolving as robotic technology improves and the experience of the surgical community grows.

## Specific Patient Populations

A number of patient populations, for example elderly patients who require intensive post discharge rehabilitation and younger patients whose employment demands heavy physical, may derive specific benefits from BHTECAB.

We previously demonstrated an improvement in quality of life and earlier return to activity following arrested heart TECAB [18]. These results can likely be extrapolated to BHTECAB. Patients with human immunodeficiency virus and other communicable diseases place the operating team at risk and a minimally invasive approach without cardiopulmonary bypass may lessen this risk [19]. Patients at risk for sternal wound complications or with conditions complicating sternotomy such as a preexisting tracheostomy [20] also benefit from sternal preservation.

## Anesthesia

In addition to standard anesthetic principles for full sternotomy OPCAB, a few modifications are necessary to ensure the success and safety of BHTECAB. The patient is positioned supine on the operative table with a roll under the left hemithorax and the legs are prepared as for an open procedure. To assist in fast-tracking patients, we utilize bispectral analysis to monitor depth of anesthesia, aiming for a target of less than 60. Near infrared spectral analysis aids in ensuring adequate brain protection [21]. External defibrillator pads are required, as internal paddles cannot be applied through limited incisions. If defibrillation is required the lungs should be inflated to improve conduction of the defibrillatory current. Single lung ventilation with controlled tension capnothorax is generally required for TECAB to increase the intrathoracic working space. These maneuvers may adversely impact the hemodynamic profile by impeding venous return, reducing cardiac filling and decreasing cardiac output. The resultant hypoxia and hypercapnia may increase pulmonary artery resistance. Unlike OPCAB, the patient's position cannot be altered with the robot docked. Judicious use of fluids, inotropes, vasopressors, vasodilators and antiarrhythmics is required to maintain the patient's hemodynamics [22]. Applying continuous positive airway pressure of 5 to 15 cm $H_2O$ or reducing the tension capnothorax and resuming bilateral ventilation at an increased respiratory rate while minimizing the tidal volumes can improve hypoxia and hypercapnia. Because the robot magnifies the excursions of the heart, it can be helpful to slow the heart rate with an intravenous esmolol drip, targeting a heart rate of 60 beats per minute to enhance myocardial stabilization when constructing the anastomosis. Although not well documented in the literature, there are anecdotal reports of unilateral lung injury in the non-ventilated lung during minimally invasive cardiac surgical procedures. The etiology of this process is not yet understood, but it is likely related to prolonged single lung ventilation. Consequently we attempt to ventilate both lungs when possible during the procedure.

## Surgical Technique

For a routine BHTECAB procedure a 12 mm camera port is placed in the fifth left intercostal space in the anterior axillary line. Carbon dioxide is insufflated to approximately 10 mmHg to increase working space and enhance visualization of the operative field. Additional ports for the left and right robotic arms are inserted under endoscopic vision into the seventh and third intercostal spaces just anterior to the anterior axillary line, forming a flat inverted triangle with the endoscope (Figure 1).

After inspecting the anatomy, paying specific attention to the location of the left phrenic nerve, harvesting of the left internal mammary artery (LIMA) begins. We prefer a skeletonized technique, which compared to a pedicled graft provides improved length, superior visualization of side branches, fewer venous bleeding sites and is easier to handle endoscopically when constructing sequential anastomoses and measuring flow. With DeBakey forceps in the left hand, the endothoracic fascia is detached from the LIMA with the spatula cautery set on 15 Watts. The LIMA is carefully teased from the chest wall, dividing most of the side branches with the cautery alone. An occasional larger branch will require the application of a hemoclip. The entire length of the LIMA can be harvested. Once completed, a hemoclip is applied at the distal end of the LIMA to allow the graft to autodilate. Topical dilating agents can be applied if required. If both the right internal mammary artery (RIMA) and LIMA are to be harvested, the mediastinal attachments to the sternum are first divided using long-tipped forceps and the cautery, and the right pleural space is opened widely to enhance visualization of the entire course of the RIMA. It is important to harvest the RIMA prior to the LIMA. If this sequence is reversed, the LIMA will hang from the thoracic wall and be at risk of injury while harvesting the RIMA.

A 1.5 cm drainage slit is made in the pericardium posterior to the left phrenic nerve to drain any blood that collects in the pericardial space during the remainder of the procedure. The cautery is set at 40 Watts and the pericardial fat pad is resected from the pulmonary artery to the diaphragm, bringing it laterally. The pericardium is opened in a large C shape from the pulmonary artery medially to the sternum, inferiorly to the diaphragm and then laterally along the diaphragm.

Preparations are now made for the anastomosis. The dynamic stabilizer is introduced through a 12 mm subcostal port placed in the left midclavicular line. An assistance port can be positioned in the fourth left intercostal space, lateral to the sternum and all bulldogs, silastic® loops and sutures can now be introduced into the thorax and parked securely in a convenient location in the mediastinal fat.

Target vessel identification is a critical aspect of the procedure and requires special attention, as the endoscopic view differs from the perspective gained through a sternotomy. A detailed comparison of the visualized anatomy can be made with the preoperative images, noting the position of curves and branches of the coronary arteries. After identifying a suitable location on the target vessel that is free of significant calcification, it is encircled with silastic® snares and the vessel is occluded proximally. Hemodynamic stability is ensured and a small arteriotomy is made using a robotic lancet blade and extended with Potts scissors. An endoluminal shunt can be used and is best placed by inserting nearly the entire shunt distally and allowing it to fall completely into the arteriotomy. Using the attached string, it is then pulled into the proximal vessel as the silastic® snare is loosened. As with open OPCAB, any ST changes from snaring the coronary target should resolve with flow through the shunt. When possible, the distal snare is not cinched to avoid post-anastomotic spasm of the target vessel.

Our preference is to construct the anastomosis using 7 cm, double armed 7-0 Pronova suture (Johnson and Johnson, Langhorne, Pa., USA). The anastomosis is started from the toe at the 10 o'clock position and carried clockwise across the back wall and around the heel to the 5 o'clock position, sewing inside out on the graft and outside in on the target vessel (Figure 2).

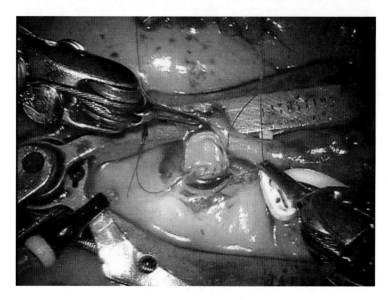

Figure 2. Intraoperative view of left internal mammary artery to the diagonal artery in a double vessel robotically assisted beating heart totally endoscopic coronary artery bypass grafting procedure. When using 7-0 Pronova suture, the back wall of the anastomosis is completed first in a clockwise direction around the heel while the robotic stabilizer exposes the vessel and limits the excursions of the contracting myocardium. An irrigator is incorporated into the stabilizer. Silastic® snares and an intraluminal shunt can be used as required.

After switching needles, the front wall of the anastomosis is completed in the opposite direction, with sutures being placed outside in on the graft and inside out on the coronary artery. Prior to completing the anastomosis, the snares are tightened as necessary and the shunt is removed. Suture tension is maintained by pulling up on both arms of the suture after every few stitches and the anastomosis is inspected for adequate tension prior to tying the suture. Intraoperative graft patency can be assessed by transit-time flow Doppler.

## Alternative Anastomotic Techniques

While sutured anastomoses can be performed comfortably and efficiently, some surgeons prefer alternative anastomotic techniques. When well selected these devices may minimize ischemic time and trauma to the vessel wall when completing anastomoses on the beating heart. A variety of devices have been developed including magnetic connectors [23], U-clips [24], and automated anastomotic devices [25]. Currently, only U-clips and the C-Port Flex A distal anastomotic device (Cardica, Redwood City, CA) are clinically relevant.

### U-Clips

Early in the development of TECAB, short suture was not available and managing a regular length suture intracorporeally is very challenging. Although suture suitable for intracorporeal use is now available, some surgeons still prefer U-clips as they maintain exposure of the anastomotic site as the anastomosis is being completed, they are self-tensioning and a new needle is used for every stitch. When using U-clips, the IMA is harvested in the standard technique. Clips are applied distally and the vessel is partially divided and spatulated, leaving the IMA attached to the chest wall. Five U-clips are passed through the IMA from outside-in, working from the heel towards the toe on the back wall of the anastomosis. Having prepared the IMA, control of the target vessel is gained with proximal and distal silastic® loops, and an arteriotomy is made. After completely transecting the IMA, it is brought into position and the clips on the back wall of the IMA are passed through the target vessel and are fully deployed. Clips are then passed through the front wall of the anastomosis and are deployed, completing the anastomosis [16]. Hemostasis is assessed and additional clips or sutures are placed as required. Internal mammary artery Y- and T-grafts can be constructed in a similar fashion. Limitations of this technique include the difficulty associated with maintaining organization of multiple clips around the anastomosis and retrieving a large number of needles from the closed chest.

## Anastomotic Devices

A number of anastomotic devices have been developed in recent years, but the Cardica distal anastomotic device is probably the most widely used in robotics, as it is deliverable through endoscopic ports and is well suited for manipulation with current robotic instrumentation. This miniature stapling device creates an arteriotomy and fires a series of twelve stainless steel clips along the edges of the two vessels creating an anastomosis. Its effectiveness has been demonstrated in open OPCAB trials [26,27].

Initial planning, preparations and setup are as per a standard BHTECAB. After IMA harvesting, the target vessel is identified and stabilized. The epicardium overlying the coronary artery is dissected away from the vessel and a silastic® snare is placed around the vessel. An adventitial U-stitch is placed at the planned anvil insertion site to facilitate closure of the arteriotomy after completing the anastomosis. A 15mm port is positioned in the second intercostal space through which the device is introduced. The distal end of the graft is first loaded onto the heel clip of the device and the right and left wing guards are then brought down over the spatulated edges of the hood of the graft. With the vessel snared, a small arteriotomy is made through the adventitial U-stitch and the anvil of the device is placed into the target vessel, paying careful attention to ensure that the anvil maintains an intraluminal path. The device is aligned with the target vessel and is deployed. Upon disengagement, the anvil stitch is tied. Approximately one in five cases requires an additional stitch at the toe. In multivessel cases requiring a T- or Y-graft, the proximal anastomosis is constructed with the anastomotic device prior to completing the distal anastomoses. If appropriate from a pathoanatomical perspective, the lateral wall is grafted prior to the anterior wall[9]. Results for this technique are discussed later in this chapter. When considering this device, it is important that the vessel be relatively free of calcification and of adequate diameter. A surgeon should have familiarity with suturing or deploying U-clips on the beating heart as the anastomosis can bleed on occasion and require either sutures or U-clips to establish hemostasis.

No large clinical studies have compared the effectiveness of various anastomotic techniques in the clinical robotic setting. Smith assessed surgical outcomes between sutured anastomoses and those constructed with U-clips in a series of 10 dogs. There was no significant difference in anastomotic time (18.0 vs. 20.2 min) and all grafts were patent by on-table angiography [28].

## Conversion to Larger Incision

As with all endoscopic procedures, a number of intraoperative conditions will necessitate conversion to a larger incision and conversion should not be considered a failure. We suggest that particularly early in the learning curve, liberal consideration should be given to conversion, rather than trying to complete an operation endoscopically and compromise the safety of the patient. When conversion is deemed necessary, surgeons with extensive experience in performing coronary surgery through a minithoracotomy advocate extending the camera port to a mini-thoracotomy [15,29]. It has been our experience that the correction of many lesions leading to conversion is more straightforward and can be undertaken most expeditiously through a sternotomy whereas conversion to a minithoracotomy can often be challenging, particularly to manage bleeding and occasionally still requires a sternotomy for definitive management. If a hybrid procedure was planned, complete surgical revascularization can be undertaken via sternotomy. We therefore discuss conversion at the time of surgical consent.

## The Role of Cardiopulmonary Bypass in BHTECAB

BHTECAB presents technical and physiological challenges inherent with both OPCAB and arrested heart TECAB, but with careful attention to patient selection, excellent outcomes can be achieved. Although this book focuses on off-pump coronary artery surgical revascularization, cardiopulmonary bypass may provide an important safety net in BHTECAB and a short pump run may overcome some intraoperative challenges that would otherwise result in conversion to sternotomy or even to the demise of the patient. Therefore, a short discussion of minimally invasive perfusion techniques is germane to this chapter. In sternotomy OPCAB, conversion to on-pump is associated with increased in-hospital mortality (10% vs. 0%, P=0.01) and morbidity [30] that extends as an increase in the hazard ratio of death for 3 years following surgery [31]. In the endoscopic setting, conversion to cardiopulmonary bypass without prophylactic cannulation requires additional steps and therefore takes much longer than in the open setting. Although not yet discussed in the literature, it would seem that conversion to on-pump in the endoscopic setting would have inferior outcomes as compared to the open setting. Consequently, although not standard practice for all robotic surgeons, we prophylactically cannulate all patients undergoing BHTECAB, but only go on pump if necessary. At a minimum, prophylactic cannulation should be considered in BHTECAB for patients with known predictors of conversion to on-pump CABG in OPCAB (limited surgeon or surgical team experience, left ventricular hypertrophy, Canadian Cardiovascular Society class 3 or 4 angina, previous CABG, urgent or emergent procedure, prior myocardial infarction and congestive heart failure) [32,33].

Reasons for conversion to sternotomy are listed in Table 1, many of which could be overcome by a short pump run.

**Table 1. Reasons for intraoperative conversion and exclusion modified from Folliguet [15], Srivastava [16] and Balkhy [9]**

| |
|---|
| Patient anatomical factors |
|     Insufficient thoracic space |
|     Enlarged heart |
|     Rotated heart |
|     Extensive pleural adhesions |
| Patient physiologic factors |
|     Inability to tolerate single lung ventilation |
|     Hemodynamic instability |
|     Acute myocardial ischemia |
|     Overt heart failure |
|     Ventricular tachycardia or fibrillation |
| Coronary anatomical factors |
|     Intramyocardial left anterior descending artery |
| Small target vessel |
| Calcified vessel |
|     Right coronary targets |
|     Posterior obtuse marginal branches of the circumflex coronary artery |
| Technical factors |
|     Anastomotic bleeding |
|     Graft dissection |
|     Graft tension |
|     Myocardial injury |
|     Pulmonary injury |
|     Robotic arm technical failure – collision |

When faced with these circumstances, the surgeon must consider whether going on cardiopulmonary bypass or completing the procedure through an alternative incision better serves the patient. Minimized extracorporeal circulation may be well suited to support the heart if required during BHTECAB [34].

# Vascular Access and Perfusion Techniques

Cardiopulmonary bypass for TECAB is most commonly achieved by femoral arterial and venous cannulation, but the choice of site should be guided by preoperative imaging. Transesophageal guidance is essential to ensure that guidewires and cannulae are positioned appropriately.

Retroaortic perfusion has been associated with a small but measureable increase in the risk of stroke [35] and retrograde aortic dissection [36], although with careful patient selection these risks can likely be minimized. Any degree of aortic, iliac or femoral atherosclerosis greater than mild should liberally direct the surgeon to seek an alternative cannulation site such as transthoracic aortic or axillary artery [37] cannulation to provide antegrade aortic perfusion.

## Hybrid Coronary Artery Revascularization

Percutaneous intervention combined with BHTECAB as a hybrid revascularization concept can be an elegant solution for patients with complex coronary disease. Hybrid procedures merge the best treatment strategies from cardiac surgery and interventional cardiology: an internal mammary artery is grafted to the left anterior descending artery and is combined with additional arterial grafts and/or percutaneous intervention with drug-eluting stents to other diseased targets vessels [12,38,39]. A detailed discussion of hybrid coronary artery revascularization strategies is beyond the scope of this chapter however a number of patient subsets are well suited for a hybrid approach. Specifically, lesion sets with a high SYNTAX score lesion of the LAD (chronic total occlusion, left main lesion, heavy calcification or complex tortuosity) and non-LAD targets with a low SYNTAX score lesion are often appropriate for hybrid revascularization. A robotic cardiac surgeon and an interventional cardiologist should carefully evaluate each patient being considered for a hybrid approach and together, determine the optimal treatment strategy. Hybrid concepts require consideration of how the procedure will be staged and the management of anticoagulants and antiplatelet agents [40].

## Outcomes

Major BHTECAB trials are summarized in Table 2. In 668 published cases, in hospital mortality was 0.6% and the stroke rate was 0.4%. Overall intraoperative conversion to a larger incision was 14.2% and decreased with increasing operator experience. Revision for bleeding was only 1.2%. Operative times are long in the early phases of program development, but as teams progress along learning curves, single vessel BHTECAB can be performed routinely in less than two-and-a-half hours. Overall short- to mid-term freedom from major adverse coronary and cerebral events, and angina are within the ranges of published studies of traditional CABG. Compared with sternotomy, patients undergoing TECAB can expect improved physical health, a shorter hospital stay and an earlier return to their daily activities [23]. Long-term follow-up studies are needed to confirm that late outcomes match those of traditional surgery.

Srivastava has the largest published series of BHTECAB to date, comprising 241 patients ranging in age from 24 – 91 years. An endoscopic procedure was completed in 214 patients who received a total of 296 grafts (single 139[65%], double 68[32%] triple 7[3%]) and 50 (17%) underwent BHTECAB as a component of a hybrid revascularization strategy. A totally endoscopic procedure could not be completed in 27 (11.2%) either because of intraoperative exclusion or conversion to a larger incision. Operative time was 177.3 (84 – 466) minutes and increased as the number of grafts increased. Intraoperative conversion to sternotomy was necessary in 2.1% of patients undergoing single vessel bypass and was 5% in patients receiving 2 grafts. No patients suffered a perioperative myocardial infarction or operative mortality. Of 239 (81%) grafts imaged with either CT or conventional angiography, there was only 1 (0.4%) graft occlusion. In follow-up (528 ± 967 days), 3 patients required reintervention (1.4%): 2 for graft failure and 1 for progression of native disease [16].

Balkhy recently reported his experience with BHTECAB using an anastomotic connector in 120 patients (65% single, 31% double and 4% triple; 17.5% as part of a hybrid strategy) over 34 months comprising 48% of all patients undergoing isolated surgical revascularization during this time period.

**Table 2. Results of totally endoscopic coronary artery bypass grafting on the beating heart without heart lung machine use**

| Author Citation | Cases | Conversion | Mortality Perioperative | Revision for Bleeding | Stroke | Renal Failure | LOS (days) |
|---|---|---|---|---|---|---|---|
| DeCannière [8] | 117 | 37 | 2 | | | | |
| Kappert [55] | 3 | 0 | 0 | | | | 6 ± 1 |
| Boyd [56] | 6 | 0 | 0 | | | | 8.6 ± 2.7 |
| Loisance [57] | 13 | 11 | 1 | | | | |
| Srivastava [58] | 108 | 15 | 0 | 1/93 | 0/93 | 1/93 | 3.4 ± 2.0 |
| Srivastava [16] | 241 | 27 | 0 | 2 | 1 | 1 | |
| Balkhy [9] | 120 | 3 | 1 | 2 | 1 | 0 | 3.3 ± 2.4 |
| Gao [29] | 60 | 2 | 0 | 1 | 0 | 0 | 5.0 ± 1.5 |
| Total | 668 | 95/668 14.2% | 4/668 0.6% | 6/514 1.2% | 2/514 0.4% | 2/514 0.4% | |

LOS – length of stay.

Conversion to a larger incision was required in only 3 (2.5%) patients and cardiopulmonary bypass was required in 1 (0.8%) patient. There was a single mortality (0.8%) and mean hospital stay was 3.3 ± 2.4 days. Graft assessment was 71% complete at 4 months and found 80 of 85 (94%) grafts patent of which one required surgical reintervention. One patient had recurrent stable angina, but the remainder of the 120 patients were alive and well at 6-10 months [9].

Gao published an initial series of 60 patients undergoing single-vessel BHTECAB with excellent results. There were only 2 intraoperative conversions to thoracotomy and one patient required re-exploration for bleeding.

All patients were alive and well at 12.7 months, but 1 patient had a gastric bleed 6 months postoperatively. Postoperative imaging was complete in all patients either by conventional coronary angiography or CT angiography prior to leaving the hospital and again at 3, 6 and 12 months postoperatively. All grafts were patent, although there was a single graft with a 50% stenosis at the anastomosis and one ITA graft was found to have a low density in the LIMA graft [29], but neither required revision.

## Steps to Successful Program Development

Slow stepwise progression towards BHTECAB with careful attention to patient selection is the key to building a safe and successful program [15]. It is also important to establish a stable operative team as each team member's learning curve will impact the success progress of the entire program. Initially, cases may take substantially longer to complete than traditional open operations, however with experience, operative times improve [29]. Consequently team member selection is also important and administrative support is required. Developing teams should first become generally acquainted with the robotic system and instrumentation in a dry lab setting and then perform simulated procedures on cadaver porcine hearts [41].

**Table 3. Suggested training track for beating heart totally endoscopic coronary artery bypass grafting**

| |
|---|
| Team selection |
| General robotic training |
|     Course on robotic basics |
|     Dry lab training |
| Wet lab training |
|     Cadaver porcine heart anastomoses |
| Team visit to centers of excellence |
| Mastery of Procedure Components |
|     Experience with open OPCAB |
|     Robotic IMA Harvesting followed by standard open CABG |
|     Robotic Pericardial fat pad resection |
|     Robotic Pericardiotomy |
|     Sternotomy with IMA harvesting followed by robotic anastomosis on arrested heart through a sternotomy |
|     Sternotomy with IMA harvesting followed by robotic anastomosis on beating heart through a sternotomy |
| Completion of entire cases |
|     Single vessel AHTECAB |
|     Single vessel BHTECAB |
|     Multivessel AHTECAB |
|     Multivessel BHTECAB |

AHTECAB – arrested heart totally endoscopic coronary artery bypass grafting; BHTECAB – beating heart totally endoscopic coronary artery bypass grafting; CABG – coronary artery bypass grafting; IMA – internal mammary artery; OPCAB – off-pump coronary artery bypass grafting.

Once generally familiar with the system, the entire team including anesthesiologists, perfusionists, assistants, nurses and surgeons should visit centers of excellence, paying close attention to all details of the procedure as well as the overall team interaction. Prior to attempting a complete BHTECAB procedure, each component of the procedure, including the anastomosis should be mastered in isolation, with the dedicated team. A suggested training protocol is outlined in Table 3.

Generally, the team should master each step before proceeding to more advanced steps. During the early phase of the learning curve, straightforward cases (LAD target, vessels greater than 2.5mm, good landing zone without calcification, non-intramyocardial coronary target vessels in low risk patients) should be selected before advancing to more complex anatomy and high-risk patients [15]. Balkhy also stresses the importance of a stepwise progression when using an anastomotic device, suggesting that the team first gain experience with the device in open on- and OPCAB cases using both arterial and venous grafts [9].

## Learning Curves

Learning curve data for arrested heart TECAB show that there is a dramatic reduction in surgical time after performing 20 cases with continued improvement to beyond a total of 100 cases. The learning curves for individual components of BHTECAB including LAD harvest, pericardial fat pad dissection, pericardiotomy and completing an LAD anastomosis follow a similar pattern [29,42]. Deliberate practice can enhance progression through the learning curve. These data suggest that BHTECAB procedures are performed best in high-volume centers where a sufficient number of cases can be performed annually. Thus the surgeon and team can be trained and maintain their collective skills.

Whether BHTECAB can be taught to residents has yet to be investigated. A structured approach has been implemented successfully in urology residency training programs [43] and although the number of open radical prostatectomies has dramatically decreased as robotics has penetrated the field of urology, graduating chief residents report performing an increased number of radical prostatectomies [44]. We have shown that focused practice using a slaughterhouse pig heart model of sutured anastomosis translates to improved procedural times clinically [41,45]. Unlike traditional open operations, a dual console system provides the trainer and trainee the same magnified visual perspective in high definition. "Push-button" instrument transfer may promote a higher comfort level for the instructor when a trainee is performing critical parts of the procedure [14] thereby providing a superior teaching environment for BHTECAB compared to traditional approaches.

## Cost Analysis

Robotic cardiac procedures have been criticized for increased costs compared with conventional procedures, although there is limited data regarding the actual costs of BHTECAB. A prospective analysis assessing robotically assisted OPCAB via minithoracotomy (Endo-ACAB) determined that total per patient hospital costs were equivalent to sternotomy OPCAB procedure, not including the acquisition cost of the robot [46]. A few limited studies consider the overall costs associated with robotic mitral valve repair. Excluding amortized capital costs, a robotic mitral repair cost AU$12328.70 compared to AU$9755.18 for a conventional procedure. The increased cost was driven primarily by the costs of robotic instruments and drapes, but was offset by a AU$1949.83 reduction in postoperative expenses. In that study, the overall cost for robotic mitral valve repair was AU$623.69 more than for conventional surgery, although this difference was not statistically significant [47]. Another study included the amortized cost of the robotic system as well as the annual maintenance charges, assuming 100 cases would be performed annually for five years and assessed the cost for robotic mitral repair to be $3444 higher than a sternotomy-based procedure. However, given that patients have both a shortened recovery and rehabilitation phase and that employed patients return to work sooner, it is likely that the societal costs are reduced with the robotic procedure [48]. With only a single commercial provider of robotic equipment for cardiac surgery, there is little competition to drive down the costs of hardware, but as more devices become available, costs of hardware and disposables may fall.

## Future Developments

BHTECAB has already reached a number of milestones including quadruple vessel bypass. However, procedural complexity and a steep learning curve have limited its penetrance through the surgical community. A number of devices are under development that may simplify BHTECAB. Exposure of coronary arteries on the lateral and posterior walls of the left ventricle on the beating heart using current commercially available robotic technology can lead to hemodynamic compromise and stabilization of the myocardium can be inadequate [49]. In addition, magnification of the operative field also magnifies any residual movement of the heart. These and other problems sometimes prevent the completion of the procedure endoscopically.

Active motion compensation aims to detect motion and either actively correct the trajectory of the instrument tips or provide the surgeon with a virtually stabilized frame of reference of the operative site by synchronizing movements of the camera with motion of the epicardium, or eliminating motion from the image in real time [50-53]. While early in development, initial reports are promising. One such device tracks 3D motion of the epicardial surface and uses an augmented reality scheme to create a virtually moving camera, rendering the surgical field of view in a moving frame of reference. Use of this system significantly improved total path length and mean error from an optimal instrument path using both a simulated data set and data from a BHTECAB procedure [54].

Using a different strategy, Riviere's group at Carnegie Mellon University is developing a miniature crawling robot that has both a camera and working arms that is introduced into the pericardial space through a port and can be guided by a surgeon to an appropriate area for intervention.

Unlike current robotic technology, which employs traditional long-stick instruments, this device is small, disposable and is attached to the control apparatus via a flexible tether. It crawls over the epicardium like an inchworm, providing exposure to all regions of the heart. Once attached to the epicardium, the frame of reference becomes that of the moving epicardium, essentially eliminating perceived motion of the heart by the surgeon.

To date, this device has been used only for developmental purposes to inject dye into the myocardium of pigs, however one can conceive that this technology could be applied to BHTECAB if additional instrument arms are incorporated.

As these concepts mature and other devices for navigating within the pericardium are developed, the learning curve for BHTECAB will flatten.

## Conclusion

Robotic BHTECAB, representing the most minimally invasive form of surgical coronary arterial revascularization, continues to evolve and mature. Early studies, though limited suggest that the procedure is safe and efficacious in well-selected patients and demonstrate fewer blood transfusions, shorter hospital stay, faster return to preoperative function levels with improved quality of life compared to patients undergoing sternotomy. These outcomes may translate into improved utilization of limited healthcare resources and overall reduced costs. However, longitudinal studies are required to determine if these early positive results are borne out in the long-term. In patients with multivessel coronary artery disease BHTECAB can be a good option for hybrid surgical revascularization. Success is highly dependent on negotiating a steep learning curve, but can be achieved by dedicated teams that adhere to a stepwise progression and methodical protocols. At this point, there has been limited adoption of these techniques, but with increased world-wide experience and if long-term outcomes remain favorable, patients and their physicians are likely to increase demand for these procedures. Stepwise progression of robotic technology and procedure development will continue to make robotic operations simpler and more efficient. Surgical scientists must continue to combine efforts with our industry partners to advance this technology and critically evaluate long-term results to extend the benefits of robotic surgery to a larger patient population.

## References

[1] Stephenson LW. History of Cardiac Surgery. In: Cohn LH, editor. Cardiac Surgery in the Adult. New York: McGraw-Hill, 2008:3–28.

[2] Cohn LH, Adams DH, Couper GS, Bichell DP. Minimally invasive aortic valve replacement. *Semin. Thorac. Cardiovasc. Surg.* 1997;9:331–336.

[3] Cosgrove DM, Sabik JF. Minimally invasive approach for aortic valve operations. *Ann. Thorac. Surg.* 1996;62:596–5977.

[4] Stevens JH, Burdon TA, Siegel LC, Peters WS, Pompili MF, St Goar FG, Berry GJ, Ribakove GH, Vierra MA, Mitchell RS, Toomasian JM, Reitz BA. Port-access coronary artery bypass with cardioplegic arrest: acute and chronic canine studies. *Ann. Thorac. Surg.* 1996;62:435–440.

[5] Vassiliades TA, Reddy VS, Puskas JD, Guyton RA. Long-Term Results of the Endoscopic Atraumatic Coronary Artery Bypass. *Ann. Thorac. Surg.* 2007;83:979–985.

[6] Loulmet D, Carpentier A, d' Attellis N, Berrebi A, Cardon C, Ponzio O, Aupecle B, Relland JY. Endoscopic coronary artery bypass grafting with the aid of robotic assisted instruments. *J. Thorac. Cardiovasc. Surg.* 1999;118:4–10.

[7] Argenziano M, Katz M, Bonatti J, Srivastava S, Murphy D, Poirier R, Loulmet D, Siwek L, Kreaden U, Ligon D. Results of the prospective multicenter trial of robotically assisted totally endoscopic coronary artery bypass grafting. *Ann. Thorac. Surg.* 2006;81:1666–1674.

[8] de Canniere D, Wimmer-Greinecker G, Cichon R, Gulielmos V, Van Praet F, Seshadri-Kreaden U, Falk V. Feasibility, safety, and efficacy of totally endoscopic coronary

artery bypass grafting: multicenter European experience. *J. Thorac. Cardiovasc. Surg.* 2007;134:710–716.

[9] Balkhy HH, Wann LS, Krienbring D, Arnsdorf SE. Integrating coronary anastomotic connectors and robotics toward a totally endoscopic beating heart approach: review of 120 cases. *Ann. Thorac. Surg.* 2011;92:821–827.

[10] Lehr EJ, Zimrin D, Vesely MR, Odonkor P, Griffith BP, Bonatti J. Axillary-coronary sequential vein graft for total endoscopic triple coronary artery bypass. *Ann. Thorac. Surg.* 2010;90:e79-81.

[11] Bonatti J, Lehr E, Vesely MR, Friedrich G, Bonaros N, Zimrin D. Hybrid coronary revascularization: which patients? when? how? *Curr. Opin. Cardiol.* 2010;25:568–574.

[12] Gao C, Yang M, Wu Y, Wang G, Xiao C, Liu H, Lu C. Hybrid coronary revascularization by endoscopic robotic coronary artery bypass grafting on beating heart and stent placement. *Ann. Thorac. Surg.* 2009;87:737–741.

[13] Katz MR, Van Praet F, de Canniere D, Murphy D, Siwek L, Seshadri-Kreaden U, Friedrich G, Bonatti J. Integrated coronary revascularization: percutaneous coronary intervention plus robotic totally endoscopic coronary artery bypass. *Circulation* 2006;114(1 Suppl):I473–1476.

[14] Lehr EJ, Grigore A, Reicher B, Zimrin D, Bartlett S, Griffith BP, Bonatti J. Dual console robotic system to teach beating heart total endoscopic coronary artery bypass grafting - a video presentation. *ICVTS* 2010;11(Supplement 2):S113–114.

[15] Folliguet TA, Dibie A, Philippe F, Larrazet F, Slama MS, Laborde F. Robotically-assisted coronary artery bypass grafting. *Cardiol. Res. Pract.* 2010;2010:175450.

[16] Srivastava S, Gadasalli S, Agusala M, Kolluru R, Barrera R, Quismundo S, Kreaden U, Jeevanandam V. Beating heart totally endoscopic coronary artery bypass. *Ann. Thorac. Surg.* 2010;89:1873–1880.

[17] Dawood MY, Lehr EJ, Bonatti J. Robotically assisted coronary endarterectomy. *Innovations*. In press.

[18] Bonaros N, Schachner T, Wiedemann D, Oehlinger A, Ruetzler E, Feuchtner G, Kolbitsch C, Velik-Salchner C, Friedrich G, Pachinger O, Laufer G, Bonatti J. Quality of life improvement after robotically assisted coronary artery bypass grafting. *Cardiology* 2009;114:59–66.

[19] van Wagenberg FS, Lehr EJ, Rehman A, Bonatti J. Is there a role for robotic totally endoscopic coronary artery bypass in HIV positive patients? *Int. J. Med. Robotics. Comput. Assist. Surg.* 2010;6:465-467.

[20] Lehr EJ, van Wagenberg FS, Haque R, Bonatti J. Robotic total endoscopic coronary artery bypass hybrid revascularization procedure in a patient with a preoperative tracheostoma. *Interact Cardiovasc. Thorac. Surg.* 2011;12:878-880.

[21] Schachner T, Bonaros N, Bonatti J, Kolbitsch C. Near infrared spectroscopy for controlling the quality of distal leg perfusion in remote access cardiopulmonary bypass. *Eur. J. Cardiothorac. Surg.* 2008;34:1253–1254.

[22] Wang G, Gao C, Zhou Q, Chen T. Anesthesia management for robotically assisted endoscopic coronary artery bypass grafting on beating heart. *Innovations* 2010;5:291–294.

[23] Falk V, Walther T, Stein H, Jacobs S, Walther C, Rastan A, Wimmer-Greinecker G, Mohr FW. Facilitated endoscopic beating heart coronary artery bypass grafting using a magnetic coupling device. *J. Thorac. Cardiovasc. Surg.* 2003;126:1575–1579.

[24] Caskey MP, Kirshner MS, Alderman EL, Hunsley SL, Daniel MA. Six-month angiographic evaluation of beating-heart coronary arterial graft interrupted anastomoses using the coalescent U-CLIP anastomotic device: a prospective clinical study. *Heart Surg. Forum* 2002;5:319–326.

[25] Kappert U, Ouda A, Virmani R, Mettler D, Matschke K, Demertzis S. The C-Port xV® vascular anastomosis system: results from an animal trial. *Thorac Cardiovasc Surg* 2011;59:222–226.

[26] Matschke KE, Gummert JF, Demertzis S, Kappert U, Anssar MB, Siclari F, Falk V, Alderman EL, Detter C, Reichenspurner H, Harringer W. The Cardica C-Port System: clinical and angiographic evaluation of a new device for automated, compliant distal anastomoses in coronary artery bypass grafting surgery--a multicenter prospective clinical trial. *J. Thorac. Cardiovasc. Surg.* 2005;130:1645–1652.

[27] Balkhy HH, Wann LS, Arnsdorf S. Early patency evaluation of new distal anastomotic device in internal mammary artery grafts using computed tomography angiography. *Innovations* 2010;5:109–113.

[28] Smith JM, Stein H, Robinson JR, Hawes J, Engel Ma AM. Influence of anastomotic techniques in totally endoscopic coronary artery bypass. *Int. J. Med. Robot.* 2006;2:197–201.

[29] Gao C, Yang M, Wu Y, Wang G, Xiao C, Zhao Y, Wang J. Early and midterm results of totally endoscopic coronary artery bypass grafting on the beating heart. *J. Thorac. Cardiovasc. Surg.* 2011;142:843–849.

[30] Légaré J-F, Buth KJ, Hirsch GM. Conversion to on pump from OPCAB is associated with increased mortality: results from a randomized controlled trial. *Eur. J. Cardiothorac. Surg.* 2005;27:296–301.

[31] Reeves BC, Ascione R, Caputo M, Angelini GD. Morbidity and mortality following acute conversion from off-pump to on-pump coronary surgery. *Eur. J. Cardiothorac. Surg.* 2006;29:941–947.

[32] Jin R, Hiratzka LF, Grunkemeier GL, Krause A, Page US. Aborted off-pump coronary artery bypass patients have much worse outcomes than on-pump or successful off-pump patients. *Circulation* 2005;112(9 Suppl):I332–337.

[33] Edgerton JR, Dewey TM, Magee MJ, Herbert MA, Prince SL, Jones KK, Mack M. Conversion in off-pump coronary artery bypass grafting: an analysis of predictors and outcomes. *Ann. Thorac. Surg.* 2003;76:1138–1142.

[34] Lehr EJ, Odonkor P, Reyes P, Bonatti J. Minimized extracorporeal circulation for the robotic totally endoscopic coronary artery bypass grafting hybrid procedure. *Can. J. Cardiol.* 2010;26:e286–287.

[35] Falk V, Cheng DCH, Martin J, Diegeler A, Folliguet TA, Nifong LW, Perier P, Raanani E, Smith JM, Seeburger J. Minimally invasive versus open mitral valve surgery. *Innovations* 2011;6:66–76.

[36] Muhs BE, Galloway AC, Lombino M, Silberstein M, Grossi EA, Colvin SB, Lamparello P, Jacobowitx G, Adelman MA, Rockman C, Gagne PJ. Arterial injuries from femoral artery cannulation with port access cardiac surgery. *Vasc. Endovascular. Surg.* 2005;39:153–158.

[37] Bonatti J, Garcia J, Rehman A, Odonkor P, Haque R, Zimrin D, Griffith B. On-pump beating-heart with axillary artery perfusion: a solution for robotic totally endoscopic coronary artery bypass grafting? *Heart Surg. Forum* 2009;12:E131–133.

[38] Bonatti J, Lehr E, Vesely MR, Friedrich G, Bonaros N, Zimrin D. Hybrid coronary revascularization: which patients? When? How? *Curr. Opin. Cardiol.* 2010;25:568–574.

[39] Narasimhan S, Srinivas VS, DeRose JJ Jr. Hybrid coronary revascularization: a review. *Cardiol. Rev.* 2011;19:101–107.

[40] Zimrin D, Bonatti J, Vesely MR, Lehr EJ. Hybrid coronary revascularization: an overview of options for anticoagulation and platelet inhibition. *Heart Surg. Forum* 2010;13:E405–408.

[41] Schachner T, Bonaros N, Ruttmann E, Höfer D, Nagiller J, Laufer G, Bonatti J. Training models for coronary surgery. *Heart Surg. Forum* 2007;10:E248–250.

[42] Schachner T, Bonaros N, Wiedemann D, Weidinger F, Feuchtner G, Friedrich G, Laufer G, Bonatti J. Training surgeons to perform robotically assisted totally endoscopic coronary surgery. *Ann. Thorac. Surg.* 2009;88:523–527.

[43] Rashid HH, Leung Y-YM, Rashid MJ, Oleyourryk G, Valvo JR, Eichel L. Robotic surgical education: a systematic approach to training urology residents to perform robotic-assisted laparoscopic radical prostatectomy. *Urology* 2006;68:75–79.

[44] Madeb R, Golijanin D, Knopf JK, Kowalczyk J, Feng C, Rashid H, Wu G, Eichel L, Valvo JR. The impact of robotics on treatment of localized prostate cancer and resident education in Rochester, New York. *J. Endourol.* 2011;25:573–537.

[45] Bonatti J, Alfadlhi J, Schachner T, Bonaros N, Rützler E, Laufer G. Do manual assisting maneuvers increase speed and technical performance in robotically sutured coronary bypass graft anastomoses? *Surg. Endosc.* 2007;21:1715–1718.

[46] Jones B, Desai P, Poston R. Establishing the case for minimally invasive, robotic-assisted CABG in the treatment of multivessel coronary artery disease. *Heart Surg. Forum* 2009;12:E147–149.

[47] Kam JK, Cooray SD, Kam JK, Smith JA, Almeida AA. A cost-analysis study of robotic versus conventional mitral valve repair. *Heart Lung Circ* 2010;19:413–8.

[48] Lehr EJ, Rodriguez E, Nifong LW, Chitwood WR. Robotic mitral valve surgery. *Eur. Surg.* doi:10.1007/s10353-011-0010-6.

[49] Falk V, Fann JI, Grünenfelder J, Daunt D, Burdon TA. Endoscopic computer-enhanced beating heart coronary artery bypass grafting. *Ann. Thorac. Surg.* 2000;70:2029–2033.

[50] Ginhou R, Gangloff J, de Mathelin M, Soler L, Sanchez A, Marescaux J. Active filtering of physiological motion in robotized surgery using predictive control. *IEEE Transactions on Robotics* 2005;21:67–79.

[51] Ortmaier T, Groger M, Boehm DH, Falk V, Hirzinger G. Motion Estimation in Beating Heart Surgery. *IEEE Transactions on Biomedical Engineering* 2005;52:1729–1740.

[52] Bebek O, Cavusoglu MC. Intelligent control algorithms for robotic-assisted beating heart surgery. *IEEE Transactions on Robotics* 2007;23:468–480.

[53] Gangloff J, Ginhoux R, de Mathelin M, Soler L, Marescaux J. Model predictive control for compensation of cyclic organ motions in teleoperated laparoscopic surgery. *IEEE Transactions on Control Systems Technology* 2006;14:235–246.

[54] Stoyanov D, Mylonas GP, Deligianni F, Darzi A, Yang GZ. Soft-tissue motion tracking and structure estimation for robotic assisted MIS procedures. *Med. Image Comput. Comput. Assist. Interv.* 2005;8(Pt 2):139–146.

[55] Kappert U, Cichon R, Gulielmos V, Schneider J, Schramm I, Nicolai J, Tugtekin SM, Schueler S. Robotic-enhanced Dresden technique for minimally invasive bilateral internal mammary artery grafting. *Heart Surg. Forum* 2000;3:319–321.

[56] Boyd WD, Rayman R, Desai ND, Menkis AH, Dobkowski W, Ganapathy S, Kiaii B, Jablonsky G, McKenzie FN, Novick RJ. Closed-chest coronary artery bypass grafting on the beating heart with the use of a computer-enhanced surgical robotic system. *J. Thorac. Cardiovasc. Surg.* 2000;120:807–809.

[57] Loisance DY, Nakashima K, Kirsch M. Computer-assisted coronary surgery: lessons from an initial experience. *Interact Cardiovasc. Thorac. Surg.* 2005;4:398–401.

[58] Srivastava S, Gadasalli S, Agusala M, Kolluru R, Barrera R, Quismundo S, Srivastava V, Seshadri-Kreaden U. Robotically assisted beating heart totally endoscopic coronary artery bypass (TECAB). Is there a future? *Innovations* 2008;3:52-58.

In: Off-Pump Coronary Artery Bypass Grafting
Editors: Shahzad G. Raja and Mohamed Amrani

ISBN: 978-1- 62081-549-6
© 2012 Nova Science Publishers, Inc.

*Chapter X*

# Technique of Reoperative Off-pump Coronary Artery Bypass Grafting

*Shahzad G. Raja[1] and Mohamed Amrani[2]*
[1]Cardiac Surgeon, Harefield Hospital, London, United Kingdom
[2]Senior Cardiac & Transplant Surgeon, Harefield Hospital, Honorary Senior Lecturer, Imperial College, London, United Kingdom

## Abstract

Despite surgical advances in coronary artery bypass grafting over the past two decades, including the routine use of arterial grafts, incomplete revascularization, progressive atherosclerotic disease of native vessels and grafts and technical failure remain the causes of recurrence of ischemia following primary surgery.

A significant proportion of patients with recurrent ischemia require reoperative coronary artery bypass grafting. Reoperative procedures pose several technical difficulties and are associated with increased operative risks which exceed those of the initial revascularization.

Traditionally, reoperative coronary artery bypass grafting has been performed on cardiopulmonary bypass. As the incidence of reoperative procedures is increasing so is the experience of reoperative coronary artery bypass grafting with resultant evolution of several alternative strategies to lower the operative risks.

These strategies include alternative techniques for reentry, strict avoidance of graft manipulation to minimize the risk of graft atheroembolism, and modification of the method of myocardial protection, depending on the status of the native coronary circulation and the patency of venous or arterial grafts. Off-pump coronary artery bypass grafting is one such technique which through avoidance of inherent risks of cardiopulmonary bypass has the potential to reduce the morbidity associated with reoperative coronary artery bypass grafting. This chapter provides an overview of the technique of reoperative off-pump coronary artery bypass grafting, evaluates the current outcomes and highlights the concerns and controversies associated with this strategy.

# Introduction

In recent decades, the incidence of reoperative coronary artery bypass grafting (CABG) has increased [1,2]. This is due to an increasing pool of patients who have already had CABG. Moreover, the increasing evidence that elderly patients can have CABG with acceptable mortality and morbidity and enjoy an excellent medium-term and long-term quality of life has led to an increase in the number of patients potentially eligible for reoperative CABG [1,3-5]. Reoperative CABG is a technically challenging operation with a high operative mortality of 5% to 16.7% [2,6-14]. There are two reasons for this. First, reoperations are technically more demanding. Sternal reentry, pericardial adhesions, in situ arterial grafts, and patent but diseased saphenous vein bypass grafts all increase the complexity and risk of coronary reoperations. Second, patients undergoing reoperation have a higher preoperative risk profile. They are older and more likely to have vascular disease, left ventricular dysfunction, and extensive coronary artery disease [6]. The mechanisms by which reoperative status influences early death are all well described and are mostly technical [1,15,16].

A variety of surgical strategies aimed at reducing the operative mortality and risks have been devised in recent years. These strategies include preoperative computed tomography scans to define cardiac proximity to the sternum, peripheral cardiopulmonary bypass (CPB) support to decompress the heart before median sternotomy, alternate incisions for access and the use of retrograde cardioplegia, which better protects areas supplied by nonfunctioning grafts and aids flushing of atheromatous debris from diseased grafts [1]. One additional strategy which has the potential to reduce the morbidity and mortality associated with reoperative CABG is off-pump technique. This chapter provides an overview of technical aspects, current outcomes, concerns and controversies associated with reoperative off-pump CABG.

# Technical Challenges Posed by Reoperative Coronary Artery Bypass Grafting and Strategies to Tackle these Challenges

Reoperative CABG presents many technical challenges not present in primary operations (Table 1). These challenges are due to both the nature of reoperations and patient characteristics. With careful preoperative planning and surgical technique, they can be managed safely.

The first challenge is sternal reentry. The pericardium is usually not closed after heart surgery, and the aorta, right ventricle, and bypass grafts may adhere to the underside of the sternum. At reoperation, these structures can be easily injured when the sternum is opened. Although using an oscillating saw decreases this risk, it does not eliminate it. Knowing the proximity of mediastinal structures to the sternum is necessary, and if preoperative imaging suggests that they may be in jeopardy, extra measures before reopening the sternum, such as peripheral cannulation and cardiopulmonary bypass (with or without hypothermic circulatory arrest), may be necessary to avoid catastrophe [6].

**Table 1. Challenges in redo coronary artery bypass grafting**

**Procedure-related**
- Sternal reentry
- Pericardial adhesions
- Patent grafts
- Atherosclerotic vein grafts
- Atherosclerotic aorta
- Availability of conduits
- Myocardial protection

**Patient-related**
- Age
- Vascular disease
- Left ventricular dysfunction
- Extensive coronary artery disease

In patients requiring limited revascularization, risk of sternal reentry can be avoided by using alternative incisions. Anterior thoracotomy has been advocated for anterior coronary artery revascularization, lateral thoracotomy for circumflex revascularization, and an epigastric approach for distal right coronary artery revascularization [6,17].

A second challenge at reoperation is managing patent atherosclerotic vein grafts. Embolization of atherosclerotic debris, resulting in coronary ischemia or myocardial infarction, may occur if these grafts are manipulated during dissection of pericardial adhesions [18]. Most common approach to deal with this situation is to avoid manipulation of atherosclerotic vein grafts before aortic clamping and arresting the heart. Limited dissection is performed to expose only enough of the heart and aorta to cannulate and clamp the aorta. After the heart is arrested and protected with cardioplegia, dissection of adhesions between the heart and pericardium is completed. If it is not possible to expose enough of the heart to cannulate safely without touching a patent atherosclerotic vein graft, peripheral cannulation is used. This is often necessary when an atherosclerotic patent vein graft to the right coronary artery is adherent to the right atrium [6].

Additional challenge is the best approach to deal with atherosclerotic vein grafts. Majority of surgeons routinely replace atherosclerotic vein grafts with another vein graft. Myocardial hypoperfusion and infarction may occur if a patent vein graft is replaced with an arterial graft [6,19]. On the other hand, all old vein grafts are not routinely divided especially if dividing an old vein graft could compromise coronary perfusion it is usually left in place. In case of atherosclerotic vein graft on the left anterior descending artery (LAD), supplementary grafting with left internal mammary artery (LIMA) is usually performed without interrupting the vein graft although concerns have been expressed regarding competititve flow [19].

At coronary reoperation, the presence of a patent LIMA graft to the LAD decreases operative mortality [20,21]. Proposed mechanisms for this salutary effect include preserved anterior wall function and the absence of atherosclerotic embolization from the LIMA graft [20,21]. However a patent LIMA–LAD graft also creates specific technical challenges at coronary reoperation. These include delivery of cardioplegia to the LAD territory and avoidance of injury to the LIMA graft. Use of retrograde cardioplegia with temporary occlusion of the LIMA graft provides adequate myocardial protection in most cases [20]. However, dissection and control of the LIMA pedicle can be challenging and hazardous, with some investigators reporting injury to the LIMA graft in 15% to 40% of coronary reoperations [21]. The risk of damage of a LIMA graft at coronary reoperation is related to the care taken at the primary operation to protect that graft. For patients who receive an in situ LIMA graft to the left coronary system, one strategy that is effective is to open the pleura and make a vertical slit in a posterior direction just lateral to the pulmonary artery at the point where the graft naturally enters the pericardial cavity [20,21]. The LIMA graft is routed into the pericardium through this slit and lies in a posterior position, just anterior to the phrenic nerve and lateral to the pulmonary artery. This approach keeps the LIMA graft from becoming adherent to the posterior sternal table or to the aorta, locations where the LIMA graft is most at risk during coronary reoperation. Other techniques for protection from injury at redo CABG include the use of a polytetrafluoroethylene graft to encase the LIMA pedicle [22], creation of a pericardial flap, and routing of the LIMA graft through a posterior hole in the pericardium [23,24].

Patients undergoing reoperation are more likely to have vascular disease, and a common challenge at reoperation is dealing with an atherosclerotic ascending aorta. If aortic atherosclerosis is detected by palpation or imaging studies, alternative cannulation sites and hypothermic circulatory arrest with or without ascending aortic replacement may be necessary. Cannulating the axillary artery when it is unsafe to cannulate the ascending aorta is a reasonable strategy because these patients usually have aortoiliac and femoral atherosclerosis as well [25,26]. Patients undergoing coronary reoperation may have multiple sources of coronary perfusion, making myocardial protection a challenge. Because antegrade cardioplegia will not reach areas of the myocardium whose coronary blood flow is supplied by in situ grafts or occluded coronary arteries, retrograde cardioplegia is extremely useful [27]. An integrated approach to myocardial protection is usually adopted to deal with this challenge. An initial single dose of antegrade cardioplegia is used to arrest the heart followed by retrograde cardioplegia administration every 15 to 20 minutes during myocardial ischemia. Antegrade cardioplegia is not repeated, to reduce risk of vein graft atheroembolism. Because retrograde cardioplegia might not perfuse the right ventricle, if a vein graft is performed to the right coronary artery, then antegrade cardioplegia is administered through the graft. Patent in situ grafts are clamped while the aorta is clamped to avoid washing out the cardioplegia and warming the heart. If in situ grafts cannot be clamped, the patient is systemically cooled.

An additional advantage of retrograde cardioplegia is that it can be used to remove vein graft atherosclerotic debris that inadvertently embolizes to a coronary artery. After the coronary arteriotomy is made, retrograde cardioplegia is administered, and the atherosclerotic debris is flushed out of the artery.

## Rationale for Reoperative Off-pump Coronary Artery Bypass Grafting

Although reoperative CABG performed with CPB has become a well-established treatment modality, there is increasing evidence that CPB may be responsible for some of the morbidity associated with redo CABG. The systemic inflammatory reaction initiated by the extracorporeal circuit results in mechanical trauma to blood, activation of various immunological cascades (complement, cytokines), impaired hemostasis, neurological, renal and gastrointestinal dysfunction. Furthermore, aortic cannulation, cross clamping and CPB can result in microembolization and macroembolization, with subsequent neurological and other end-organ injury, including global myocardial ischemia/reperfusion injury [28].

Off-pump coronary artery bypass grafting eliminates morbidity associated with CPB. Evidence is growing that avoidance of CPB is advantageous [28-33]. A large number of randomized controlled trials (RCTs) have been conducted over the last decade comparing outcomes of off-pump CABG and CABG on CPB [34-40]. In these RCTs, several important outcome measures have repeatedly favored off-pump CABG, including lower rates of blood transfusion, decreased postoperative ventilator time, intensive care unit length-of-stay (LOS), and hospital LOS. Serum markers of myocardial injury [35], systemic inflammation, and neuronal injury [37] have also been found to be lowered in patients undergoing off-pump CBAG. In addition, several trials have demonstrated a benefit in terms of cost savings and resource utilization [36,37].

It is intuitively obvious that high-risk patients for whom CPB is likely to be deleterious constitute the group of patients for whom avoidance of CPB will be most beneficial during coronary revascularization [41]. There is abundant evidence from large retrospective studies for reduced morbidity and mortality following off-pump CABG in high-risk patients including patients with poor ventricular function, advanced age, renal dysfunction, severe atherosclerosis and previous history of stroke [42-45]. Since patients undergoing reoperative CABG usually have these aforementioned comorbidities and as reoperative CABG has been reported to be associated with relatively higher mortality and morbidity, and long CPB time has been identified as the most powerful independent predictor of mortality after reoperative CABG [8] therefore adoption of off-pump strategy for myocardial revascularization may be considered a valuable alternative in these patients [46].

# Approaches for Reoperative Off-pump Coronary Artery Bypass Grafting

Reoperative off-pump coronary artery bypass grafting can be performed through repeat median sternotomy [47], thoracotomy [17] or minimally invasive direct coronary artery bypass (MIDCAB) approach [48]. Repeat median sternotomy offers the advantage of full cardiac mobilization with the intention of complete multivessel revascularization. It is a safe and feasible approach for multivessel off-pump CABG [47,49-53]. However, in patients with an absolute or relative contraindication to sternotomy or CPB (Table 2), a posterolateral thoracotomy provides excellent access to the circumflex system but only limited access to the LAD and right **coronary** systems. This is the most common approach used for redo off-pump one or two grafts to the circumflex system [17,54-63]. For single vessel redo CABG involving the LAD territory, MIDCAB is a feasible approach [48,62,64,65] with minimal morbidity due to avoidance of resternotomy, extensive dissection of the heart, aortic clamping, and incomplete myocardial protection.

## Table 2. Indications for redo off-pump CABG by thoracotomy

- Sternotomy dangerous
- Patent bypass graft(s) at risk
- Cardiac structure adherent to sternum
- Previous sternal wound infection/mediastinitis
- Previous mediastinal irradiation
- Calcified ascending aorta
- Diffuse atherosclerosis
- Blood conservation

Occasionally, in patients undergoing coronary reoperations with patent mammary graft to the LAD and with the need for isolated surgical revascularization of the right coronary artery or posterior descending artery a small laparotomy approach using right gastroepiploic artery allows avoidance of both resternotomy and CPB [66,67].

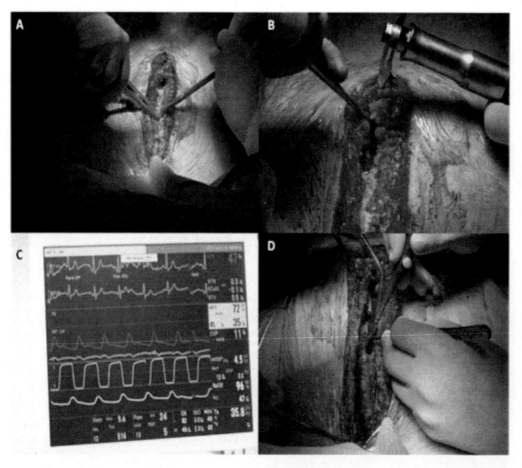

Figure 1. Steps for safe re-entry into chest during reoperative off-pump coronary artery bypass grafting. (A) Removal of sternal wires; (B&C) Systolic blood pressure < 80 at the time of opening the chest; (D) Use of diathermy for dissection to minimize blood loss.

## Technical Aspects

### Median Sternotomy

Median sternotomy is our surgical approach of choice for multivessel revascularization. External defibrillation pads are placed before skin prepping. Normothermia is maintained with warm intravenous fluids, a heating mattress, a humidified airway and a warm operating theatre. Standard intraoperative monitoring techniques are used. A CPB circuit is on stand-by for all cases. We no longer routinely expose femoral vessels (a reflection of our experience) however recommend this as an essential initial step for novice and less experienced surgeons particularly at the start of their careers. The redo sternotomy and mediastinal dissection are performed essentially by using an oscillating saw, initial exposure of the aorta and right atrium, the "no-touch" technique for previously placed grafts, and careful progression of the dissection on the left ventricle to identify and preserve previously placed internal mammary artery graft(s). The entire heart is mobilized in all cases. Prior to opening the chest we ask for controlled hypotension (systolic blood pressure < 80 mmHg), if tolerated, in order to decompress the right ventricle and aorta. We predominantly use diathermy for dissection as in our experience this achieves bloodless field without the need for prolonged hemostasis at the end of the operation (Figure 1). Indications for conversion to cardiopulmonary bypass include major bleeding at sternal re-entry, hemodynamic instability during mediastinal dissection, or injury to internal mammary artery or other patent graft(s), rendering off-pump methods technically difficult.

A cell-saving device for blood salvage is used. To minimize hemodynamic compromise, the right pleural space is opened to create a space for the rotated and vertically positioned heart. Suction-type (Octopus® 3; Medtronic, Inc, USA) mechanical stabiliser is used to stabilise the target coronary artery. One deep pericardial retraction suture is placed at the posterior fibrous pericardium very close and medial to the most proximal part of the inferior vena cava. Another retraction suture is placed in the fibrous pericardium very close to the left superior pulmonary vein avoiding the left phrenic nerve. These act as levers to help the surgeon manipulate and rotate the heart to vertical and lateral positions along with the stabiliser. Anticoagulation is achieved with 150 U/kg of heparin. If required, heparin is supplemented to maintain the activated clotting time above 250 s and is reversed by protamine at the end of the procedure. To facilitate distal anastomoses, a $CO_2$ blower mister or a fine coronary suction is used routinely. We have not used coronary shunts for the past 5 years however recommend their use particularly during grafting of the main body of the dominant right coronary artery. We routinely use soft bulldog clamps for local vascular control of the target vessel in order to achieve a bloodless field. Blood pressure is continually optimised during the procedure, and the mean arterial pressure is maintained above 50 mmHg by repositioning the heart and by intravenous fluids, selective use of vasoconstrictors or both. The distal anastomoses are constructed using 8-0 polypropylene (Figures 2). Right internal mammary artery (RIMA) is our conduit of choice for grafting the left anterior descending (LAD) artery in cases where the left internal mammary artery (LIMA) is already occluded. For all other territories, depending on availability of conduit(s), either long saphenous vein or radial artery is preferred. The proximal aortic anastomoses are performed by using a partial, side-biting, atraumatic vascular clamp. Occasionally, the proximal anastomoses may be constructed on a vein graft (Figure 2) or internal mammary artery especially if the native aorta is atherosclerotic or the length of the graft conduit is short. Aspirin 300 mg is administered 6 h postoperatively or once bleeding has settled.

## Anterolateral Thoracotomy

After institution of double-lumen endotracheal intubation, the patient is placed in the right lateral decubitus position with the pelvis externally rotated to 45° to allow access to the femoral artery. A small skin incision is made along the fifth intercostal space and the fifth intercostal space is opened. The thoracotomy is extended anteriorly or posteriorly to facilitate the operation. With the lung deflated, the LIMA is harvested under direct vision in a pedicled fashion using a Finocchietto retractor starting from the lower space of the incision until the origin of the first intercostal branch. The RIMA also can be dissected from this approach after the pericardial fat and the thymus are carefully removed. The pericardium is then opened anterior to the phrenic nerve. Limited adhesiolysis, sufficient to expose the target vessels, is performed, and then the anastomosis is performed by using standard techniques.

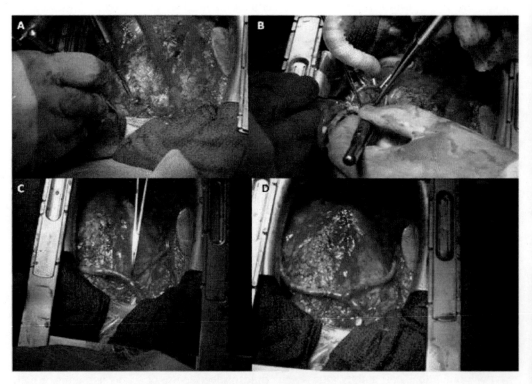

Figure 2. Construction of distal and proximal anastomosis during reoperative off-pump coronary artery bypass grafting. (A) Forceps pointing to blocked previously placed left internal mammary artery to left anterior descending artery; (B) Anastomosis of saphenous vein graft to distal left anterior descending artery; (C) Determining the length of right coronary artery vein graft for proximal anastomosis to the left anterior descending artery vein graft; (D) Completed proximal anastomosis of right coronary artery vein graft.

## Posterolateral Thoracotomy

The fifth intercostal space is used to enter the chest. The pericardium is palpated to locate and avoid old vein grafts if present and is opened posterior to the phrenic nerve. After the target coronary is identified, the distal anastomosis is then performed using 8-0 polypropylene in a manner similar to that previously described. The graft is then tailored according to the required length and proximal anastomosis is performed. The descending aorta is generally chosen as the source of inflow. A side-biting clamp is used to help in completion of the proximal anastomosis on the descending aorta. In cases where the descending aorta is severely atherosclerotic, the left subclavian artery is used for inflow. Proximally, the vessel is dissected circumferentially and occluded with a side-biting clamp or with vessel loops. Anastomosis is fashioned proximal to the origin of LIMA. With a patent LIMA to LAD graft, if a test occlusion of the subclavian artery did not result in ECG changes or clinical ischemia, only then the arteriotomy is performed and proximal anastomosis completed. Grafts originating from the left subclavian artery as well as the descending aorta are routed anterior to the hilum. Before chest closure, grafts are examined with the lung inflated to ensure that they are neither kinked nor under tension. Chest tubes are placed, intercostal block with bupivicaine 0.25% is performed and full expansion of the lung ensured before routine chest closure.

## Small Laparotomy Approach

The patients are placed in the standard supine position. General setup is the same as for multivessel grafting. Above the xiphoid, an 8- to 10-cm median incision is made on the scar of the previous sternotomy. This incision is long enough to divide or excise the xiphoid process, position a standard sternal retractor, obtain adequate exposure of the inferior wall of the heart, and allow for easy access to the upper abdomen for harvesting the gastroepiploic artery (GEA), making an additional lower sternotomy superfluous in all cases. The diaphragmatic surface of the heart is then dissected free from the diaphragm to facilitate exposure of the inferior wall of the heart. The right coronary artery (RCA) and posterior descending artery (PDA) are identified to choose the target coronary artery for the anastomosis. Dissection of adhesions is limited, just enough to permit exposure of the target coronary artery. The remaining adhesions are kept intact, because such adhesions act as stabilizers.

At this stage, the peritoneum is opened, the stomach is pulled gently out of the abdomen, and harvesting of the GEA is performed. GEA harvesting is performed either by using hemoclips or an ultrasonic scalpel (Harmonic Scalpel; Ethicon, Johnson & Johnson, New Brunswick, NJ) to separate its branches from the stomach and omentum. After heparinization, the distal part of the GEA is divided and 3 to 4 mL of a nitroprusside hydrochloride solution (20 mg of nitroprusside hydrochloride diluted in 50 mL of physiologic saline) is injected intraluminally to relieve spasm. A hemoclip is placed at the distal end of the GEA; the graft is put in a warm gauze imbedded in dilute nitroprusside and is then placed back into the abdominal cavity, together with the stomach. This handling of the GEA allows the artery to vasodilate both by the pharmacologic effect of the nitroprusside and by its own blood pressure.

Next, a hole in the right hemidiaphragm is made to route the GEA intrapericardially. The site of the opening is chosen according to the intended location of the anastomosis. The GEA is always routed antegastrically and in front of the liver. Once the GEA is placed intrapericardially, an Octopus suction stabilizer® (Medtronic, Minneapolis, MN) is fixed cranially on the retractor, and the suction branches are placed as close as possible to the target coronary artery. The suction device acts not only as a coronary stabilizer, but also allows us to push back and to pull up the inferior wall of the heart for an optimal surgical view. In patients with deep chests, exposure of the surgical field is improved by either suturing the diaphragm to the caudal end of the skin incision or placing a deep abdominal retractor, pulling caudally the diaphragm, liver, and other abdominal organs.

An incision of approximately 4 mm in the target coronary artery is made and the anastomosis is performed with a continuous 8-0 polypropylene suture on the beating heart. At the end of the procedure, a small drainage tube is placed into the pericardium, and the incision is routinely closed. It is advisable to place a nasogastric tube to deal with possible gastroparesis after the procedure.

## Current Outcomes

Mishra et al. [49] recently reported their 10-year experience using various techniques of single and multivessel reoperative off-pump CABG. From January 1996 until December 2005, 332 underwent redo off-pump CABG, of whom 296 (89.2%) were male and 36 (10.8%) were female. Out of these 265 (79.8%) patients underwent bypass through a median sternotomy, 63 (19%) patients underwent bypass though an anterolateral thoracotomy, and 4 (1.2%) patients had CABG through posterolateral thoracotomy. 35.5% of the study population required urgent operations, 7.6% had an intra-aortic balloon pump, and 16% had significant left main disease. Preoperatively planned redo off-pump CABG required intraoperative conversion to redo CABG in only 11% of cases, and in only 8% of cases was institution of intra-aortic balloon pump support needed. There was no difference in outcome between patients requiring intraoperative conversion to redo CABG and those preoperatively selected for redo CABG. An average of 2.17 grafts per patient could be placed in those requiring multivessel bypass, with 57% receiving LIMA–LAD anastomoses. In the group undergoing anterolateral thoracotomy, all 68 patients received LIMA–LAD grafts without the need for cardiopulmonary bypass. Hospital mortality was 3.3% (11 patients) in the median sternotomy group, and 1 patient died after anterolateral thoracotomy. In the multivessel redo off-pump CABG group, morbidity also was low: postoperative myocardial infarction, 4.8%; renal failure, 0.6%; cerebrovascular accident, 0%; and prolonged ventilation, 7.5%. This largest and most comprehensive experience of the use of off-pump techniques for reoperative coronary artery bypass surgery validates the safety and efficacy of routine reoperative off-pump CABG.

Vohra et al. in a recent publication reported their experience of reoperative off-pump CABG over a 5-year period [50]. This study is unique as it is the first in the literature comparing reoperative CABG on CPB and reoperative off-pump CABG by the propensity score analysis. Applying the propensity score, 43 off-pump CABG patients were matched with 43 CABG on CPB patients. All these patients had previously undergone CABG on CPB.

The number of diseased coronary arteries was 3 ± 0.5 and 2 ± 0.8 in reoperative CABG on CPB and reoperative off-pump CABG, respectively ($p < 0.01$). There were no differences in other preoperative risk factors between the two groups.

Twelve patients underwent reoperative off-pump CABG through anterior thoracotomy (1 double and 11 single grafts). The remaining patients underwent median sternotomy. In one patient off-pump CABG was converted to CABG on CPB because of hemodynamic instability. The mean number of grafts performed was 3 ± 0.8 in reoperative CABG on CPB and 2 ± 0.6 in reoperative off-pump CABG ($p < 0.05$). The 30-day mortality rate was 6.9% for reoperative CABG on CPB ($n = 3$) and 2.3% reoperative off-pump CABG ($n = 1$; $p =$ NS) with an overall mortality of 4.6%. The mean follow-up for redo CABG on CPB was 30 ± 21.3 months (range 0.1–63 months) and that of redo off-pump CABG was 37 ± 19.2 months (0.1–62.5 months). Actuarial survival at 5 years was 87 ± 5.5% for redo CABG on CPB and 95 ± 3.2% for redo off-pump CABG ($p = 0.17$). Event-free survival (death, myocardial infarction and repeat intervention) was 71 ± 8.0% for redo CABG on CPB and 78 ± 7.2% for redo off-pump CABG ($p = 0.32$).

Several other reports suggest similar or improved outcomes after redo multivessel off-pump CABG (Table 3).

Although a tailored approach for selected patients, the prevalence of off-pump coronary reoperation through a thoracotomy is increasing [16,53-61]. This growing popularity is explained by the increased need for reoperation in patients who have undergone previous CABG through median sternotomy, the growing familiarity and confidence with off-pump techniques, and recognition that the thoracotomy approach is advantageous in patients at particular risk for resternotomy. Unlike median sternotomy approach, the inflow vessel is usually the left subclavian artery [17], left axillary artery [57], or descending thoracic aorta [58].

Azoury et al. [17] from Cleveland clinic have reported their experience of redo off-pump CABG in 21 patients through a posterolateral thoracotomy who had contraindications to conventional redo CABG. The specific indications to perform reoperative CABG through thoracotomy without CPB included patent graft at particular risk for resternotomy (n = 17), calcified ascending aorta (n = 3), serious comorbidities (n = 5), and diffuse atherosclerosis (n = 4). Several patients had more than one indication for this approach.

There were a total of 24 distal anastomoses performed for a mean of 1.1 grafts/patient. Targets approached included branches of the circumflex coronary artery (n = 23) and the LAD diagonal (n = 1). Fourteen conduits (67%) were venous (12 greater and 2 lesser saphenous veins), and 10 (48%) were arterial (radial artery). Inflow was obtained from the descending aorta in 15 patients and the left subclavian artery in 6 patients. The left subclavian artery was used for inflow when the descending aorta was severely atherosclerotic; 5 such patients had a patent LIMA-LAD graft, and temporary occlusion of the left subclavian artery caused no hemodynamic compromise. Complete revascularization was the goal and was achieved in all but 1 patient.

Ngaage et al. [62] from Mayo clinic reported similar outcomes for 26 patients who underwent redo off-pump CABG through left posterolateral thoracotomy. These results have been replicated by several other institutions [51-60,63,64,68] (Table 3).

## Table 3. Current outcomes of redo off-pump CABG[Δ]

| Study | Number of patients | Access | Operative mortality | Morbidity | Follow-up | Late survival | Reoperation | Ref. |
|---|---|---|---|---|---|---|---|---|
| Azoury et al. (2001) | 21 | PLT | Nil | Non-Q MI (5%) IABP (5%) AF (5%) | 15 ± 13 months | 95% at 2 years | Nil | [17] |
| Hirose et al. (2005) | 27 | RMS | Nil | Q-wave MI (3.7%) | 2.5 ± 0.6 years | 100% | 1 | [47] |
| Jacobs et al. (2005) | 46 | MIDCAB | 4.6% | Perianastomotic hematoma (2.3%) | 37 ± 21 months | 74.8% | 1 | [48] |
| Mishra et al.* (2008) | 332 | RMS (265) ALT (63) PLT (4) | 3.3% | MI (4.8%) Bleeding (2.8%) AF (3.6%) RF (0.6%) | NR | NR | Nil | [49] |
| Vohra et al.[†] (2008) | 43 | RMS (31) ALT (12) | 2.3% | IABP (2.3%) AF (14%) RF (9.3%) Stroke (2.3%) | 37 ± 19.2 months | 95 ± 3.2% | 2 | [50] |
| Trehan et al. (2000) | 50 | RMS (21) ALT (25) PLT (4) | 4% | MI (4%) Transfusion (24%) | NR | NR | NR | [52] |
| Ngaage et al. (2007) | 84 | RMS (48) ALT (10) PLT (26) | 1% | RF (11%) IABP (14%) Stroke (4%) | 3.6 years | 77% | NR | [62] |

AF, atrial fibrillation; ALT, anterolateral thoracotomy; IABP, intra-aortic balloon pump; MI, myocardial infarction; MIDCAB, minimally invasive direct coronary artery bypass; NR, not reported; PLT, posterolateral thoracotomy; RMS, repeat median sternotomy; RF, renal failure.
[Δ] Studies with at least 20 patients.
* Retrospective comparison with on-pump group.
[†] Propensity-matched analysis

Performing a MIDCAB procedure using the LIMA without requiring a sternotomy and avoiding CPB as well as extensive dissection of the heart may present a valuable treatment alternative in selected patients who require redo CABG of the anterior wall. Jacobs et al. [48] have reported the largest experience to date of redo MIDCAB. From January 1997 to October 2003, 46 patients (age, 66 ± 7.4 years) underwent reoperative MIDCAB using the LIMA to the LAD on the beating heart. Included were patients who had a previous cardiac operation through a sternotomy without the use of the LIMA and a stenosis of an LAD that was regarded as the major target vessel ("culprit lesion") for revascularization. The mean interval between the first operation and reoperation was 9.4 ± 3.5 years.

Forty-three patients successfully received the MIDCAB procedure. In 3 patients, the MIDCAB procedure was not completed for the following reasons. In 1 patient with a large anterior wall aneurysm the LAD was completely occluded. An endarterectomy was not considered feasible (not an access-related problem), and no bypass graft was performed. This patient received a transplantation successfully 13 months later. In another patient, as a result of excessive cardiomyopathy with an ejection fraction of only 0.10 and no tolerance for single-lung ventilation, harvesting of the LIMA through a minithoracotomy was not possible. This patient underwent a sternotomy and off-pump single bypass grafting. The third patient had massive pleural adhesions, rendering an operation through a minithoracotomy rather difficult.

In-hospital mortality was 2 of 43 patients (4.7%). Twenty-three patients underwent postoperative angiography, which demonstrated Fitzgibbon type A graft patency in all patients. In 1 patient, however, routine angiography on postoperative day 6 demonstrated a small anastomotic leakage. The patient was reoperated on through the same access, giving a reoperation rate of 2.3%.

Morishita et al. [61] in an earlier publication had reported their results of redo MIDCAB in seven patients. The target sites were as follows: LAD, 7; first diagonal branch, 1; and the conduit was the LIMA, 7; and saphenous vein graft (SVG), 1. Complete revascularization was accomplished in all patients, by including hybrid therapy in three patients and axillocoronary bypass grafting with SVGs in two patients. Postoperative angiography showed all patent grafts and all patients were discharged. During a mean follow-up period of 2.4 years (range: 0.5 to 3.5 years), all were free from cardiac events, except for one patient who had recurrent angina due to failure of a previously patent graft 3 years after redo MIDCAB. These results for the first time highlighted that MIDCABG via left anterolateral thoracotomy is an effective and safe technique in redo cases, as well as an alternative procedure for hybrid revascularization that combines minimally invasive revascularization of LAD with additional catheter interventional therapy.

## Concerns and Controversies

The two most important concern regarding redo off-pump CABG are the completeness of revascularization and graft patency. Complete revascularization is the main goal of primary coronary bypass, and it is reasonable to assume the same is true of coronary reoperation. Studies have demonstrated that incomplete myocardial revascularization negatively affects outcome after primary operations [69]. In the setting of coronary reoperation, Di Mauro and associates [16] found higher rates of incomplete revascularization in patients undergoing redo off-pump CABG (17.7% vs 5.9%, $P < .01$) when compared with redo CABG on CPB and showed that incomplete revascularization was an independent risk factor for cardiac death and cardiac mortality at 5 years. Tugtekin and coworkers [70] used the index of completeness of revascularization (preoperative planned/performed anastomosis) to compare redo CABG on CPB and redo off-pump CABG. They found a higher incidence of complete revascularization in their redo CABG on CPB group (86.9% for redo CABG vs 48.6% for redo OPCABG, $P < .01$). In the study by Czerny and colleagues [71], in which redo off-pump CABG was targeted to culprit coronary targets (target vessel revascularization), because of significant difference in completeness of revascularization, a higher incidence of recurrent angina was noted during a 5-year follow-up period. From these studies, there is some evidence of less complete revascularization when performing coronary reoperations by using off-pump techniques.

Graft patency after off-pump CABG has been questioned in the past, but evaluation of current best available evidence suggest that early patency rates are comparable to those after on-pump CABG for primary procedures [72]. In patients undergoing repeated off-pump CABG, there are few studies that report graft patency. In their select group of high-risk patients, Ngaage et al. [62] found a late patency rate of 76% in a subgroup reinvestigated for recurrent symptoms. Therefore, it is self-evident that this patency rate is an under-estimation. The selection of patients with a greater propensity to graft occlusion for repeated angiography underpins the low late graft patency rate observed in this cohort of patients. Also, early postoperative angiography, which was performed to diagnose 5 of 6 occluded grafts, can be misleading, especially for arterial grafts. On the other hand, Jacobs and coworkers reported that twenty-three patients that underwent postoperative angiography out of a total of 43 redo MIDCAB patients all had patent grafts [48].

Graft patency verification is increasingly recognized as an important component of surgical myocardial revascularization. Intuitively, eliminating intraoperative graft failure should reduce cardiac mortality and morbidity in the short term and improve clinical outcome in the long term. Although conventional angiography remains the gold standard technique for assessing graft patency, it is rarely available in the operating room and consequently several other less invasive approaches have been advocated [73]. The 2 most commonly used are the transit time flow measurement (TTFM) and the intraoperative fluorescence imaging (IFI). The TTFM is a quantitative volume flow technique, whereas the IFI is based on the fluorescent properties of indocyanine green. TTFM cannot define the degree of graft stenosis nor discriminate between the influence of the graft conduit and the coronary arteriolar bed on the mean graft flow. IFI provides a "semiquantitative" assessment of the graft patency with images that provide some details about the quality of coronary anastomoses. Both methods are valuable in identifying only at the extremes, that is, either patent or occluded grafts, and can confirm very good grafts; however, neither method is sensitive or specific enough in identifying more subtle abnormalities. These abnormal grafts most likely have poor long-term patency and are predestined to fail [74,75]. Although at present the current standard of care in CABG surgery does not require intraoperative imaging however one could argue that there is a strong case to adopt routine intraoperative graft patency assessment at least in the setting of reoperative off-pump CABG.

Last but not the least, it is important to be aware of the technical problem of graft kinking with resultant occlusion that can jeopardise the early and late outcome of any coronary revascularization operation in general and in particular grafting of the circumflex territory through a left thoracotomy. One of the strategies, described by Ricci et al. [76] to tackle this issue, consists of bringing coronary grafts to the descending thoracic aorta through a tunnel made between the inferior and superior pulmonary veins, underneath the left lower lobe of the lung. By using this technique, coronary grafts to the circumflex system are allowed to lie in a straight line, and are not affected by respiratory excursions. Subsequently, proximal anastomoses on the descending aorta are constructed in the usual manner, after lateral-occlusion clamping has been accomplished.

## Conclusion

Repeat CABG provides several technical challenges that distinguish it from primary CABG. It is of the utmost importance that this operation be carefully planned. We have developed a safe approach over the years for performing off-pump reoperative CABG. Off-pump CABG may be suitable, safe alternative in patients with an excessive risk who require one or two grafts. Its selective use in experienced hands can mitigate operative mortality with satisfactory short- as well as mid-term outcomes. However, currently the published experience with this strategy is limited and there is need for further studies to validate the safety and efficacy of reoperative off-pump CABG beyond doubt.

## References

[1] Yap CH, Sposato L, Akowuah E, et al. Contemporary results show repeat coronary artery bypass grafting remains a risk factor for operative mortality. *Ann Thorac Surg* 2009; 87:1386-91.

[2] Yau TM, Borger MA, Weisel RD, Ivanov J. The changing pattern of reoperative coronary surgery: trends in 1230 consecutive reoperations. *J Thorac Cardiovasc Surg* 2000;120:156-163.

[3] Ferguson B, Hammill BG, Peterson ED, DeLong ER, Grover FL. A decade of change—risk profiles and outcomes for isolated coronary artery bypass grafting procedures, 1990–1999: a report from the STS National Database Committee and the Duke Clinical Research Institute. *Ann Thorac Surg* 2002;73:480-489.

[4] Abramov D, Tamariz MG, Fremes SE, et al. Trends in coronary artery bypass surgery results: a recent, 9-year study. *Ann Thorac Surg* 2000;70:84-90.

[5] Van Eck FM, Noyez L, Verheugt FW, Brouwer RM. Preoperative prediction of early mortality in redo coronary artery surgery. *Eur J Cardiothorac Surg* 2002;21:1031-1036.

[6] Sabik JF, Blackstone EH, Houghtaling PL, Walts PA, Lytle BW. Is reoperation still a risk factor in coronary artery bypass surgery? *Ann Thorac Surg* 2005;80:1719-1727.

[7] Christenson JT, Simonet F, Schmuziger M. The impact of a short interval (≤1 year) between primary and reoperative coronary artery bypass grafting procedures. *Cardiovasc Surg* 1996;4:801-807.

[8] He GW, Acuff TE, Ryan WH, He YH, Mack MJ. Determinants of operative mortality in reoperative coronary artery bypass grafting. *J Thorac Cardiovasc Surg* 1995;110:971-978.

[9] Noyez L, van Eck FM. Long-term cardiac survival after reoperative coronary artery bypass grafting. Eur J Cardiothorac Surg 2004;25:59-64.

[10] Reid CM, Rockell M, Skillington PD, et al. Initial twelve months experience and analysis for 2001–2002 from the Australasian Society of Cardiac and Thoracic Surgeons–Victorian database project. *Heart Lung Circ* 2004;13:291-297.

[11] Dinh DT, Lee GA, Billah B, Smith JA, Shardey GC, Reid CM. Trends in coronary artery bypass graft surgery in Victoria, 2001–2006: findings from the Australasian Society of Cardiac and Thoracic Surgeons database project. *Med J Aust* 2008;188:214-217.

[12] Allen KB, Matheny RG, Robison RJ, Heimansohn DA, Shaar CJ. Minimally invasive versus conventional reoperative coronary artery bypass. *Ann Thorac Surg* 1997; 64:616-622.

[13] Teodori G, Iaco AL, Di Mauro M, et al. Reoperative coronary surgery with and without cardiopulmonary bypass. *J Card Surg* 2000;15:303-308.

[14] Akins CW, Buckley MJ, Daggett WM. Reoperative coronary grafting: Changing patient profiles, operative indications, techniques, and results. *Ann Thorac Surg* 1994;58:359-364.

[15] Cosgrove 3rd DM. Is coronary reoperation without the pump an advantage? *Ann Thorac Surg* 1993;55:329.

[16] Di Mauro M, Iaco AL, Contini M, et al. Reoperative coronary artery bypass grafting: analysis of early and late outcomes. *Ann Thorac Surg* 2005;79:81-87.

[17] Azoury FM, Gillinov AM, Lytle BW, Smedira NG, Sabik JF. Off-pump reoperative coronary artery bypass grafting by thoracotomy: patient selection and operative technique. *Ann Thorac Surg* 2001;71:1959-1963.

[18] Keon WJ, Heggtveit HA, Leduc J. Perioperative myocardial infarction caused by atheroembolism. *J Thorac Cardiovasc Surg* 1982;84:849-855.

[19] Navia D, Cosgrove 3rd DM, Lytle BW, et al. Is the internal thoracic artery the conduit of choice to replace a stenotic vein graft? *Ann Thorac Surg* 1994;57:40-44.

[20] Lytle BW, McElroy D, McCarthy P, et al. Influence of arterial coronary bypass grafts on the mortality in coronary reoperations. *J Thorac Cardiovasc Surg* 1994;107:675-683.

[21] Gillinov AM, Casselman FP, Lytle BW, et al. Injury to a patent left internal thoracic artery graft at coronary reoperation. *Ann Thorac Surg* 1999;67:382-6.

[22] Zehr KJ, Lee PC, Poston RS, Gillinov AM, Hruban RH, Cameron DE. Protection of the internal mammary artery pedicle with polytetrafluoroethylene membrane. *J Card Surg* 1993;8:650-655.

[23] Pacifico AD, Sears NJ, Burgos C. Harvesting, routing, and anastomosing the left internal mammary artery graft. *Ann Thorac Surg* 1986;42:708-710.

[24] Berry BE, Davis DJ, Sheely CH 2nd, Hackler MT. Protection and expanded use of the left internal mammary artery graft by pericardial flap technique. *J Thorac Cardiovasc Surg* 1988;95:346-350.

[25] Sabik JF, Lytle BW, McCarthy PM, Cosgrove DM. Axillary artery an alternative site of arterial cannulation for patients with extensive aortic and peripheral vascular disease. *J Thorac Cardiovasc Surg* 1995;109:885-891.

[26] Sabik JF, Nemeh H, Lytle BW, et al. Cannulation of the axillary artery with a side graft reduces morbidity. *Ann Thorac Surg* 2004;77:1315-1320.

[27] Borger MA, Rao V, Weisel RD, et al. Reoperative coronary bypass surgery: effect of patent grafts and retrograde cardioplegia. *J Thorac Cardiovasc Surg* 2001;121:83-90.

[28] Raja SG, Dreyfus GD. Current status of off-pump coronary artery bypass surgery. *Asian Cardiovasc Thorac Ann* 2008;16:164-78.

[29] Raja SG, Berg GA. Impact of off-pump coronary artery bypass grafting on systemic inflammation: current best available evidence. *J Card Surg* 2007;22:445-55.

[30] Raja SG, Dreyfus GD. Impact of off-pump coronary artery bypass grafting on postoperative bleeding: current best available evidence. *J Card Surg* 2006;21:35-41.

[31] Raja SG, Dreyfus GD. Impact of off-pump coronary artery bypass grafting on postoperative pulmonary dysfunction: current best available evidence. *Ann Card Anaesth* 2006;9:17-24.

[32] Raja SG, Dreyfus GD. Impact of off-pump coronary artery bypass grafting on postoperative renal dysfunction: current best available evidence. *Nephrology (Carlton)* 2006;11:269-73.

[33] Raja SG, Dreyfus GD. Off-pump coronary artery bypass surgery: to do or not to do? Current best available evidence. *J Cardiothorac Vasc Anesth* 2004;18:486-505.

[34] Angelini GD, Taylor FC, Reeves BC, Ascione R. Early and midterm outcome after off-pump and on-pump surgery in Beating Heart Against Cardioplegic Arrest Studies (BHACAS 1 and 2): a pooled analysis of two randomised controlled trials. *Lancet* 2002;359:1194-1199.

[35] Gerola LR, Buffolo E, Jasbik W, et al. Off-pump versus on-pump myocardial revascularization in low-risk patients with one or two vessel disease: perioperative results in a multicenter randomized controlled trial. *Ann Thorac Surg* 2004;77:569-573.

[36] Puskas JD, Williams WH, Duke PG, et al. Off-pump coronary artery bypass grafting provides complete revascularization with reduced myocardial injury, transfusion requirements, and length of stay: a prospective randomized comparison of two hundred unselected patients undergoing off-pump versus conventional coronary artery bypass grafting. *J Thorac Cardiovasc Surg* 2003;125:797-808.

[37] Kobayashi J, Tashiro T, Ochi M, et al. Early outcome of a randomized comparison of off-pump and on-pump multiple arterial coronary revascularization. *Circulation* 2005;112(Suppl 9):I338-I343.

[38] Muneretto C, Bisleri G, Negri A, et al. Off-pump coronary artery bypass surgery technique for total arterial myocardial revascularization: a prospective randomized study. *Ann Thorac Surg* 2003;76:778-782.

[39] van Dijk D, Nierich AP, Jansen EWL, et al. Early outcome after off-pump versus on-pump coronary bypass surgery – results from a randomized study. *Circulation* 2001;104:1761-1766.

[40] Widimsky P, Straka Z, Stros P, et al. One-year coronary bypass graft patency: a randomized comparison between off-pump and on-pump surgery angiographic results of the PRAGUE-4 trial. *Circulation* 2004;110:3418-3423.

[41] Puskas JD, Thourani VH, Kilgo P, et al. Off-pump coronary artery bypass disproportionately benefits high-risk patients. *Ann Thorac Surg* 2009;88:1142-7.

[42] Meharwal ZS, Mishra YK, Kohli V, Bapna R, Singh S, Trehan N. Off-pump multivessel coronary artery surgery in high-risk patients. *Ann Thorac Surg* 2002;74,S1353-7.

[43] Demaria RG, Carrier M, Fortier S, et al. Reduced mortality and strokes with off-pump coronary artery bypass grafting surgery in octogenarians. *Circulation* 2002;106:I5-10.

[44] D'Ancona G, Karamanoukian H, Kawaguchi AT, Ricci M, Salerno TA, Bergsland J. Myocardial revascularization of the beating heart in high-risk patients. *J Card Surg* 2001;16:132-9.

[45] Al-Ruzzeh S, Nakamura K, Athanasiou T, et al. Does off-pump coronary artery bypass (OPCAB) surgery improve the outcome in high-risk patients?: a comparative study of 1398 high-risk patients. *Eur J Cardiothorac Surg* 2003;23:50-5.

[46] Bergsland J, Hasnain S, Lajos TZ, Salerno TA. Elimination of cardiopulmonary bypass: a prime goal in reoperative coronary artery bypass surgery. *Eur J Cardiothorac Surg* 1998;14:59-62.

[47] Hirose H, Amano A, Ruzheng L, Xiang Z. Routine reoperative off-pump coronary artery bypass grafting via midline sternotomy: is it feasible? *Angiology* 2005;56:243-8.

[48] Jacobs S, Holzhey D, Walther T, Falk V, Mohr FW. Redo minimally invasive direct coronary artery bypass grafting. *Ann Thorac Surg* 2005;80:1336-9.

[49] Mishra YK, Collison SP, Malhotra R, Kohli V, Mehta Y, Trehan N. Ten-year experience with single-vessel and multivessel reoperative off-pump coronary artery bypass grafting. *J Thorac Cardiovasc Surg* 2008;135:527-32.

[50] Vohra HA, Bahrami T, Farid S, et al. Propensity score analysis of early and late outcome after redo off-pump and on-pump coronary artery bypass grafting. *Eur J Cardiothorac Surg* 2008;33:209-14.

[51] Mishra Y, Wasir H, Kohli V, et al. Beating heart versus conventional reoperative coronary artery bypass surgery. *Indian Heart J* 2002;54:159-63.

[52] Trehan N, Mishra YK, Malhotra R, Sharma KK, Mehta Y, Shrivastava S. Off-pump redo coronary artery bypass grafting. *Ann Thorac Surg* 2000;70:1026-9.

[53] Fanning WJ, Kakos GS, Williams TE Jr. Reoperative coronary artery bypass grafting without cardiopulmonary bypass. *Ann Thorac Surg* 1993;55:486-9.

[54] Byrne JG, Aklog L, Adams DH, Cohn LH, Aranki SF. Reoperative CABG using left thoracotomy: a tailored strategy. *Ann Thorac Surg* 2001;71:196-200.

[55] Lajos TZ, Akhter M, Bergsland J, et al. Limited access left thoracotomy for reoperative coronary artery disease: on or off pump. *J Card Surg* 2000;15:291-5.

[56] Dewey TM, Magee MJ, Acuff T, et al. Beating heart surgery reduces mortality in the reoperative bypass patient. *Heart Surg Forum* 2002;5 Suppl 4:S301-16.

[57] Minakawa M, Takahashi K, Kondo N, Hatakeyama M, Kuga T, Fukuda I. Left thoracotomy approach in reoperative off-pump coronary revascularization: bypass grafting from the left axillary artery or descending thoracic aorta. *Jpn J Thorac Cardiovasc Surg* 2003;51:582-7.

[58] Kuniyoshi Y, Yamashiro S, Miyagi K, Uezu T, Arakaki K, Koja K. Off-pump redo coronary artery bypass grafting via left thoracotomy. *Ann Thorac Cardiovasc Surg* 2003;9:378-83.

[59] Shapira OM, Natarajan V, Kaushik S, DeAndrade KM, Shemin RJ. Off-pump versus on-pump reoperative CABG via a left thoracotomy for circumflex coronary artery revascularization. *J Card Surg* 2004;19:113-8.

[60] Mack MJ. Off-pump surgery and alternatives to standard operation in redo coronary surgery. *J Card Surg* 2004;19:313-9.

[61] Morishita A, Shimakura T, Miyagishima M, Kawamoto J, Morimoto H. Minimally invasive direct redo coronary artery bypass grafting. *Ann Thorac Cardiovasc Surg* 2002;8:209-12.

[62] Ngaage DL, Zehr KJ, Daly RC, et al. Off-pump strategy in high-risk coronary artery bypass reoperations. *Mayo Clin Proc* 2007;82:567-71.

[63] D'Ancona G, Karamanoukian H, Lajos T, Ricci M, Bergsland J, Salerno T. Posterior thoracotomy for reoperative coronary artery bypass grafting without cardiopulmonary bypass: perioperative results. *Heart Surg Forum* 2000;3:18-22.

[64] Ricci M, Bergsland J, D'Ancona G, Salerno TA, Karamanoukian HL. Reoperative grafting of the LAD system using the LAST approach: technical details. *J Card Surg* 2000;15:383-4.

[65] Kerr PC, Ricci M, Abraham R, D'Ancona, Salerno TA. Redo left anterior descending artery grafting via left anterior small thoracotomy. An alternative approach. *Ann Thorac Surg* 2001;71:384-5.

[66] Grandjean JG, Mariani MA, Ebels T. Coronary reoperation via small laparotomy using right gastroepiploic artery without CPB. *Ann Thorac Surg* 1996;61:1853-5.

[67] Akther M, Lajos TZ, Grosner G, Bergsland J, Salerno TA. Reoperations with the right gastroepiploic artery without cardiopulmonary bypass. *J Cardiac Surg* 1997;12: 210-4.

[68] D'Ancona G, Karamanoukian HL, Lajos T, Ricci M, Bergsland J, Salerno TA. Reoperative coronary artery bypass grafting without cardiopulmonary bypass: determinants of perioperative morbidity and mortality. *Heart Surg Forum* 2001;4:152-8.

[69] Caputo M, Reeves BC, Rajkaruna C, Awair H, Angelini GD. Incomplete revascularization during OPCAB surgery is associated with reduced mid-term event-free survival. *Ann Thorac Surg* 2005;80:2141-2147.

[70] Tugtekin SM, Alexiou K, Kappert U, et al. Coronary reoperation with and without cardiopulmonary bypass. *Clin Res Cardiol* 2006;95:93-98.

[71] Czerny M, Zimpfer D, Kilo J, et al. Coronary reoperations: recurrence of angina and clinical outcome with and without cardiopulmonary bypass. *Ann Thorac Surg* 2003;75:847-852.

[72] Raja SG, Dreyfus GD. Impact of off-pump coronary artery bypass grafting on graft patency: current best available evidence. *J Card Surg* 2007;22:165-9.

[73] Balacumaraswami L, Taggart DP. Intraoperative imaging techniques to assess coronary artery bypass graft patency. *Ann Thorac Surg* 2007;83:2251-7.

[74] Leacche M, Balaguer JM, Byrne JG. Intraoperative grafts assessment. *Semin Thorac Cardiovasc Surg* 2009;21:207-12.

[75] Ricci M, Karamanoukian HL, Salerno TA, Dancona G, Bergsland J. Role of coronary graft flow measurement during reoperations for early graft failure after off-pump coronary revascularization. *J Card Surg* 1999;14:342-7.

[76] Ricci M, Karamanoukian HL, D'Ancona G, Salerno TA, Bergsland J. Reoperative "off-pump" circumflex revascularization via left thoracotomy: how to prevent graft kinking. *Ann Thorac Surg* 2000;70:309-10.

*Chapter XI*

# Technique of Hybrid Coronary Revascularization

### Shahzad G. Raja[1] and Charles D. Ilsley[2]
[1]Cardiac Surgeon, Harefield Hospital, London, United Kingdom
[2]Senior Cardiologist, Clinical Director, Harefield Hospital,
London, United Kingdom

## Abstract

The search for the optimal strategy for myocardial revascularization is still in progress, more than 40 years after the first coronary artery bypass graft operation and nearly 30 years after the first percutaneous coronary angioplasty. The ideal revascularization strategy should be safe and effective, provide the best immediate and long-term result, be associated with minimal morbidity and invasiveness, be inexpensive, and require a short hospitalization. Hybrid coronary revascularization is one such strategy that involves combining minimally invasive coronary artery bypass grafting and percutaneous coronary intervention.

The main principle of the technique includes placement of left internal mammary artery graft to the left anterior descending coronary artery and performance of percutaenous coronary intervention in non- left anterior descending target vessels. This principle is based on increasing data showing equivalent results of percutaneous coronary intervention with coronary revascularization using saphenous vein grafts in selected patients.

Hybrid coronary revascularization has been designed to allow rapid rehabilitation and minimize periprocedural pain under concomitant preservation of the patient's body integrity. Providing that perioperative and long-term results are as good as the results of conventional surgical revascularization, this option seems to be quite appealing for patients and referring cardiologists. This chapter provides an overview of the technique of hybrid coronary revascularization, evaluates the current outcomes and highlights the concerns and controversies associated with this strategy.

# Introduction

In the past few years a rapid expansion of the available options for myocardial revascularization has occurred both in the interventional cardiology and in the cardiac surgery field; as a result, the gap between percutaneous and surgical coronary revascularization is narrowing, as percutaneous techniques move from "plain old balloon angioplasty" to more invasive and costly techniques [1] and surgery is moving toward less invasive and less expensive approaches [2]. In the current era of minimally invasive approaches to treat coronary artery disease, hybrid coronary revascularization (HCR) of patients with multivessel coronary artery disease is emerging as an option that is believed to offer "the best of both worlds", minimally invasive direct coronary artery bypass (MIDCAB) and stenting. MIDCAB will diminish noncardiac complications associated with classical coronary artery bypass grafting (CABG) and provide "gold standard" left internal mammary artery to left anterior descending artery (LIMA-to-LAD) graft while percutaneous intervention (PCI) will minimize major adverse cardiac and cerebral events [3]. This chapter focuses on the concept, technique and current status of hybrid coronary revascularization.

# Concept of Hybrid Coronary Revascularization

Hybrid coronary revascularization also termed integrated coronary revascularization is a combination between surgical and catheter-based intervention on the diseased coronary arteries. Most commonly a LIMA bypass graft placed on the LAD in a minimally invasive or endoscopic fashion is combined with PCI and stenting of the right coronary artery or circumflex artery system. The idea for HCR was floated for the first time in mid 1990 following the discovery of the MIDCAB operation [4]. Angelini and associates [5] were the first to report outcomes for HCR in 1996. A series of 6 patients received placement of a LIMA on the LAD on the beating heart through left anterior minithoracotomy and PCI or PCI + stent on other coronary vessels. Two of these operations were carried out simultaneously in the cardiac catheterization laboratory. There was no postoperative mortality. Ever since then increasing experience has been reported with this technique.

The rationale for HCR is based on the evidence that successful LIMA-to-LAD offers tremendous mortality advantage [6] while percutaneous interventional treatment of coronary lesions of the circumflex system or the right coronary artery are less frequently associated with subsequent restenosis than treatment of LAD lesions [7,8]. Furthermore, as the mortality rates of minimally invasive single LIMA to LAD procedures are also reported in the near zero percent range [9-11], MIDCAB LIMA-to-LAD grafting is likely to reduce the morbidity rates compared with conventional CABG on cardiopulmonary bypass (CPB), since it does not necessitate the cross-clamping of the aorta with its attendant stroke rate, has a lower chance of hemodynamic shifts when going on and off CBP, has a superior cosmetic result, and avoids the pulmonary embarrassment of the sternotomy [12]. Patients may thus recover faster with shorter lengths of stay in the hospital and return to work more quickly than with conventional CABG [13]. In addition, the perioperative need for blood transfusion in patients undergoing minimally invasive LIMA-to-LAD grafting is reduced when compared to conventional CABG [14,15]. Hence, HCR (with its potential life-extending benefit of LIMA-to-LAD grafting) has emerged as an attractive option for multivessel coronary artery disease patients with LAD disease not ideal for catheter-based intervention but with other vessels amenable to catheter-based intervention, who would otherwise be referred for conventional CABG, thus avoiding the side effects from CPB and median sternotomy. HCR allows the interventionalist to revascularize non-LAD lesions percutaneously and the surgeon to provide the benefits of the LIMA-to-LAD graft to the patient.

# Indications and Contraindications of Hybrid Coronary Revascularization

Basically any patient with multivessel coronary artery disease who is suitable for minimally invasive LIMA to LAD placement and whose coronary arteries other than the LAD are suitable for catheter-based intervention is suitable for HCR. HCR may be especially useful in complex LAD lesions, restenotic lesions in LAD, acute myocardial infarction in "non-LAD" territory, high-risk elderly patients with multiple comorbidities who are poor surgical candidates for conventional CABG and who are not likely to tolerate CPB well and patients with severe left ventricular systolic dysfunction who are not ideal candidates for conventional bypass surgery [15].

## Patient Selection

Selecting patients for HCR involves close consultation between cardiac surgeon and interventional cardiologist. Surgeon and cardiologist must address specific concerns regarding the suitability of coronary anatomy as well as clinical characteristics as they relate to the specifics of minimally invasive LIMA-to-LAD revascularization.

The angiogram should be carefully reviewed for the suitability of the LAD for surgical grafting. A large distal LAD will provide the best incremental advantage to LIMA-to-LAD revascularization as compared with multivessel stenting [16]. Very small LAD targets or obvious long intramyocardial LAD segments may pose significant technical challenges to the minimally invasive surgeon and should be approached carefully. Total chronic occlusions of the LAD can be safely approached with minimally invasive LIMA-LAD. However, anterior wall viability and myocardium at risk should be assessed preoperatively. Diffuse anterior wall thinning, or limited anterior wall myocardial viability will limit the effectiveness of the surgical portion of a hybrid revascularization strategy [16].

The non-LAD targets should be reviewed in detail for PCI options. An estimation of both the technical considerations and the possible long-term success of the PCI should be considered. Decisions regarding the possible aggressiveness of PCI should be based on the HCR strategy, as the presence of a patent LIMA-LAD graft may change the safety margin for the interventional cardiologist. In general, a suitable LAD with focal proximal lesions in the right coronary artery and/or circumflex distribution provides the best situations for HCR [16].

The need for single-lung ventilation and chest cavity insufflation raises important considerations when selecting patients for minimally invasive CABG. The ideal patients will have a small cardiac silhouette and a large left pleural space. Absolute exclusion criteria for robotic or thoracoscopic CABG include patients with severe chronic obstructive pulmonary disease who cannot tolerate single-lung ventilation and those patients who have had prior left chest surgery. Patients with severe pulmonary hypertension also provide a relative contraindication as rapid desaturation and hemodynamic compromise can occur with single-lung ventilation and thoracic cavity insufflation. Actively ischemic patients also pose a challenge. The chest insufflation can exacerbate ischemia and result in malignant arrhythmias that can be challenging to handle [16].

Patients who are deemed poor candidates for MIDCAB type approaches can still have strategies designed to take advantage of an HCR approach. In especially high-risk patients, off-pump LIMA-to-LAD through a sternotomy remains an option with plans for stenting of the non-LAD targets [16].

Contraindications for HCR can be derived from contraindications for a minimally invasive LIMA-to-LAD procedure and those for catheter-based intervention, which are listed in Table 1 [17].

**Table 1. Contraindications for Hybrid Coronary Revascularization**

*General Contraindications for minimally invasive LIMA to LAD*
    Subclavian artery stenosis
    Known damage to the LIMA
    Previous chest irradiation (relative)
    Pleural adhesions (relative)
    Intramyocardial LAD (relative)
    Severe lung disease precluding single lung ventilation
    Additional valve disease
**MIDCAB Specific Contraindications**
    Massive obesity (relative)
**AH-TECAB Specific Contraindications**
    Contraindications for remote access perfusion
    (aortoiliac atherosclerotic disease, ascending aortic diameter > 3.7 mm)
*BH-TECAB Specific Contraindications*
    Severe abdominal adhesions precluding subxiphoid placement of endostabilizer
*Contraindications for PCI/Stent to the RCA and Cx System*
    Chronic total occlusions (relative)
    Complex lesions
    (recurrent restenosis, angled lesions, bifurcation lesions, calcified lesions, Type C stenosis)

MIDCAB = minimally invasive direct coronary artery bypass grafting; LIMA = left internal mammary artery; LAD = left anterior descending artery; AH-TECAB = arrested heart totally endoscopic coronary artery bypass grafting; BH-TECAB = beating heart totally endoscopic coronary artery bypass grafting; PCI = percutaneous coronary intervention; RCA = right coronary artery; Cx = circumflex coronary artery.

# Surgical Options for Minimally Invasive LIMA-to-LAD Procedure

The minimally invasive revascularization strategies primarily used for LIMA-to-LAD revascularization all aim to ameliorate 2 potentially invasive surgical components: the CPB machine and the sternotomy incision. Currently used strategies include MIDCAB, Endoscopic Atraumatic Coronary Artery Bypass (Endo-ACAB), and Totally Endoscopic Coronary Artery Bypass Grafting (TECAB).

## MIDCAB

Minimally invasive direct coronary artery bypass grafting (MIDCAB) refers to a minimally invasive LIMA-to-LAD revascularization which is performed on the beating heart through a small left-sided thoracotomy in the fourth or fifth interspace. Costal cartilage removal or disarticulation is sometimes necessary and a special chest wall retractor is used to allow for open-LIMA takedown [16]. Cardiac stabilization can be accomplished with a stabilizer that is delivered directly through the wound. MIDCAB has the advantage of not requiring any special endoscopic or robotic skills to master the LIMA takedown. Although single-lung ventilation improves exposure, chest cavity insufflation is not necessary. However, the degree of chest wall retraction necessary to allow for open-LIMA mobilization is quite extensive and postoperative pain control can be a challenge [18].

Clinical and angiographic studies validating the safety and efficacy of MIDCAB have been reported in the literature as early as 1994. However, it is clear that a comfort level with off-pump surgery is important with this procedure and experience with sternal-sparing incisions is likewise beneficial. Short-term patency rates with respect to LIMA-to-LAD grafts in both the earliest series and the more contemporary series range from 95% to 97% [19-22]. The advantages of MIDCAB over conventional CABG are rooted in the avoidance of CPB and the absence of aortic manipulation or cross-clamping. It appears that open MIDCAB can decrease bleeding and infection rates when compared with off-pump CABG × 1 through a sternotomy [16]. However, it is not clear that there is a significant difference in pulmonary complications or postoperative pain between open MIDCAB and traditional off-pump CABG × 1. To avoid the significant chest wall manipulation associated with open MIDCAB and to improve postoperative pain control, thoracoscopic and robotic techniques have been employed for LIMA mobilization.

## Endo-ACAB

Endo-ACAB refers to the thoracoscopic or robotic identification of the LAD and complete mobilization of the LIMA without compromising the integrity of the chest wall. A directed, nonrib-spreading or limited-rib spreading thoracotomy then allows for a hand-sewn LIMA-LAD anastomosis on the beating heart. Robotic and thoracoscopic techniques can also be used to mobilize both the internal thoracic arteries. With this technique, a more complete surgical revascularization can be performed [23,24].

Robotic LIMA mobilization requires single-lung ventilation and chest cavity insufflation to develop the virtual space of the anterior mediastinum in which the LIMA lies. Insufflation of the chest is performed using carbon dioxide at pressures ranging from 8 to 15 mm Hg. During insufflation, a controlled pneumothorax is induced. The resultant cardiac displacement results in rising central venous pressure, decreased right and left heart filling, a drop in blood pressure, and an alteration in oxygenation [25]. Adequate volume loading and peripheral vasoconstriction are necessary to maintain appropriate hemodynamics. After the pericardiotomy, LAD identification, LIMA takedown, and distal transection, a small (4-5 cm) anterior thoracotomy is performed without costal cartilage disarticulation. The LAD is stabilized with an endoscopic stabilizer delivered into the wound through the left arm port. This approach significantly decreases the pain and wound complications of conventional MIDCAB, yet retains the reliability of a hand-sewn anastomosis.

## TECAB

Robotically assisted TECAB has emerged as another viable option for closed chest coronary artery bypass surgery. The first TECAB surgeries were performed robotically on the arrested heart during CPB. Peripheral CPB with an intra-aortic balloon occluder for cardioplegic arrest is a critical component to the arrested heart TECAB [26,27]. The complications associated with intra-aortic balloon occlusion and the inflammatory response of CPB have led most minimally invasive surgeons to opt for beating-heart off-pump revascularization in lieu of a TECAB approach.

The beating-heart TECAB was the next extension of the arrested heart TECAB. The beating-heart TECAB is performed in an identical way as the robotic Endo-ACAB, with the exception of the 4-cm thoracotomy for open, hand-sewn anastomosis. Instead, the anastomosis is performed intracorporeally with the robot. The TECAB has proved to be an incredibly challenging operation that only a few have mastered. Early results are encouraging from a small number of skilled operators, but widespread adoption of this operation has not occurred [28,29].

# Technical Issues

The single most important technical issue in HCR is the timing of the two coronary revascularization procedures. There are 3 basic HCR approaches, all with their potential advantages and disadvantages: PCI can be performed first followed by minimally invasive LIMA-to-LAD anastomosis; minimally invasive LIMA-to-LAD anastomosis can be performed first followed by PCI; and minimally invasive LIMA-to-LAD anastomosis and PCI can be performed in the same sitting in a hybrid operative suite.

## PCI First Followed by Minimally Invasive LIMA-to-LAD Anastomosis

The potential advantages of a strategy that employs PCI before LIMA-to-LAD anastomosis are 3-fold. First, revascularization of non-LAD targets provides excellent collateral circulation, thereby minimizing the potential risk of ischemia during the LAD occlusion of surgical intervention. This provides a safety net of collateral flow during the LAD occlusion at the time of surgery [16]. Second, it allows the interventional cardiologist the fallback position of conventional CABG if a suboptimal PCI result be obtained. Finally, this approach allows for HCR in the setting of acute myocardial infarction in which the target lesion is in a non-LAD vessel. The acute lesion can be treated and the LAD can be revascularized surgically a later sitting [16]. In addition, in case of any interventional complication, surgery will effectively treat the underlying coronary disease as well as the interventional complication in one procedure [15,17,30,31]. However, improvements in the combined balloon/ device/pharmacologic approach to coronary intervention in elective procedures has resulted in angiographic success rates of 96–99%, with Q-wave MI rates of 1–3%, emergency coronary bypass surgery rates of 0.2–3% and unadjusted in-hospital mortality rates of 0.5–1.4% [15,32].

Although this approach was used fairly commonly in the era of percutaneous transluminal coronary angioplasty and bare metal stents (BMS), the risk of acute stent thrombosis with drug eluting stents (DES) has raised serious concern about such an approach [16]. With this strategy, in-hospital patients need to be maintained on eptifibatide (Integrilin; Schering Plough, Kenilworth, NJ), which can be stopped for surgery. Clopidogrel (Plavix; Bristol Myers Squibb, Bridgewater, NJ) can be administered once the patient is extubated in the postoperative period. However, it is clear that the risk of stent thrombosis with both BMS within 1 month and DES for up to 1 year is related to both brief discontinuation of glycoprotein IIIa/IIb inhibitors and the inflammatory reaction of both noncardiac and cardiac surgery [33]. Some surgeons have performed surgery on clopidogrel, but this approach is plagued by an increased incidence of bleeding (9.6% vs. 7.5%) [34]. Furthermore, such an approach does not eliminate the risk of stent thrombosis in the setting of inflammatory mediator release from the trauma of surgery or administration of protamine to reverse heparin.

This approach can still be used in selected situations. It should be kept in mind, especially in the setting of BMS placement for acute myocardial infarction. Brief discontinuation of Plavix after 1 month of therapy or surgery on Plavix remain viable options in these patients.

## Minimally Invasive LIMA-to-LAD Anastomosis First Followed by PCI

The advantages of performing the LAD revascularization first would be:

(1) an opportunity for verification of the LIMA-to-LAD short-term patency;
(2) the patient could be pre-treated with clopidrogel and it would not have to be discontinued due to the CABG procedure; and
(3) catheter-based intervention being performed at a reduced risk as LAD is already revascularized with functioning LIMA [15]. Left main lesions and diagonal bifurcation lesions are just two such lesions that can be more safely treated through PCI with a protected LAD [16].

The minimally invasive surgeon should be cognizant of possible intraoperative ischemia with this HCR approach because the collateral, non-LAD vessels are unrevascularized. Judicious use of intracoronary shunts, careful attention to cardiac-filling pressures and systemic blood pressure during insufflation, and the use of peripheral CPB when necessary are all critical to success in this setting. This HCR approach also makes the determination paramount that PCI has a very high chance of success and a low chance of procedural complications with the non-LAD lesions assigned for treatment [16].

It remains unclear at present what is the optimal timing for PCI following Mid-CAB. A period of waiting after surgery seems prudent to allow the patient to resolve the potential inflammatory milieu which exists immediately after the operation. This response is quite brief and usually has resolved within 3 to 5 days, making it possible to perform PCI on the index hospitalization or days to weeks later. Patients may need 7 to 10 days of mental and physical recovery before undergoing a second procedure. However, some physicians may feel uneasy discharging certain patients with an incomplete revascularization, prompting PCI before discharge. Economic issues also bear on the hospital system, as a single diagnosis-related group is typically used to reimburse 2 separate costly procedures. As HCR becomes more common, these issues will likely be addressed to provide a fuller hospital reimbursement [16].

### Simultaneous Minimally Invasive LIMA-to-LAD Anastomosis

With the advent of endovascular surgical procedures and percutaneous valvular therapy, operating suites have been created that have the capability of both minimally invasive surgical procedures and PCI. This has led some investigators to favor a combined surgery with completion angiography and stenting of non-LAD vessels in the same operative sitting [35]. The potential advantages of such an approach include the ability to perform routine imaging of the LIMA-to-LAD before closure to confirm an anatomically acceptable anastamosis. Complete revascularization before leaving the operating suite is the other major advantage of such an approach. The emotional and psychologic benefit to the patient of a complete "fix" in 1 anesthetic sitting also has its merits [16]. Finally, PCI performed in the setting of a completed LIMA-LAD allows a more aggressive percutaneous approach to otherwise challenging lesions. The security of general anesthesia and the operating room likewise provide a safety net if a PCI failure occurs.

The timing of the two procedures evokes considerable debate with no definite consensus at the current time and perhaps a case-by-case basis would be most appropriate [15]. It is expected that simultaneous intervention in the near future, once purpose built catheter-lab operating rooms are available, will put an end to this debate.

## Outcomes

Following the first ever publication of Angelini and coworkers [5] on HCR, several nonrandomized studies have looked at the early and mid-term outcomes of HCR (Table 2). Lloyd et al. [36] reported on 18 patients, of which 14 were first treated with MIDCAB followed by catheter-based intervention 1–3 days later and 4 underwent simultaneous MIDCAB and catheter-based intervention. All patients were extubated early, with a mean intensive care stay of 14.7 ± 9.4 hours. The mean primary hospital stay was 5 ± 1.5 days (range, 3–7 days). There were no post-operative complications or deaths. At 18-month follow-up, all but 1 patient remained asymptomatic and on no anti-anginal treatment.

In a series of 31 HCR patients where PTCA was, in general, performed prior to MIDCAB, 38 of 39 vessels (97%) were successfully treated with PTCA, with the exception of 1 failure in a chronic total occlusion [37]. All 31 patients were asymptomatic at a mean follow-up of 7 months. The average length of stay after MIDCAB was 2.79 ± 1.05 days. There were 2 adverse clinical events, both related to PTCA and not to MIDCAB. Postoperative angiography in 84% of patients revealed a patent anastomosis and normal flow in the graft and bypassed vessel. At a longer follow-up of 10.8 ± 3.8 months, three patients (9.6%) in this series required repeat target vessel revascularization in the distribution of the previous percutaneous coronary intervention [38].

Wittwer et al. [39] reported no procedure related complications for 35 patients (29 male, 6 female), mean age 56.7 years who underwent a hybrid revascularization performed as a primary MIDCAB procedure for grafting of the LAD with LIMA, followed by staged angioplasty and stenting of additional coronary lesions. All patients remained free from angina and no stress ECG changes were recorded. Several other series report similar results [40-46].

## Emerging Developments

The last 5 years have seen the advancement of endoscopic and, finally, robotic endoscopic LIMA mobilization through 3-mm and 5-mm port access. No spreading of the rib cage or removal of rib is required for this approach. Totally endoscopic robotic closed chest coronary bypass is being carried out in a few centers in the world and is the least invasive surgical procedure to accomplish the goal of LIMA-to-LAD graft construction. Recently, early experiences with HCR using a combined approach of catheter-based intervention and robotically-assisted MIDCAB have been published [47-49]. Stahl et al. [47] were the first to use robotics for HCR. They reported their experience of HCR in 54 consecutive patients from four institutions in whom LIMA grafts were endoscopically harvested with robotic assistance using either the Aesop or Zeus system. However, all anastomoses in this series were manually constructed through a 4- to 6-cm anterior thoracotomy incision. Lee et al. [48] have also reported using this technique with mixed results.

Davidavicius et al. [49] published 1-year follow-up of patients with multivessel disease in whom combined LIMA-to-LAD grafting by robotically enhanced MIDCAB and PCI of the lesions located in the right coronary artery and left circumflex coronary artery was performed. In this study, twenty patients with multivessel disease were selected to undergo combined PCI and robotically enhanced MIDCAB because they had a lesion amenable to PCI in the right and/or the left circumflex coronary artery and a lesion in the LAD and/or the first diagonal branch that was considered less than ideal for PCI. PCI was actually performed only when fractional flow reserve (FFR) was <0.80 ("provisional PCI"). In 7 stenoses, FFR was >0.80 and the planned PCI was not performed. Surgery was performed before provisional PCI in 6 cases. An angiogram was obtained in all patients before discharge, and a complete clinical follow-up including a stress test was obtained in all patients after a mean of 12 months. There were no significant intraoperative complications, conversions to cardiopulmonary bypass, or reinterventions for bleeding. At early control angiogram, 2 moderate stenoses just proximal to anastomosis were observed, both with normal run-off. After 12 months there were no objective signs of ischemia at stress testing. After an average follow-up of 19 ± 10 months there were no deaths, myocardial infarctions, or repeat revascularizations.

## Table 2. Outcomes of Hybrid Coronary Revascularization

| Author | Number | Age (years) (mean ± SD) | Initial Procedure | Vessels Grafted | Vessels PCI/Stented | Mortality | Follow-up (Months) | TLR[a] (%) | Event-free survival |
|---|---|---|---|---|---|---|---|---|---|
| Lloyd et al.[36] | 18 | 63 | Mixed | 18 | 21/10 | 0 | 18 | 6 | 89% |
| Zenati et al.[38] | 31 | 69 | PCI | 32 | 39/23 | 0 | 11 | 10 | 90% |
| Wittwer et al.[39] | 35 | 57 ± 7 | MIDCAB | 35 | 47/14 | 0 | NR | NR | NR |
| Riess et al.[43] | 57 | 66 ± 8 | MIDCAB | 57 | 72/53 | 0 | 24 | 14[b] | NR |
| Cisowski et al.[44] | 50 | 54 ± 20 | MIDCAB | 50 | 50/39 | 0 | 6-24 | 13[b] | 87% |
| Lewis et al.[46] | 14 | 72 ± 9 | PCI | 14 | 28/20 | 0 | 1-44 | 0 | 93% |
| Stahl et al.[47] | 54 | 62 | Mixed | 63 | 58 | 0 | 12 | NR | 87% |

SD = standard deviation; PCI = percutaneous coronary intervention; TLR = target lesion revascularization; MIDCAB = minimally invasive direct coronary artery bypass; NR = not reported.
[a] Calculated on a per patient basis (more than one reintervention occurred in some patients).
[b] Included revision or stenting of LIMA graft.

In: Off-Pump Coronary Artery Bypass Grafting
Editors: Shahzad G. Raja and Mohamed Amrani

ISBN: 978-1- 62081-549-6
© 2012 Nova Science Publishers, Inc.

*Chapter XII*

# Technique of Awake Off-pump Coronary Artery Bypass Grafting

*Kaan Kırali*
Department of Cardiovascular Surgery,
Kartal Koşuyolu Heart Education & Research Hospital,
Istanbul, Turkey

## Abstract

In order to reduce the adverse effects of general anesthesia, awake coronary artery bypass (ACAB) surgery has emerged as a new and unique technique in the treatment of coronary artery disease. This new surgical modality of coronary revascularization combines the minimal invasive nature of off-pump coronary bypass surgery with epidural anesthesia avoiding endotracheal intubation and mechanic ventilation. Particularly, it extends also the limits of coronary surgery where patients are deemed unfit for conventional surgery or general anesthesia. Due to its nature, ACAB offers several advantages over general anesthesia, including better analgesia, decreased myocardial ischemia, improved ventricular function, avoidance from tracheal intubation and mechanical ventilation, improved pulmonary function, reduced stress response and preservation of fibrinolytic system. ACAB also promotes modern trends in perioperative care including early mobilization and recovery, daycare and outpatient surgery. The clear advantage of ACAB is a more rapid recovery from surgery, allowing the patient to leave home on the day of surgery.

A perfect understanding and co-operation between patient and anesthesiologist is necessary for ACAB, while an excellent collaboration between cardiac surgeon and anesthesiologist provides an uneventful procedure. Cardiac sympatholysis achieves bradycardia, dilates coronary arteries and in situ arterial grafts, improves left ventricular function, and prevents arrhythmia thereby making coronary anastomosis less challenging using ACAB technique. Single or multiple vessels revascularization can be performed with ACAB through different incisions, whereas mechanic stabilizer and apical holder enable surgical revascularization of coronary arteries on the lateral and/or inferior surface of the heart without hemodynamic deterioration during repositioning of the heart. Thoracic sympatholysis allows complete arterial revascularization via harvesting bilateral internal mammary arteries with or without radial artery, but if using vein grafts is mandatory they are harvested via combined peripheral regional anesthesia. Avoidance of pneumothorax seems to be an important issue in carrying out ACAB, which occurs most commonly during sternotomy or harvesting internal mammary artery, but surgeon may try to manage it by primary repair or leave pleural space fully open to avoid tension pneumothorax. Adequate epidural anesthesia helps to perform single or multiple bypass grafts on the beating heart easily and quickly.

Although ACAB procedures require advanced anesthetic technique and high-level surgical competence in terms of skill and speed, this novel approach in coronary revascularization opens the door of surgical treatment for high-risk patients in whom general anesthesia is not feasible, as well as allows patients who opt for early recovery after surgery to return to daily life with markedly improved quality of life. This chapter provides a comprehensive account of the technique and outcomes of ACAB.

## Introduction

Cardiopulmonary bypass (CPB) and general anesthesia through standard full median sternotomy have been preferred applications since the early days of coronary artery bypass surgery. Every cardiac surgeon with varying degree of technical skills around the world can perform coronary artery bypass grafting (CABG) with acceptable outcomes. The known benefits of conventional CABG are complete revascularization on the arrested heart, using arterial grafts, performing associated cardiovascular procedures, and reduction of coronary dependent morbidity and mortality.

On the contrary, several scientific studies have observed a strong correlation between conventional CABG and various early postoperative complications. Renewed interest in off-pump coronary artery bypass (OPCAB) and minimal invasive operations has initiated a new era in CABG surgery by proposing to avoid side effects of extracorporeal circulation and median sternotomy. Combination of high thoracic epidural anesthesia (HTEA) with general anesthesia has improved early postoperative results by reduction of systemic stress response, superior pain control, improvement of diaphragmatic and pulmonary function, decreasing heart rate and myocardial oxygen demand, dilatation of stenotic coronary vessels, and maintenance of hemodynamic stability.

Furthermore, adequate postoperative analgesia prevents patient discomfort, and HTEA decreases postoperative morbidity and hospital length of stay. Cardiac surgery in awake patients has additional benefits on top of the advantages of HTEA like avoidance of mechanical ventilation, monitoring of neurologic vigilance, avoidance of intensive care unit stay, providing cost effectiveness due to shorter hospital length of stay and less overall charges.

Not only returning to daily activities is comparable with benefits of percutaneous interventions, but also patients would benefit utilization of arterial grafts through a less invasive procedure.

Awake cardiac surgery can also extend the limits of cardiac procedures by eliminating contraindications for general anesthesia and endotracheal intubation.

# Evolution of Awake Coronary Artery Bypass Surgery

Cardiac surgeons have tried to minimize the operative trauma of cardiac operations, especially CABG, since modern cardiac surgery was introduced in 1950's. The first step was to avoid extracorporeal circulation and perform coronary revascularization using off-pump techniques, which have been widely acknowledged during the last two decades [1-3]. The second step was to minimize surgical incisions and to avoid median sternotomy. Several types of minimal incision have been introduced to harvest internal mammary artery (IMA) and to revascularize the left anterior descending (LAD) artery [4-6]. The third step was advances in off-pump surgical technology and adoption of creative techniques which rendered possible revascularization of circumflex and right coronary systems through standard median sternotomy [7]. The OPCAB techniques are constantly undergoing refinement and many areas of potential benefit are being vigorously explored [8]. These procedures are more useful in high risk patients including those with severe left ventricular dysfunction, severe obstructive pulmonary disease, renal insufficiency, and diabetes mellitus [9-12]. Encouragingly, off-pump revascularization does not have any negative effect on the myocardium [13]. The last step is to prefer only arterial grafts for off-pump coronary artery revascularization in patients with multi-vessel disease [14,15]. Furthermore, early and midterm angiographic studies have showed that graft patency after OPCAB is comparable with conventional on-pump technique, especially patency of arterial grafts [16-18].

The first description of HTEA and analgesia in cardiac surgery was published in mid 1950's [19]. However, clinical application of HTEA in cardiac surgery during the modern surgical era could be realized after two decades when it was routinely utilized in the immediate postoperative period for treating systemic hypertension [20]. Practical and modernized usage of HTEA was performed in 1987 and the authors suggested the insertion of thoracic epidural catheters in patients before cardiac operation [21]. Since that time, HTEA has been used mostly for providing analgesia, stress response attenuation, or thoracic cardiac sympathectomy in cardiac surgery. It was only at the end of $20^{th}$ century, that the quality of analgesia obtained with HTEA had been observed as sufficient enough to allow ACAB without general endotracheal anesthesia.

Whereas the main progress in cardiac surgery was avoidance of cardiopulmonary bypass in the $20^{th}$ century, the new millennium allowed us to avoid general anesthesia and mechanical ventilation during cardiac operations. A new strategy to reduce the invasiveness of cardiac surgery via avoidance of general anesthesia was described at the beginning of this century [22]. The authors' basic idea behind this procedure was to facilitate CABG in the least invasive manner and to perpetuate surgical revascularization as a serious competitive approach against percutaneous revascularization. They used only HTEA without general anesthesia to shorten postoperative care and hospital stay. In a few years, several reports were published in the literature to show the applicability of this technique in different cardiac centers with the same success as the conventional CABG techniques [23-28]. Several transthoracic incisional approaches have been developed for awake coronary artery bypass (ACAB) surgery, especially in single vessel disease: mini-thoracotomy [29], rib cage lifting technique [30], full median sternotomy [31], reversed J inferior sternotomy [32], and subxiphiodal approach [33]. Left or right coronary arteries can be revascularized with these techniques, whereas multivessel revascularization on the anterior surface of the heart (left anterior descending artery, diagonal branches, high lateral circumflex artery) can be also performed through the same incision. Arterial grafts (internal mammary artery, radial artery, right gastro-epiploic artery) are favored for coronary revascularization and thoracic sympatholysis covers all possible incisions for arterial grafts during ACAB. However, as saphenous vein graft remains the most acceptable graft for multivessel CABG therefore different regional anesthetic techniques can be combined to harvest saphenous vein graft during ACAB [34-36]. On the other hand, hybrid revascularization provides minimally invasive options for high risk patients with multivessel coronary artery disease [37]. The last two steps of ACAB are complete revascularization of lateral or inferior heart surfaces by utilizing arterial grafts. Harvesting bilateral IMAs is the pinnacle of HTEA technique which allows utilization of bilateral IMAs in situ [38]. New technical devices like epicardial stabilization devices (mechanical or vacuum assisted) with or without apical heart repositioning devices enable to immobilize the heart and to pull it up for posterolateral wall revascularization with preserved hemodynamic parameters [39].

## Physiologic Effects of High Thoracic Epidural Anesthesia

General anesthesia is the most commonly used anesthetic technique and considered to be the gold standard for all kinds of cardiac operations. The main advantages are complete anesthesia and analgesia, fully paralyzed body without any agitation and efficient control of respiratory and cardiovascular systems intraoperatively. Furthermore, adequate postoperative analgesia prevents unnecessary patient discomfort and decreases morbidity, hospital length of stay and cost [40]. Despite the well-known advantages of general anesthesia it has also several risks, which can be very serious or fatal (Table 1). Additionally, inadequate analgesia during early postoperative period and stress response hormones (norepinephrine, epinephrine) increased by CPB aggravate sympathetic activity and cause disruption of the balance between coronary blood flow and myocardial oxygen demand aggravating ischemia. In order to avoid these adverse effects of general anesthesia, HTEA has been introduced as a supplemental or sole anesthetic approach in cardiac surgery procedures with several positive effects (Table 2). It has been used for two types of cardiac surgical procedures: awake/paralyzed off-pump or on-pump procedures, where its major usage is supplemental to general anesthesia. Inhibition of thoracal sympathetic system has two main effects: adequate analgesia after sensory and motor blockade at the thoracal level (complete control of pain and stress response) and cardiac sympathetectomy (Table3). Thoracic epidural anesthesia causes segmental thoracic sympathetectomy, which has direct effects on the heart, pulmonary vascular tone, renal and splanchnic perfusion regulation, and venous return. Other than providing cardiovascular stability, the potential benefits of using HTEA in combination with general anesthesia are attenuation of stress response, superior analgesia, and reduction of total amount of intravenous narcotics, improved pulmonary function, early extubation and mobilization [40]. Moreover, IMA dilatation with sympathetic blockage at the C6 level provides excellent graft flow. There is also provocation of fibrinolytic cascade that might counterbalance the procoagulant state observed after beating heart surgery and this may also improve graft patency. The cumulative effect of HTEA increases coronary perfusion in ischemic myocardium and improves left ventricular function in patients undergoing CABG. Combination of general anesthesia with HTEA provides the usage of a regional anesthesia in cardiac surgery, whereas ACAB enables the usage of HTEA as sole anesthetic method in cardiac surgery.

## Cardiac Innervation

The heart is supplied with branches of the sympathetic and parasympathetic autonomic nervous systems which have major regulatory actions on healthy and diseased humans. The sympathetic fibers end on vascular smooth muscle cells, while parasympathetic fibers end in the adventitia of coronary vessels.

**Table 1. Risks of general anesthesia**

**Mechanical ventilation**
- barotrauma (airway pressure-induced injury)
- volotrauma (lung inflation-induced injury)
- atelectrauma (injury due to cyclic opening / closing of small airways/lung units)
- biotrauma (release of a variety of proinflamatory mediators)

**Endothraceal intubation**
- trauma to teeth
- vocal cords edema
- peri-intubational hypoxia

**Pulmonary**
- atelectasis
- collapse of the lung(s)
- pneumonia
- aspiration

**Cardiovascular**
- significant increase in stress-response hormones (norepinephrine, epinephrine, etc)
- coronary artery vasoconstriction and decreasing the myocardial oxygen supply
- tachycardia, dysrhythmias
- perioperative myocardial ischemia
- hypotension – hypertension attacks (immobile hemodynamic status)

**Neuromuscular**
- perioperative neuropathy

**Others**
- postoperative nausea and vomiting
- hypothermia and hyperthermia
- adverse drug reactions
- complications of positioning

The sympathetic nerves to the heart and coronary vessels arise from the superior, middle, and inferior cervical sympathetic ganglia and the first four thoracic ganglia. The satellite ganglion (inferior cervical + first thoracic ganglia) is a major source of cardiac sympathetic innervation. Stimulation of sympathetic efferent nerves increases chronotropy and inotropy of the heart, cardiac output, arterial vasoconstriction and systemic vascular resistance.

Parasympathetic stimulation causes bradycardia, decreases contractility, and lowers blood pressure. These effects can be abolished by atropine. Parasympathetic stimulation normally causes vasoconstriction by the activation of muscarinic receptors on vascular smooth muscle cells, but it can cause coronary vasodilatation due to increasing endothelial nitric oxide level. Parasympathetic control has not been shown to be important in the initiation of myocardial ischemia.

## Coronary Innervation

All coronary arteries are dominated by adrenergic receptors, and as a rule, β-receptors cause dilatation whereas α-receptors engender constriction. If both $α_1$ (large epicardial vessels) and $α_2$ (small coronary arteries < 100 μm in diameter) adrenoceptors are activated by neuronally released (sympathetic activation) or circulating (iv infusion) norepinephrine coronary vasoconstriction occurs. On the other hand, $β_2$ adrenoceptors in the large and small coronary arteries mediate vasodilatation. Besides sympathetic innervations, the intact endothelium also plays an important role in the vascular tone (autoregulatory response). Circulating metabolites stimulate release of different endothelium-derived relaxing or contracting substances which have modulating effects on the coronary endothelium. The endothelium can also act to limit the effect of norepinephrine by metabolizing it. In a normal heart, the direct effect of sympathetic stimulation is coronary vasoconstriction which is in competition with the metabolically mediated dilatation of exercise or excitement, and the net effect is a marked increase in coronary flow. Once coronary arteries are damaged by atherosclerosis, the vascular response to hormonal and physical properties changes dramatically. Coronary α-adrenergic activation in normal heart results in vasoconstriction maintaining transmural blood flow during periods of increased demand (for example operation-stress) by preventing epicardial coronary flow steal, but in atherosclerotic disease it reduces arterial lumen diameter at the stenotic segment and produces a significant increasing in flow resistance that causes a greater shunting of blood to the epicardium. In patients with coronary stenosis, sympathetic vasoconstrictor activation can precipitate myocardial ischemia by further narrowing of stenotic segments. Dysfunction of the diseased endothelium may also predispose to excessive α-adrenergic constriction due to restricted autoregulatory response. Sympathetic blockade causes vasodilatation at the stenotic segments of coronary arteries and increases myocardial blood flow in ischemic regions which overall improves myocardial function.

## Effects on the Conduction System

HTEA has a clear effect on cardiac electrophysiology due to sympathetic system activation. Stimulating sympathetic system increases excitability and conductivity of the heart both of which cause tachycardia or dysrhythmia. The main effect of HTEA is significant reduction of heart rate due to extended repolarization time and prolonged refractory period which is more pronounced at ventricular level than the atrium [41]. The atrio-ventricular nodal conduction time and functional refractory period are also lengthened. A further reduction of the heart rate can occur if any β-blocker, which is used commonly in OPCAB to slow the heart, is added to HTEA intravenously. Although perioperative dysrhythmia is reduced, HTEA does not decrease the incidence of postoperative atrial fibrillation. However, ACAB may be associated with a lower incidence of postoperative atrial fibrillation because not only is there an inhibition of sympathetic innervations, but also vagal nervous system is dominant after surgery [42].

**Table 2. Physiologic advantages of HTEA**

| |
|---|
| **Cardiac sympathicolysis** |
| • Anti-ischemic and anti-anginal (optimal redistribution of coronary blood flow) |
| • Anti-vasoconstrictor (paradoxical vasoconstrictor response) |
| • Anti-chronotropic (small, but significant bradycardia) |
| • Anti-arrhythmic (preventing dysrhythmias) |
| • Improvement of left ventricular function |
| **Thoracic sympathicolysis** |
| • Motor blockage of intercostal muscles |
| • Adequate intra- and postoperative analgesia |
| • Decreasing systemic response to surgery |
| • Anti-catabolic (decreasing metabolic activity) |
| • Anti-thrombogenic (preserving fibrinolytic system) |
| • Immunologic (preserving immune response) |
| • Increasing gastrointestinal motility and perfusion |
| **Spontaneous ventilation** |
| • Avoidance of endotracheal intubation |
| • Avoidance of mechanical ventilation |
| • Avoidance of pulmonary complications |
| • Neurologic monitoring |

## Effects on the Cardiovascular System

Activation of the sympathetic system is one of the important factors in the development of myocardial infarction, angina pectoris, and fatal cardiac arrhythmias in patients with coronary heart disease. HTEA reduces myocardial oxygen consumption by lowering pre- and after-load, and heart rate. All these changes cause an effective relief even in unstable angina.

HTEA with local anesthetics influences various aspects of the cardiac functions via loss of sympathetic tone to the myocardium, the epicardial coronary arteries, and the small resistance vessels. The main effects of HTEA can be opposite in healthy state and patients with coronary artery disease. In healthy state, HTEA decreases contractility and cardiac output without a reduction in left ventricular ejection and diastolic filling performance after the loss of sympathetic innervations[43]. In patients with coronary artery disease, HTEA does preserve left ventricular systolic function via a reduced incidence of regional wall motion abnormalities [44]. In contrast to healthy state, HTEA improves left ventricular diastolic dysfunction, which is more frequent than systolic dysfunction and the earliest hemodynamic manifestation in coronary artery disease.

The cardiac sympathetic stimulation has a vasoconstrictor influence on both normal and diseased coronary segments. Cardioselective epidural block can improve oxygen supply in ischemic myocardium due to dilatation of stenotic coronary arteries (while not affecting the diameter of the nonstenotic segments), redistribution of coronary blood flow in favoring the endocardium (whereas total coronary blood flow is unaltered), reduction of myocardial oxygen consumption by lowering arterial systolic and pulmonary capillary wedge pressures (no significant changes in coronary perfusion pressure) and a favorable alteration of the myocardial supply/demand ratio (significant reduction of myocardial oxygen consumption), and reduction of catecholamine levels [45].

The main adverse hemodynamic effect of HTEA is hypotension due to cardiodepressing action and vasodilatation (arterial and venous) by diminishing sympathetic counter-regulation in a substantial vascular reservoir [46]. In fact, HTEA does not produce any change in intravascular volume or its components, but the inhibitory effect of HTEA on the vasoconstrictor sympathetic outflow causes functional hypovolemia which can be avoided by administration of plasma expanders. If the sympathetic block is not extensive, circulating cathecolamines can also augment sympathetic activity below the block and avoid functional hypovolemia, but if the block is extensive vasopressors must be preferred in the treatment.

### Effects on Lung Function

General anesthesia may lead to myocardial ischemia because of adverse hemodynamic responses to tracheal intubation, suction of the endotracheal tube, and extubation. Endotracheal intubation can also cause mucosal injury, reduced mucociliary function, bypassing upper airway defenses, and reduced effectiveness of cough. On the other hand, epidural motor blockage of thoracic respiratory muscles and the potentially detrimental effects of sympatheticolysis which leads to an unopposed vagal tone and increased bronchial tone and reactivity, are the most serious side effects of HTEA. Combination with general anesthesia is a good strategy to avoid these risks, but at the same time complications of mechanical ventilation are also hazardous. The avoidance of mechanical ventilation in awake patients improves pulmonary function via better diaphragmatic contractile function and cough activity, which prevents atelectasis and pulmonary infections, maintains upper airway defenses, and better controls postoperative pain. Patients with chronic obstructive pulmonary disease or laryngeal stenosis, which are main contraindication for general anesthesia with endotracheal intubation and mechanical ventilation, can also undergo operation safely with this approach. Using HTEA can induce hypercapnia, particularly in patients with severe chronic obstructive pulmonary disease, and the severity of hypercapnia might be correlated with operative time. Administration of oxygen through a Venturi mask can simply prevent hypoxemia, whereas hypercapnia can only be prevented via deep and periodic diaphragmatic respiration. On the other hand, neither the arterial-alveolar partial oxygen difference nor the direct measurement of shunt will be negatively affected by HTEA [47].

## Technique of High Thoracic Epidural Anesthesia

As a general rule, most anesthesiologists using regional techniques in patients undergoing CABG with subsequent heparinization (vascular or cardiac surgery) demand at least one hour interval between insertion of the epidural catheter and administration of heparin. Insertion of HTEA on the day of surgery seems logistically simpler, because it does not takes more than 20 minutes and the patient can be supervised in the operating room, and the period between insertion and heparinization gives adequate time to check the full efficiency of HTEA and to provide required monitoring during ACAB. The operating room is kept warm (22-24°C) and quite. It is important to prevent heat loss rather than actively re-warm patients. Maintenance of normothermia is essential to prevent shivering. First of all, basic monitoring before HTEA should be carried out using electrocardiogram, noninvasive blood pressure measurement, and pulse oxymetry. Local anesthetic ointments can be used before insertion of all invasive and epidural catheters. Two venous catheters are utilized peripherally to infuse only isothermic intravenous fluids. Usually during this period sedation is not necessary, but if the patient is apprehensive in the operating room a small dose of midazolam (0.07 mg/kg) can be administered. Monitoring after HTEA includes continuous electrocardiogram, direct arterial pressure, central venous pressure, pulse oxymetry, and body temperature. A Foley catheter or rectal probe is not necessary. A conscious patient also allows anesthesiologists to assess neurologic monitoring. Epidural insertion can be applied with median or paramedian approaches, but median approach lowers the risk of inadvertent puncture of a vessel and should therefore be preferred for HTEA [48]. Upper intervertebral spaces are clearly identifiable with median approach, which usually is a straight line perpendicular to the skin with an angel of 90° for insertion. More important than the catheter and needle specifics, HTEA for ACAB should not be attempted by inexperienced anesthesiologists because of the inherent risk of epidural hematoma. Either the hanging drop or the loss of resistance technique can be utilized. In majority of cases the loss of resistance technique is preferred. The patient is positioned sitting upright on the operating table and inspected one more time whether there is an anatomical contraindication for insertion of the epidural catheter, especially between intervertebral spaces C7 and T3. First, local anesthesia with lidocaine (2-4 mL) is applied and then a 16-gauge flexible-tip catheter is inserted through a Tuohy needle at the intervertebral space between T1 and T2. The catheter is cephally directed and advanced no more than 3-4 cm inside the epidural space, otherwise migration and knotting of catheter may occur. Tingling and numbness during the passage of catheter occurs frequently, but this may not necessarily indicate the onset of a neurologic deficit [49]. The epidural catheter is fixed on the skin. The whole procedure should be almost painless, a forceful needle insertion should be avoided, and no more than several attempts should be undertaken to localize the epidural space. If a bloody tap occurs or blood comes into syringe, elective surgery is cancelled until the next day and CABG should be planned with general anesthesia. Patients with very tight or calcified intervertebral spaces may be declined the procedure due to access related problems. The block level is tested after epidural administration of 5 mL lidocaine (2%) as a bolus to confirm the absence of untoward effects. Once level is confirmed, full dose of epidural anesthetic infusion is started epidurally after 10 mL epidural anesthesia solution is administered as a bolus. Patient lies in supine position on operation table which stands in horizontal plane. Fifteen minutes later, the analgesic level of the block is tested by assessing both temperature and pin prick discrimination. Loss of temperature discrimination is deemed necessary to continue the operation with epidural anesthesia. Motor block of the intercostal muscles is assessed visually by monitoring the loss of intercostal movement. An additional bolus dose of epidural anesthesia solution should be administered if motor block of the intercostal muscles is not adequate. Absence of an adequate level of analgesia or presence of patchy analgesia 45 minutes after infusion of epidural anesthetic solution is termed "failed epidural". In this situation, HTEA is aborted and procedure is converted to general anesthesia.

Observation of the new onset Horner's syndrome is a very important sign of the successfully conducted HTEA, which indicates the upper tolerable level of epidural anesthesia in awake patients. The objective of HTEA is to achieve somatosensory block at C7 to T8 levels, and motor block of the intercostal muscles while preserving diaphragmatic respiration. Internal mammary artery dilatation can be achieved when the block level raises to the C6 level. On the other hand, if the block level raises above C4 level, diaphragm paralysis ensues. Because diaphragmatic respiration is vital for adequate respiratory function, the upper permissible level of block should be C6. An epidural anesthesia solution is used for the entire operation, which includes bupivacaine hydrochloride, lidocaine, fentanyl, and bicarbonate (Table 4). The continuous administration of this solution rather than the intermittent bolus application provides a very stable hemodynamic profile. It is important to use HTEA to its maximum strength to benefit from its full potential effect, which prevents any additional sedative or muscle-paralyzing agent. Inadequate analgesia can be managed with more specific calculation of epidural infusion rate (normal infusion rate 15-25 mL/h) or a small bolus of 3-5 mL. A small dose of propofol (0.5 mg/kg) would suffice if patient is excited. Since T1 is the upper part of full median sternotomy skin incision, this area needs to be covered by HTEA. If patient has pain in the upper or lower wound, a small dose of local anesthetic can be injected, especially during full median sternotomy. It is not necessary to use local anesthesia during the partial lower median sternotomy techniques, and pain around the xiphoid can be avoided by lifting up the head of the operation table (< 30°) so as to spread sensory blockade to cover upper abdominal region. Operation table is leveled back in horizontal plane during the surgical prep. Throughout the operation, patients spontaneously breathe oxygen (4 L/min) through a Venturi mask. After a successful HTEA, most patients can sleep without any sedative medication. Diaphragmatic respiration is adequate to maintain sufficient levels of oxygenation and a moderate carbon dioxide retention is not clinically significant. If anesthesiologist observes hypoventilation or hypercapnia, patients are stimulated to breathe more deeply and frequently. Decreasing the dose of epidural anesthetic solution is also sufficient to deal with hypercarbia. It is not necessary to monitor tidal volume, minute volume or lung compliance. On the other hand, there is also no need to use a facemask, positive airway pressure ventilation, naso-pharyngeal or laryngeal mask airway, and nasogastric tube. Facemask of the mechanical ventilator with continuous positive airway pressure support is reserved only for patients who develop hemodynamic instability, hypoventilation or irritability. If patients cannot tolerate HTEA, epidural anesthesia is aborted and the procedure is converted to general anesthesia with endotracheal intubation.

Adequate space must be provided at the head of patients for monitoring respiration, communication with patients, and any intervention if necessary. Patients are draped allowing free and unrestricted access for the anesthesiologist to manipulate the head and neck of patients, in case an urgent endotracheal intubation should be necessary. We cover only the thorax and, if necessary, the left arm with a sterile drape and the whole body except the head is covered with sterile operation cloths. In all emergency situations, patients are intubated with an endotracheal tube directly and mechanical ventilation support is started immediately. When adequate analgesia, sedation or anxiolysis is not produced during ACAB operation agitation, hypercapnia and hypoventilation can be prevented with an administration of midazolam (0.07 mg/kg) intravenously and the assisted ventilation.

### Table 3. Cardiovascular effects of HTEA

**Coronary blood flow**
- increased diameter of stenosed epicardial coronary arteries
- no influence on nonstenotic and resistance coronary vessels
- increased regional flow favoring the endocardium
- no effect on coronary perfusion pressure

**Conduction system**
- decreased heart rate
- lengthening of repolarization
- prolongation of ventricular refractory time
- delayed AV nodal conduction and refractory period
- decreased baroreflexes' sensitivity
- decreased dysrhythmias

**Ventricular function***
- improvement in global and regional wall motion
- increased left ventricular function
- decreased extent of ischemia

**Vascular blood flow**
- arterial vasodilatation (decreasing afterload)
- venous vasodilatation (decreasing preload)
- hypovolemia
- interference with renin-angiotensin system
- increased vasopressin plasma concentration

* Patients with coronary artery disease.

### Table 4. Composition of HTEA

| Agent | Concentration | Dose | Volume |
| --- | --- | --- | --- |
| Bupivacaine | 0.5% | 100 mg | 20 mL |
| Lidocaine | 2% | 400 mg | 20 mL |
| Fentanyl | 0.005% | 0.25 mg | 5 mL |
| Bicarbonate | 8.4% | 42 mg | 5 mL |

Careful timing with anticoagulation and HTEA catheter removal is essential in all patients. At least two hours must be elapsed between epidural catheter insertion and the last dose of heparin or one hour between catheter insertion and heparinization for ACAB. Only one dose of heparin (5000 IU) is given for anticoagulation at the beginning of IMA harvesting, which is not reversed with protamine at the end of the operation. A recent activated coagulation time (ACT) and international normalized ratio (INR) status should be obtained before removal of HTEA, and heparin must be started at least two hours after removal of the HTEA catheter. It is not necessary to discontinue anticoagulation with acetylsalicylic acid or clopidogrel preoperatively, which cannot cause any bleeding during HTEA. Administration of acetylsalicylic acid, clopidogrel or warfarin can be commenced immediately after surgery, and HTEA is continued for 24 hours to prevent postoperative pain and epidural catheter can be removed after 24 hours.

## Complications of High Thoracic Epidural Anesthesia

Potential complications of HTEA may reduce acceptance and enthusiasm for this technique in cardiac surgery (Table 5). Neurological or hemorrhagic complications can be fatal because of the risk of vertebral canal hematoma. Local anesthetic neurotoxicity is a well-known phenomenon related to the type and concentration of anesthetic and systemic absorption. Hemodynamic complications can be dangerous if the treatment gets delayed or combines with cardiac decompensation during anastomosis. The later complications can be prevented or treated by decreasing the rate or holding the epidural infusion.

**Table 5. Complications of HTEA**

**Neurological**
- spinal cord injury
- dural puncture
- damage by irritant drugs
- epidural infection or abscess
- transient deficits (paresis, paralysis)
- cervical myelitis
- hemorrhagic
- bleeding
- epidural hematoma
- spinal hematoma
- neurotoxicity
- seizure
- loss of airway protective reflexes
- coma
- motor autonomic blockade (urinary retention, weakness)
- phrenic nerve palsy

**Hemodynamic**
- hypotension
- bradycardia
- arrhythmias
- myocardial depression

**Respiratory (silent)**
- bronchospasm
- bronchial hyperactivity
- respiratory depression
- hypercapnia
- diaphragm paralysis

There can be two problems after surgery: paresthesia in the arms and motor blockade of hand or forearm. Since T1 is the upper part of the full median sternotomy incision, HTEA must cover this area which also shares the same dermatome for sensitivity of the arm. If partial inferior sternotomy is preferred it is not necessary for HTEA to cover this region and lowering the level of HTEA resolves this problem. But, paresthesia or motor blockade of the lower extremities should alert the team until an epidural hematoma is excluded in diagnosis.

## Patient Selection for Awake Off-pump CABG

### Patient Approval

The initial selection criterion for ACAB is patient approval. In spite of the fact that patients undergoing CABG have major anxiety against general anesthesia, they also refrain from awake cardiac surgery. It may be better to begin the ACAB program with well-motivated patients, because they will be conscious throughout the entire operation and aware of what is being done to them and around them. Patients should be well informed about the pros and cons of this new surgical procedure, and early- and mid-term results which are comparable to conventional CABG. Preoperative information of the procedure eliminates or relieves operation anxiety. Exercise of the diaphragmatic respiration is the other key leading to successful CABG on the conscious patient. These basic efforts help to maintain epidural anesthesia which is necessary to continue awake operation without any difficulty. Furthermore, patients must be assured that the operative procedure will be converted immediately to the conventional technique in case of any unexpected problem. The benefits of HTEA listed in Table 6 should also be explained and documented, followed by a written informed consent obtained from every patient. The first and main contraindication of ACAB is inadequate communication skills or failure of the patient to comprehend the needs of the operation, because these patients cannot coordinate with anesthesiologist for the critical steps of ACAB (hyper- or hypoventilation, cough, moving, more speaking, etc). The first indication to convert to general anesthesia at the beginning of the operation is persistent anxiety or feeling pain which engenders patient discomfort.

## Indications and Contraindications for ACAB

The surgical indications and contraindications for ACAB have broadened over the last ten years (Table 7). At the beginning, only single vessel ACAB was offered to patients without any risk factors. But now, patients with multivessel disease and more co-morbidities are undergoing ACAB operation with an excellent quality of anastomosis and increased comfort of the operation procedure. Revascularization of coronary arteries on the anterior wall of the heart is the easiest stage of ACAB, but revascularization of lateral or inferior wall is more complicated. All vascular situations causing extension of anastomotic period, failure of appropriate positions for circumflex artery (Cx) or right coronary artery (RCA) anastomosis, new onset acute myocardial ischemia or hemodynamic instability are relative indication to convert to conventional CABG under general anesthesia if simple maneuvers can not salvage the planned surgical procedure. Essentially, surgical revascularization should be performed as quick as possible to prevent patient discomfort which is the most common reason to sedate patients with central anesthetics or to convert to general anesthesia during ACAB. Both coronary anatomy and cardiac status should be taken into account when selecting patients for ACAB procedures (Table 8).

### Table 6. Benefits of HTEA in ACAB

**Intraoperatively**
- Attenuation of stress response
- Superior analgesia
- Hemodynamic stability
- Cardiac sympathicolysis
- Release angina (optimal redistribution of coronary blood flow)
- Reduced oxygen demand
- Neurologic monitoring (communication with operating team)

**Postoperatively**
*Early postoperative period*
- pain free rest
- avoidance from late complications of general anesthesia (no vomiting, no delirium, no hypercapnia, etc)
- improved pulmonary function and pain-free cough (aproblematic upper and lower respiratory tracts)
- stress free period (no anxiety)
- consciously active interest around (read news or books, watch television, listen to music, etc)
- early orally contact with relations or friends
- early drink or eat something (aproblematic mouth and nasopharynx)

*Return to physical activities*
- early mobilization (in hours)
- early discharge to the ward (in hours) or no stay in the intensive care unit
- early discharge from the hospital (≥ in same day)
- early return to daily life (≥ in same week)
- early return to work (≥ in same week)
- early return to heavy physical work (> 2 weeks)
- earlier sexual activity or sport (> 2 weeks)

**Lower hospital cost**

## Coronary Anatomy

*Coronary artery size* > 1 mm is acceptable to perform surgical revascularization while HTEA slows the heart rate and mechanical stabilizer achieves an immobile anastomotic area. Intracoronary shunts must be avoided due to potential risk and time consuming effects while positioning. *Total occluded coronary lesions*, especially on the LAD, are preferable for ACAB because the retrograde collateral circulation better supplies the anterior wall. After the left IMA (LIMA) is anastomosed to the LAD, the rest of the coronary targets can be revascularized easily and with more stability while the antegrade flow of the LAD reverses collateral circulation. *The structure and characteristics* of coronary artery lesion, which is going to be bypassed and the target vessel quality can alter the decision of ACAB procedure pre- and intraoperatively. Coronary arteries requiring long anastomosis (> 1 cm) or endarterectomy (> 2 cm) are not suitable for ACAB. On the other hand both approaches can be performed if LAD is totally occluded and supplied by the retrograde blood flow. *Complicated course of epicardial coronary arteries* is an important relative indication to convert to conventional technique. Because coronary revascularization should be performed efficiently, coronary artery walls must be visible and accessible for a quick anastomosis. Aggressive dissection of intramyocardial vessel as well as redundant adipose tissue to find coronary arteries is a waste of time and increases the risk of ACAB. Visible epicardial coronary artery with a healthy segment for anastomosis must be preferred at the beginning of this new surgical procedure, with time and experience more complicated coronary arteries could be revascularized.

**Table 7. Indication and contraindication for ACAB**

**Indications**
*Anatomic*
- tracheal stenosis, previous tracheal operation
- general posture (kyphoscoliosis, immobile neck, etc without a risk for insertion of a needle into vertebral space)

*Contraindication for general anesthetics with mechanical ventilation*
- severe chronic obstructive pulmonary disease
- hepatic insufficiency

*Patient preference*

**Contraindications**
*Patient refusal*
*Anatomic*
- high risk during insertion of needle (previous operations or infections of the cervical and upper thoracic spinal cord, osteosclerosis, etc)
- congenital anomaly of spinal cord

*Cardiac*
- inappropriate coronary anatomy
- left ventricular dilatation (CHF, LVD, LVA, etc) for multivessel bypass
- acute myocardial infarction
- hemodynamic instability
- severe bradycardia or atrioventricular block
- presence of any valvular pathology
- concomitant procedures except carotid endarterectomy

*Neurologic*
*Hematologic*
- risk for hemorrhage
- bleeding disorders
- heparin induced thrombocytopenia
- contraindication to discontinue anticoagulant therapy (heparin, low-molecular-weight heparin, warfarin, ticlopidine)
- thrombolytic treatment

*Infection at the local site of injection*
*Language barriers*

CHF = congestive heart failure; LVA = left ventricular aneurysm; LVD = left ventricular dysfunction.

**Table 8. Selection criteria of coronary and cardiac status for ACAB**

**Coronary anatomy**
*Suitable for anastomosis*
- diameter > 1 mm
- healthy vessel wall on the anastomotic side
- subepicardial coronary vessel
- no intra-myocardial course
- no intra-adiposal course
- no intra-adhesional course

*Plaque structure*
- non-long segment lesion (discrete occlusion)
- non-complicated lesion (no calcification, no atherosclerotic plaque)
- non-consecutive lesions (single stenosis)

*Adequate myocardial perfusion*
- preferably retrograde collateral circulation
- suitable anastomotic area on the distal healthy coronary segment

**Cardiac functions**
*Ventricular function*
- normal left ventricular function (LVEF > 50%)
- limited regional left ventricular dysfunction
- limited global left ventricular dysfunction (LVEF > 35% with hibernation)

*Valvular function*
- absence of aortic regurgitation
- absence of mitral regurgitation
- absence any other valvular stenotic pathology

*Sinus rhythm*

## Cardiac Function

Patients with preserved left ventricular function are the best candidates for ACAB. Single vessel revascularization (LIMA-LAD) can be performed even in the presence of severe left ventricular dysfunction.

If cardiac chambers' size is preserved, circumflex and/or RCA can be revascularized comfortably.

Patients with left ventricular dysfunction can undergo multivessel revascularization safely if the left ventricle has not been enlarged. Patients with left ventricular enlargement with or without mitral valve insufficiency should undergo conventional CABG for multivessel revascularization.

It is not reasonable to take patients with left ventricular dysfunction to ACAB operation with the support of any left ventricular assist device.

**Table 9. Thoracic incisions in ACAB surgery**

**Anterior approach**
*Full median sternotomy*
- through standard skin incision
- through limited skin incision

*Partial lower median ministernotomy*
- reversed J-inferior sternotomy (one-side)
- mini T-sternotomy (double-side)

**Anterolateral approach**
anterior minithoracotomy

**Anteroinferior approach**
rib cage lifting technique
subxiphoid approach

**Single vessel ACAB**
- full median sternotomy
- reversed J-inferior sternotomy
- anterior minithoracotomy
- rib cage lifting technique
- subxyphoid approach

**Multivessel ACAB**
- full median sternotomy
- mini T-sternotomy
- rib cage lifting technique
- subxyphoid approach

# Operative Techniques

## Thoracic Incisions

Access to surgical field is achieved via different thoracic incisions depending on the selected ACAB procedure (Table 9). Multivessel revascularization is performed mostly through full median sternotomy, whereas single vessel revascularization can be performed through partial inferior sternotomy or left anterior mini-thoracotomy (Table 10). However, the reversed-J sternotomy is the preferred approach for single vessel disease because it has a beneficial effect on pulmonary function as a result of well preserved superior thoracic aperture, especially intra-operatively. This may not be so apparent in patients undergoing intubation and general anesthesia but it is important in patients who would spontaneously breath throughout the operation.

## Median Sternotomy

Median sternotomy remains the most widely used incision in coronary artery bypass surgery because it provides ideal access to all coronary arteries and appropriate manipulation of the heart, which enables the surgeon to perform complete revascularization. It is also suitable for multivessel bypass surgery using bilateral IMAs. This technique is also the preferred approach in repeat sternotomies. There are several types of median sternotomy in coronary bypass surgery, and full median sternotomy through full midline incision is the main approach.

**Table 10. Recommendations for ACAB surgery in different situations**

| Surgical approach | Revascularization strategy | Population | Efficiency |
|---|---|---|---|
| Full median sternotomy | Complete revascularization with proximal anastomoses on the ascending aorta | all patients | suitable |
| Mini-T median ministernotomy | Complete revascularization with in situ arterial grafts (bilateral IMAs) | all patients | suitable |
| Reversed-J partial lower sternotomy | Single vessel revascularization using in situ arterial graft (LIMA-LAD) or (RIMA-RCA) | all patients | suitable |
| H-graft technique through anterior mini thoracotomy | Single vessel revascularization using in situ arterial graft (LIMA-RA-LAD) | high-risk patients | alternative (faster procedure) |
| Rib cage lifting technique | Complete revascularization with in situ arterial grafts (bilateral IMA's) | female patients | alternative (cosmetic) |
| Subxyphoid approach | Single vessel revascularization using in situ arterial graft (RGEA-LAD) | patients with severe pulmonary disease | alternative |

IMA = internal mammary artery; LAD = left anterior descending artery; LIMA = left internal mammary artery; RA = radial artery; RCA = right coronary artery; RGEA = right gastro-epiploic artery; RIMA = right internal mammary artery.

## Full Median Sternotomy

Full median sternotomy *through full midline skin incision* is the basic approach in ACAB surgery. The skin incision is initiated approximately 2 cm below the jugular notch and stops just above the xiphoid process. Full median sternotomy *through a limited midline skin incision* is a cosmetic approach where the midline skin incision starts at the level of sternomanubrial junction (the angle of Louis) and extends down to sternoxiphoidal junction for approximately 8 to 10 cm. Analgesia around the jugulum is achieved by HTEA whereas at the lower part (xiphoid area) can be achieved using local anesthetic injection. After the subcutaneous tissues and presternal fascia are incised with the electrocautery, the periostium of the sternum is cut straight in the midline. Using blunt finger dissection, a pathway is created beneath manubrium and xiphoid to avoid pneumothorax. The patient may feel pain and agitation during this maneuver, and a small additional dosage of general anesthetic can be used. It can also help the patient not to hear saw-noise during sternotomy. Sternotomy can be performed during the inspiratory phase of the respiration because both pleura are pulled out underneath the sternum (opposite general anesthesia). The nose plate of the sternal saw is hooked underneath the suprasternal ligament and the sternum is divided superior to inferior (in a cephalad to caudad direction). Upward lifting on the sternal saw allows safe passage and helps avoiding injury to the underlying pleura. After hemostasis of the sternum, a sternal retractor is used to spread the two halves of the sternum and the blades are opened very gently to judge the pain tolerance of the patient. If the patient does not feel pain operation can be continued awake, but if the patient has agitation low dose sedation can be given. Before initiating IMA harvest, careful examination should be applied to observe any disruption on the both pleura causing pneumothorax. If there is a small hole it should be repaired primarily with or without catheter aspiration of the air in the pleural space. If the hole is irreparable the left pleura must be left open widely, which would cause total collapse of the left lung, but prevent the tension pneumothorax. An awake patient can tolerate the single lung respiration in absence of the tension pneumothorax. If the hole in the right pleura is irreparable the patient should be converted to the mechanical ventilation under the general anesthesia because of the additive risk of a new pneumothorax occurrence on the left side. If both pleura are opened the patient should be converted to the general anesthesia with no question. After harvesting of uni- or bilateral IMAs, a small sternal retractor is used to spread the two edges of the sternum and the pericardium is opened using longitudinal reverse Y-shaped incision. If pedicled graft(s) will be used, the pericardium must be left intact over the aorta. To place stay sutures at the both edges of the pericardium for exposure of the heart is advisable to avoid the displacement of the heart during respiration. However, caution must be exercised as deep pericardial sutures can cause pneumothorax.

## Partial Lower Median Sternotomy

These techniques are used only with in situ arterial grafts, because it is very difficult to perform any proximal anastomosis on the ascending aorta. Different ministernotomy approaches aim to preserve the stability of the thoracic aperture for early and better postoperative recovery. Partial lower median sternotomy techniques avoid the invasiveness of full median sternotomy by preserving the upper part of the sternum and the continuity of the superior thoracic aperture, which are the basic components of the chest stability. The perceived advantages of these ministernotomy approaches include comfortable spontaneous breathing during surgery, better oxygenation due to sternal stability, and need for less amount of analgesia. Furthermore, these techniques also cause less chest tube drainage and transfusion requirements, shorter intensive care unit and hospital length of stay, cost effectiveness, quicky recovery and early return to work. Last but not the least most ministernotomy approaches are easily reproducible, with no need for learning curve. Furthermore, conversion to full sternotomy is more practical than the other small thoracotomy approaches. The incision can be easily and rapidly extended to a full sternotomy if technical problems are encountered or the exposure is not adequate.

*Reversed-J inferior sternotomy (one-side partial lower median ministernotomy)* is the best alternative for single vessel ACAB surgery. This approach provides good access to the entire course of the LIMA. The pleural cavity is not opened, so spontaneous respiration during surgery is not impaired. It is not necessary to use local anesthetics during sternotomy, and pain around the xiphoid can be prevented while the head of operation table is lifted upwards (< 30°) so as to spread sensory blockade covering lower part of sternum. The midline skin incision begins at the level of sternomanubrial junction (second rib; angle of Louis) and extends down to the xiphoid process accounting for approximately 10 to 12 cm. Using blunt finger dissection, a pathway is created below the xiphoid following which the nose plate of the sternal saw is hooked underneath it. If this maneuver causes pain or agitation an additional anesthetic can be given, but it is usually uneventful. The sternum is divided from xiphoid to the second intercostal space in a down to up (caudad to cephalad) direction, and the sternum is transected obliquely to the left side at the level of the second intercostal space with great caution not to damage the LIMA. Upward lifting on the sternal saw allows safe passage and helps to avoid any injury to the underlying pleura. After hemostasis of the sternum, an IMA retractor is used to retract the left half of the sternum. The surgeon should act very gently on the left pleura and more importantly the mid-part of the LIMA. During lifting the left hemithorax, the LIMA may be stretched at the second and third intercostal spaces which can damage the artery and both the second and third side branches of the LIMA should be divided first to mobilize the graft and to avoid stretch injury. Because heart occupies more space in the left hemithorax, it is more difficult to injure the left pleura during the reverse J sternotomy. If there is a hole in the left pleura it should be repaired primarily or it must be left open widely. However, if the right pleura is already disrupted and it is impossible to repair it, then the rest of operation should be completed under general anesthesia. After harvesting the LIMA, a small sternal retractor is used to spread the two halves of the sternum and the pericardium is opened above the course of the LAD. It is not necessary to place any pericardial stay suture for exposure of the heart.

*Mini T-sternotomy (double-side partial lower median ministernotomy)* is a new alternative to full median sternotomy with good exposure of all coronary arteries and bilateral IMAs in ACAB surgery [50]. Continuity of the upper sternum is helpful to the patient during spontaneous breathing. The vertical skin incision is extended from the angle of Louis to the xiphoid process. Using blunt finger dissection, a plane is created below the xiphoid and the nose plate of the sternal saw is hooked underneath the xiphoid. If this maneuver causes pain or agitation an additional anesthetic can be given, but it is mostly uneventful. It is not necessary to use local anesthetics during sternotomy, sensory blockade covering lower part of the sternum is achieved while the head of operation table is lifted upwards (< 30°). The midline sternotomy is started from the xiphoid process and extended to the level of the second intercostal space. Manubrium is left intact and sternum is cut bilaterally (in a T-shaped manner) at the second intercostal space level. The conduct of the remaining procedure is similar to operating via full median sternotomy approach. After harvesting of bilateral IMAs, a small sternal retractor is used to spread the two halves of the sternum and the pericardium is opened using longitudinal reverse Y-shaped incision. It is unadvisable to place any pericardial stay sutures.

## Anterior Mini-Thoracotomy

The most important goal of the left anterior mini-thoracotomy is to avoid sternotomy and its related complications. But in ACAB surgery, classic mini-thoracotomy is not the preferred method because the left pleura can be injured frequently and the left lung collapses in most of the cases. To begin the ACAB operation with single lung respiration is not a feasible and preferable approach in spite of the fact that most patients can tolerate it. If this approach is preferred a 6 to 8 cm left anterolateral mini-thoracotomy through the left fourth intercostal space is performed. Excessive rib spreading must be avoided to prevent dislocation or fracture of the ribs, and also resection of any costal cartilage with/without a small part of the fourth rib is unnecessary. Every effort should be made not to open the left pleura. Very gentle blunt finger dissection can help to peel the attached left pleura backwards and to prevent any openings in the pleura. Secondly, using a radial artery to construct a composite graft can simplify the procedure and prevent pneumothorax. Thirdly, the fat pad over the pericardium is displaced backwards to prevent any tension on the pleura. Finally, harvesting LIMA must be limited proximally until the second intercostal branch to avoid pneumothorax. After harvesting LIMA, a small costal retractor or a self-retaining retractor is used to spread the upper and lower ribs and the pericardium is opened above the course of the LAD. Different from the other ACAB techniques, traction sutures are placed on the pericardium and pulled through the incision to avoid the displacement of the heart during respiration.

Another alternative is the H-graft technique through the anterior mini-thoracotomy. H-graft technique is considered to be suitable in the awake setting because there is no necessity for complete IMA dissection and thus opening of the pleural cavity. The operative time also seems to be shorter, which is an important factor in ACAB surgery. The disadvantages of this approach are a second incision for harvesting the left radial artery, a second anastomosis for the attachment of the free arterial graft onto the LIMA, and the potential for diversion of significant LIMA flow to noncoronary vascular beds (steal syndrome). A 5 to 6 cm left anterior skin incision above the fourth rib is performed, and the pectoralis muscle is divided and the exposed costal cartilage is removed by extrapleural disarticulation at the chondrosternal joint. The removed rib is never reimplanted.

## Rib-cage Lifting Technique

This alternative technique preserves whole chest wall integrity while it permits bilateral IMA harvest and the target vessel anastomosis. This technique is risk-free for pneumothorax and it can be used in patients with severe pulmonary dysfunction. However, it is a technically demanding procedure and requires considerable experience. Rib cage retraction may cause increased pain in upper abdomen through traction of the muscles in the spontaneously breathing patient, which limits the use of this approach. The best advantage is superior cosmetic result, especially female patients. As Karagoz et al. [30] first described, an 8-10 cm skin incision is made 1 cm above the level of the xiphoid process and coursing parallel and 1 cm above the left (or bilateral for multivessel bypass) costal margin. A few centimeters of skin are undermined above and below the incision. The linea alba is left intact and the rib cage is freed from its attachments to the rectus abdominis muscle. An inferior ministernotomy is performed, which starts from the edge of the xiphoid process and ends at the fifth intercostal space. A single Favaloro retractor is used to lift the left rib cage, pulling the left rib cage toward the patient's left shoulder. The left IMA (or bilateral) can be harvested up to the level of the subclavian vein. The first branch can be left intact to prevent aggressive dissection and pneumothorax. This technique allows extrapleural dissection of the LIMA. The space to handle the pericardial cavity is large enough to perform coronary anastomosis with any kind of stabilization. While this technique is suitable for revascularization of LAD or RCA, revascularization of diagonal and the circumflex branches seems to be difficult.

## Subxiphoid Approach

Another alternative technique has been developed by Watanabe et al. [33] for patients with severe pulmonary dysfunction, which involves absolutely no sternotomy and eliminates the risk of intraoperatively pneumothorax. The right gastro-epiploic artery (RGEA) is used as the pedicled arterial graft. After approximately 8 cm subxiphoid vertical incision is made, only the xiphoid process at the lower end of the sternum is excised. Then, a mini-laparotomy is performed under the same surgical field and a hole through the diaphragm is made as small as possible. Harvesting the RGEA graft through this incision in the upper abdomen is painless and obviates the possible problem of respiratory depression. The pericardium over the LAD is incised for anastomosis. While this technique is suitable for revascularization of the LAD and RCA, revascularization of the other coronary arteries seems to be difficult.

# Harvesting Bypass Conduits

## Internal Mammary Artery

The IMA has proven to be the gold standard conduit in CABG and it is the best available arterial graft in ACAB surgery. The patency of the in situ IMA graft is better than 90% at 20 years, whereas a free IMA graft has lower patency rate. The LIMA or right IMA (RIMA) should be used as the graft of choice to LAD while the second IMA can be used as the second arterial graft to circumflex or RCA. Harvesting IMA without significant injury is the main goal in ACAB surgery, because IMA is a very delicate vessel and it can be injured easily during harvesting. The technique is similar through sternotomy or anterior mini-thoracotomy with some technical variations. In all operations, 5,000 IU of heparin is given for anticoagulation at the beginning of IMA harvest, which is not reversed with protamine at the end of the operation.

Harvesting LIMA through full median sternotomy in ACAB surgery is similar in conventional technique with some differences. First, the spontaneous respiration and cough can make harvesting challenging because of rhythmic motion of pleura and diaphragm. Pleural surface moves toward the midline during inspiration in mechanical ventilation, whereas the reverse occurs during spontaneous respiration. The surgeon must be an expert for harvesting LIMA in paralyzed patients, because harvesting IMA in a spontaneously breathing patient needs a learning curve. Second, collapse of a single lung or tension pneumothorax after sternotomy can hinder harvesting LIMA in awake patients. In case of a hole in the pleura, repair of the pleural injury must be attempted first. However, if it is not possible the pleura is opened widely. These maneuvers can prevent hypoxia and hypercapnia, and the patient can tolerate rest of the procedure very well. Third, the surgeon must preserve the left pleura intact and an extra-pleural approach should be applied very diligently. Fourth, a nontraumatized LIMA should be harvested without any injury (hematoma, dissection, rupture) caused by electrocautery, scissors or any dissector. Excessive traction, stretching, clamping or misplaced metal clips during harvesting should be avoided. Fifth, skeletonization or semiskeletonization techniques should be preferred in spite of these techniques being technically more demanding and time-consuming. The advantages are increasing luminal diameter with better flow, providing a longer graft, allowing more distal anastomoses and sequential grafting. Furthermore, the degree of sternal ischemia produced by LIMA harvest is decreased after skeletonization technique and especially when the distal bifurcation is preserved.

Through full median sternotomy, a Favaloro retractor is used to elevate the left sternal half. The left sternal half is elevated partially followed by the lose areolar tissue with pleural reflection immediately posterior to the sternum being dissected away and pushed down using a low thermal cautery setting until the course of the LIMA is identified from its origin near the first intercostal space to its bifurcation (lateral musculophrenic and superior epigastric branches) at the sixth intercostal space. These tissues must never be peeled from the chest wall with a sterile gauze, because this maneuver can cause wide pleural opening. After full elevation of the left sternal half, the LIMA is palpated and an initial small incision ($\approx$ 1 cm) of the endothoracic fascia is performed using electrocautery along the medial side of the accompanying internal thoracic vein at the fourth rib. Then the endothoracic fascia is taken down and incised by the electrocautery or a scissors proximally and distally along the full length of the LIMA. The lateral incision is not necessary. The edge of the endothoracic fascia is then grasped with a forceps and the LIMA is harvested using the tip of the cold cautery as a dissector to depress and dissect the graft. Major branches are ligated with double hemostatic clips and divided by a scissors, and the small branches are divided by electrocautery. Then the LIMA with surrounding thin tissue is easily separated from the endothoracic fascia while both internal thoracic veins are left intact at the chest wall. Surrounding thin tissue can facilitate handling the LIMA. The LIMA is left intact and wrapped in a papaverine-soaked sponge until distal anastomosis is performed.

Through the lower reversed-J median sternotomy, harvesting of the LIMA takes a few minutes without any difficulty (Figure 1). A Favaloro retractor is used to elevate the left hemisternum partially until the course of the LIMA is identified near the second intercostal space (Figure 2). Continuation of elevating the left hemisternum over stretches the LIMA and may cause rupture or dissection. Before the retractor is elevated completely, the lose areolar tissue with pleural reflection immediately posterior to the sternum is dissected away and pushed down using a low cautery setting. The second side-branch of the LIMA should be divided first to prevent stretching, rupture or dissection of the LIMA during the elevation of the left hemisternum (Figure 3). After full elevation of the left sternal half, the LIMA is palpated and an initial small incision ($\approx$ 1 cm) of the endothoracic fascia is performed by electrocautery along the medial side of the accompanying internal thoracic vein at the fourth rib. The edge of the endothoracic fascia is then grasped with a forceps and the LIMA is harvested using the tip of the cold cautery as a dissector to depress and dissect the graft (Figure 4). Major branches are ligated with double hemostatic clips and divided by a scissors, and the small branches are divided by electrocautery (Figure 5). The LIMA is mobilized distally as described above without any risk of pneumothorax because the parietal pleura is far from the sternum above the left heart (Figure 6). The first side-branch can also be divided to avoid any possible steal phenomenon from the LIMA flow.

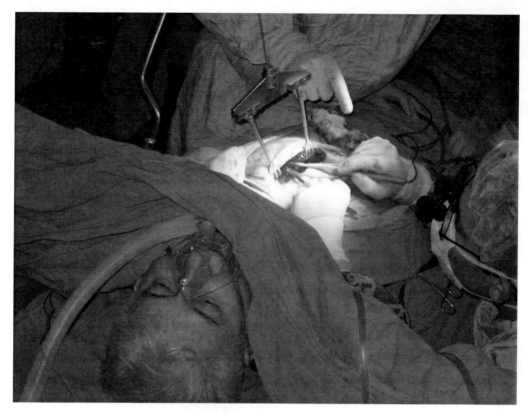

Figure 1. Intraoperative view of the surgical team during harvesting of the left internal mammary artery via reversed-J partial lower sternotomy technique.

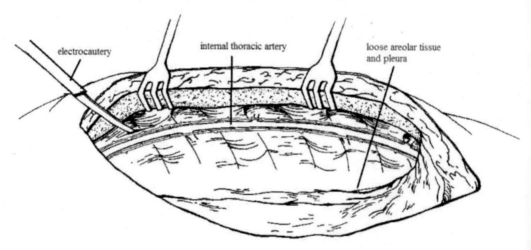

Figure 2. After the loose areolar tissue with pleural reflection immediately posterior to the sternum are dissected away and pushed down, the course of the left internal mammary artery is identified.

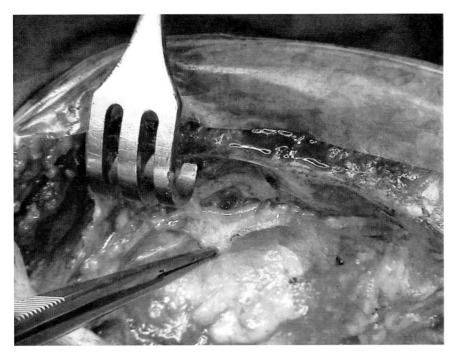

Figure 3. The second side-branch of the left internal mammary artery (LIMA) should be divided first to prevent stretching, rupture or dissection of the LIMA during the elevation of the left hemisternum.

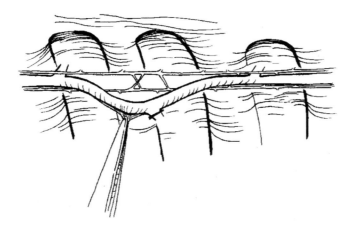

Figure 4. The edge of the endothoracic fascia is grasped with a forceps and the left internal mammary artery is harvested using the tip of the cold cautery as a dissector to depress and dissect the graft.

Through the anterior mini-thoracotomy, LIMA can be harvested as in the median sternotomy approach or it is left untouched to be used as an inflow for H-graft technique. In classic technique, the surgeon exposes the left pleural space to the atmosphere and the left lung collapses totally, which cannot have adverse effect on the spontaneous respiration and ACAB procedure is to be continued complication-free. On the other hand, the H-graft technique avoids pneumothorax because of the extra-pleural nature of this approach. The LIMA lies immediately deep to the cartilage such that a 1.5 to 2 cm segment of the vessel is thereby exposed. All branches of the LIMA are left intact because there is no dissection of the LIMA from the thoracic wall. In the original technique, a 3 to 8 cm segment of the right inferior epigastric artery is attached proximally end-to-side to the LIMA. [51] But, a short segment of the left radial artery is the best alternative for this technique in ACAB surgery because HTEA covers both arms. The left radial artery is dissected through a small 5 cm incision with standard technique and a 6 to 7 cm long radial artery is harvested and preserved in a special solution. After completion of the distal anastomosis, the radial artery is bridged to the side of the in situ LIMA at the area exposed.

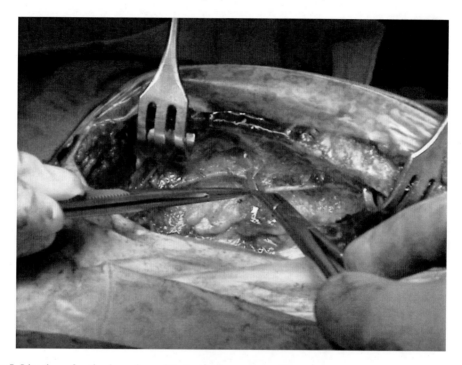

Figure 5. Ligation of major branches with double hemostatic clips.

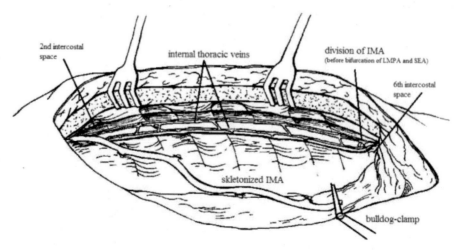

Figure 6. Harvesting of full length of the left internal mammary artery until its bifurcation (lateral musculophrenic and superior epigastric branches) at the sixth intercostal space.

## Harvesting Radial Artery

Extension of sensory and motor block provided by HTEA to C5 level is sufficient to harvest the radial artery without additional subcutaneous infiltration of local anesthetic agent or regional block. If it is necessary musculocutaneous nerve block, axillary block or local anesthetic agents can be used. If motor blockade is insufficient patients may move their arms/forearms during harvesting. Advising the patient to keep the hand still and reassuring him are quite effective in preventing further movements. The arm is abducted to 80 degrees and under sterile conditions prepared and draped. Radial artery is dissected through a small or conventional incision with standard technique depending on the ACAB procedure and preserved in verapamil-nitroglycerin solution. [52]

## Saphenous Vein

If there is a clear contraindication to harvest an arterial graft, saphenous vein can be used as an alternative or additional graft in ACAB surgery. Combined HTEA with local or regional anesthetics is an effective approach for saphenous vein harvest. Use of lumbar epidural anesthesia, lumbar subarachnoid block, or femoral block in addition to HTEA can be chosen to facilitate harvesting of vein graft. If the leg incision is made after harvesting arterial grafts, sensory block in the lower limbs may be sufficient due to diffusion of local anesthetic agents across the dural membrane, which allows vein harvesting without any additional anesthesia. Conventional technique is preferred to harvest saphenous vein graft.

# Coronary Anastomosis

Using a mechanical or suction stabilizer is the best choice to stabilize the heart during ACAB. Pericardial stay sutures can be used to lift the heart and get better access. Sponges are also placed under the heart, but this maneuver can cause discomfort to patients with signs of cough, agitation and dyspnea. All anastomoses are performed with the standard beating heart bypass technique using a blower system to visualize the anastomosis site. All anastomoses are carried out with 7-0 or 8-0 polypropylene sutures in a continuous fashion, which should not take more than 10 minutes. A mechanical or vacuum assisted stabilizer and soft silicone elastomer tapes can be used to stabilize and occlude coronary arteries. Exposure of the postero-lateral and inferior walls of the heart is accomplished by apical stabilization devices. First the LAD artery is revascularized, and than the others. In situ arterial grafts are anastomozed and coronary blood flow is restored before free graft anastomoses. Usage of any intraluminal shunt is unnecessary.

## Single Vessel Revascularization

In single vessel revascularization (LIMA-LAD) through full sternotomy, the sternum is spread with a retractor and the pericardium is opened to expose the LAD leaving the pericardium over the aorta intact. It is not proposed to use any traction suture to avoid the displacement of the heart and to get better exposure of the LAD. The pericardium does not usually block the exposure because it moves both laterally during spontaneously breathing. A sterile gauze may be put under the heart to move it anteriorly for better exposure of the LAD, but this maneuver causes a mild discomfort to the patient. The most comfortable way is to use a stabilizer, which holds the LAD area immobile and visible during LIMA-LAD anastomosis.

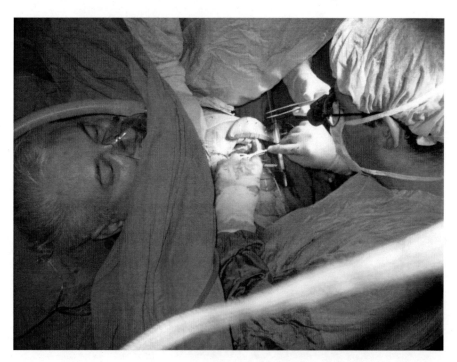

Figure 7. Positioning a mechanical stabilizer for left internal mammary artery to left anterior descending artery anastomosis through the reversed-J partial lower sternotomy.

In single vessel revascularization (LIMA-LAD) through the reversed-J inferior sternotomy, the sternum is spread with a small retractor. Because the left hemisternum is pushed to the left, the left ventricle lies directly under the exposure area through the sternal retractor and it is very easy to open the pericardium for 6 to 8 cm only above the LAD. A traction suture can be placed deeply on the left pericardium and pulled through the incision to avoid the displacement of the heart during respiration. The LIMA-LAD anastomosis can be performed with or without the aid of a stabilizer, which holds the LAD area immobile and visible during LIMA-LAD anastomosis (Figure 7).

In single vessel revascularization (LIMA-LAD) through anterior mini-thoracotomy, a self-retaining retractor or a small thoracic retractor is used to spread both upper and lower ribs. The pericardium is opened just enough to expose the LAD. Traction sutures are placed on the pericardium and pulled through the incision to avoid the displacement of the heart during respiration. The heart can be stabilized with a stabilizer or epicardial pledget-armed sutures or only LAD is immobilized using two heavy U sutures buttressed with Teflon felt, which are placed at 1.5 to 2 cm apart and at either side of the LAD. These sutures are pulled through incision appropriately, to pull the anastomosis territory into sight, and to diminish cardiac displacement. With these sutures pulled up, the heart becomes wedged to the thoracotomy and stabilizes itself. In conventional technique, the LIMA is anastomozed directly to the LAD in end-to-side fashion. In H-graft technique, the distal end of the radial artery graft is anastomozed end-to-side to the LAD and its proximal end is anastomozed end-to-side to the in situ LIMA at the thorax.

In single vessel revascularization (LIMA-LAD) with rib cage lifting technique, a small pediatric sternal retractor is used to lift the rib cage. After the pericardium is opened stay sutures are placed into the left cavity of the pericardium and pulled upward and anteriorly through the incision to elevate the heart and to expose the middle and distal parts of the LAD.

## Multivessel Revascularization

After completion of the LAD revascularization with the in situ IMA, both native LAD and graft flows are restored by releasing the occluded LAD and the microvascular bulldog clamp on the IMA. If the second in situ IMA graft is used for the next dominant coronary artery revascularization, the free arterial and/or venous grafts are anastomozed to the third or other coronary arteries. Except LAD and RCA double vessel revascularization, the LIMA should be directed to the circumflex territory whereas the RIMA is anastomozed to the LAD in the multivessel revascularization procedures (because the patency rate of the IMA is better in circumflex territory than RCA). Most of the time, it is not suitable to take the RIMA through the transverse sinus to the circumflex branches.

After completion of the RIMA-LAD anastomosis in patients with double vessel disease (LAD and circumflex), the patient is placed in a mild Trendelenburg position to facilitate rotation of the heart as well as to increase venous filling to maintain cardiac output just before circumflex anastomosis. Moderate right lateral decubitus positioning at 30 degree of the operation table allows for gravity-assisted rotation of the heart rightward. Exposure of the postero-lateral wall is then accomplished by apical stabilization devices. The apex of the heart is rotated toward the patient's right and hold just above the right arm of the sternal retractor. Manipulation and rotation of the heart can cause discomfort with varying degrees. Positioning of the heart for the LIMA-circumflex anastomosis is less problematic. A metal stabilizer with or without soft silicone elastomer tapes is used to stabilize and occlude the circumflex-branch, and distal anastomosis is performed with the standard beating heart technique. The RIMA is suitable on RCA in patients with double vessel disease (LAD and RCA), but it cannot be long enough to access the distal branches, like posterior descending artery (PDA). If these patients have distal RCA lesion, it is better to choose a free graft to revascularize the PDA or left ventricular branch of the RCA.

A free graft is anastomozed to the RCA in patients with triple vessel disease after completion of RIMA-LAD and LIMA-circumflex anastomoses. Exposure of the inferior wall is accomplished by pulling up the apex of the heart. The apex of the heart is rotated toward the patient's left shoulder and placed just above the left arm of the sternal retractor. A metal stabilizer and soft silicone elastomer tapes are used to stabilize and occlude the PDA and anastomosis is performed with the standard beating heart bypass technique. Proximal anastomosis is performed with or without new technical devices.

## Finishing the Operation

After all anastomoses, a careful inspection should be made to control any anastomotic bleeding, correct graft kinking or stretching, assess arterial graft flow, possible spasm, and myocardial dysfunction (Figure 8). If there is no problem, then the sternum or thoracotomy incision can be closed. Chest drainage tubes are inserted. The important point is not to leave any pneumothorax. The rest of the operation is similar to the conventional technique.

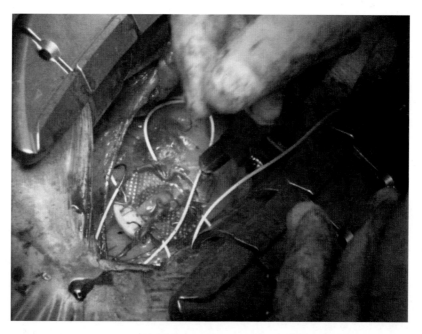

Figure 8. Careful assessment for any minimal anastomotic bleeding, graft kinking or stretching, arterial graft flow and possible spasm, and myocardial dysfunction.

## Management of Intraoperative Complications

### Intraoperative Irritability

Adequate analgesia, good sedation, and anxiolysis are important components of a successful HTEA. It is preferable to have an awake calm patient who is pain-free. The discomfort of patients causes hyperventilation, cough, body movements, and irritability which affect surgeons as well and make procedure difficult. The discomfort can be prevented with administration of midazolam (0.07 mg/kg) intravenously with/without assisted ventilation.

### Intraoperative Pneumothorax

Maintaining the intact pleura is the most important issue during ACAB procedure and pneumothorax caused by pleural damage is the biggest obstacle. Pneumothorax prevents spontaneous breathing and causes respiratory distress due to retention of carbon dioxide, paradoxical thoracic movement and restricted lung expansion. The thoracic movements related to tachypnea further complicate the surgical procedures. Several stages of awake revascularization have the risk of iatrogenic pleural damage or spontaneous opening of pleura. It occurs most commonly during sternotomy, while harvesting uni- or bilateral IMA, and placing pericardial traction sutures. Because of the anatomical position of the heart deviated more to the left in the thorax, it is more difficult to open the left pleura during the reverse-J sternotomy as the left pleura is not attached to the lower part of the sternum. The other important step to avoid iatrogenic pneumothorax is to limit using deep pericardial traction sutures, which may cause unexpected small hole on the pleura. If pleural damage occurs, purse string suturing and closure of the hole on the pleura may be tried while simple aspiration with continuous negative pressure is administered through pleural tear. However, suturing is very difficult because the damaged pleura is very thin and delicate, besides challenging due to respiratory movements. A novel closure method using polyglycolic acid nonwoven fabric and fibrin glue has been offered to prevent intra-operative pneumothorax in ACAB surgery, which achieves a strong closure with sufficient durability on the moving thin pleura regardless of the defect size. [53] If repair of the breach in the pleura may not be possible, opening the damaged pleura completely is the only way to avoid tension pneumothorax. The last suggestion is to do nothing to treat pneumothorax if oxygen saturation and hemodynamic performance are unaffected. Unilateral widely opened pleura is not necessarily a reason for conversion to general anesthesia, but bilateral opened pleurae cannot be tolerated by a conscious patient. Endotracheal intubation and mechanical ventilation is required if pneumothorax cannot be managed effectively and if adequate oxygenation and carbon dioxide elimination is not possible.

## Stretching or Distortion of Pedicled Arterial Grafts

After anastomoses of both IMAs, all thymic and adipose tissues are cut off to imbed both grafts under the apical part of the left lung. The LIMA reaches the LAD easily without the incision of the left pericardium. The length of the RIMA is also adequate to revascularize LAD, and it is not necessary to incise the right pericardium.

If the LIMA is anastomozed to the circumflex territory, the left pericardium is incised 10 mm left of the pulmonary artery and the incision is carefully lengthened 4-5 cm down parallel to the left phrenic nerve. This maneuver increases the usable length of the LIMA and allows the LIMA to lie intrapericardially as its courses to the circumflex branches. Because the LIMA now lies medial and posterior to the lung, altered respiration does not produce any distortion or stretching of the LIMA.

If the RIMA is utilized for the right coronary system, the pericardium is wedged 10 mm right of the aorta and the incision is carefully lengthened 4-5 cm down parallel to the right phrenic nerve and vena cava superior. This maneuver allows the RIMA to lie intrapericardially as it courses onto the right coronary artery branches. Because the RIMA now lies medial and posterior to the lung, altered respiration does not cause any distortion or stretching of the RIMA.

## Conversion to General Anesthesia

Patients experiencing significant hypoxia or discomfort during ACAB procedures will require ventilator assistance. Due to complete epidural block, intercostal muscles are denervated and respiratory effort is only through the diaphragm. Patients with severe chronic obstructive pulmonary disease are more likely tolerate HTEA better because they are accustomed to hypercapnia and hypoxia. The main reasons to convert to general anesthesia are ineffective HTEA, respiratory distress caused by pneumothorax, hemodynamic instability, and difficult anatomy of coronary arteries (Table 11). Noninvasive ventilation like continuous positive airway pressure support is administered first. If clinical improvement is not observed conversion to general anesthesia is performed and an endotracheal tube is inserted. Tube insertion is carried out in a similar manner as in elective cases as upper airway and cough reflexes are intact.

## Conversion to Full Median Sternotomy

Partial lower sternotomy techniques can minimize surgical trauma while providing optimum exposure to coronary arteries, whereas the main drawback is access to the ascending aorta. Conversion to full median sternotomy becomes unavoidable if cardiopulmonary support is required due to technical problems or a proximal anastomosis is necessary. The incision can be easily and rapidly extended to a full sternotomy if technical problems are encountered or the exposure is inadequate. Surgeons should keep in mind that the sternal saw should be preserved sterile until the end of the operation because it is not suitable and safe to wait for the second to extend the mini-sternotomy.

Table 11. Reasons of conversion to general anesthesia

- Inadequate epidural anesthesia
- Diaphragmatic paralysis
- Bilateral pneumothorax
- Respiratory distress caused by pneumothorax
- Inability to harvest internal mammary artery
- Inadequate anatomy of coronary arteries
- Deteriorating hemodynamic parameters
- Uncontrolled arrhythmias
- Uncontrolled hypoventilation
- Uncontrolled coughing
- Uncontrolled irritability
- Signs of hypercapnia or dyspnea
- Local anesthesia intoxication

## Postoperative Fast-track Recovery

Patients can be mobilized immediately after arrival to intensive care unit and allowed to speak, drink or walk much earlier compared to conventional technique. Since there is no pharyngeal pain or trauma associated with endotracheal intubation, aspiration would not be observed during early postoperative period. Patients may be managed in an intermediate care unit before being discharged to the ward. After an uneventful operation, hemodynamically stable patients can also be transferred to the ward directly. Patients are able to return to normal daily activities a few days after surgery, and they can be discharged from hospital in a shorter time, even on the same day of surgery. Generally, it seems more feasible to discharge patients from the hospital on the second postoperative day. Avoidance of intensive care unit stay and shorter hospital stay translates into significant reduction in hospital costs. Patients can return to normal daily life more quickly than patients operated on with conventional CABG procedure. Especially, this recovery is more obvious for patients operated with reversed-J mini-sternotomy or anterior mini-thoracotomy. They can continue to perform normal daily life activities and return to work one week after the operation. These minimal invasive approaches provide better intraoperative oxygenation, less mediastinal drainage, and almost negligible transfusion requirements.

## Early Clinical Results

Clinical studies including different ACAB approaches show that the early postoperative course is very smooth and flawless. None of the investigators have observed any intraoperative electrocardiographic changes, myocardial ischemia or infarction, or conversion to the conventional technique because of incomplete or unsuccessful coronary artery anastomosis. Requiring unplanned coronary endarterectomy is very seldom, but it can be performed without any myocardial ischemia and/or arrhythmia. The intraoperative heart rate decreases significantly to the levels (55-65 beats/min) where distal anastomoses can be performed comfortably. Mean systolic arterial pressure is generally maintained at the optimal level (100-120 mmHg) and it only decreases during manipulation of the heart.

During surgery, patients are provided with oxygen through a face mask to maintain oxygen saturation level consistently more than 95% as measured by pulse oxymetry. Patients, who are operated on without full median sternotomy for single vessel disease, can tolerate the procedure without hypoxia, and only mild hypercapnia (45-50 mmHg) may be observed intraoperatively which resolves immediately after sternal closure. Partial arterial carbon dioxide level can be higher (45-55 mmHg) during full sternotomy for multivessel revascularization, but it is not a reason for conversion to the general anesthesia. The main reason for intraoperative respiratory distress is pneumothorax, which may develop due to injury of the pleura iatrogenically or spontaneously. A hole in the pleura may occur in approximately one-third (30% - 35%) of the patients, but a half of these defects can be repaired easily. The pleura can be left wide open without any difficulty approximately in one-sixth of the patients (15% - 20%), while conversion to general anesthesia is observed infrequently (0% - 5%).

Once learning curve is over, operation times decrease significantly to the levels similar for conventional techniques. The operation time skin to skin can be approximately 90 minutes for single vessel revascularization and 180 minutes for multivessel revascularization. If patients get transferred directly to ward, they can be discharged as early as the same day of surgery (range 0 to 3 days for single vessel revascularization through ministernotomy or minithoracotomy, but it can be longer for full sternotomy or multivessel revascularization). The main rule is to shorten all stages of the procedure as much as possible without any fear.

These techniques include all minimal invasive maneuvers and surgeons should stay focused and very careful during the entire procedure. Attention to detail and precision results in lowering chest tube drainage and requirement for blood products, which in return shortens hospital length of stay and also prevents possible complications related to mediastinal drainage or transfusion. The mean drainage may be as low as 300 mL and chest tubes may be removed in 12 hours.

## Conclusion

Combining advanced anesthetic and high-level surgical competence, this alternative surgical revascularization opens the door of surgical treatment for patients in whom conventional general anesthesia is not suitable. Like every new technique, ACAB surgery introduces new challenges into routine practice of anesthesiologists, surgeons, and other operating room staff. The program of ACAB surgery should be developed step-by-step. ACAB like any other surgical procedure has a learning curve. Once it is successfully negotiated, it can be safely offered to a vast array of patient subgroups.

## Acknowledgement

The author wishes to thank to Başar Sareyyüpoğlu, M.D., a successful cardiovascular surgeon working in the USA, for assistance with language editing and improvement in the content of this chapter.

## References

[1] Benetti FJ, Naselli C, Wood M, Geffner L. Direct myocardial revascularization without extracorporeal circulation. Experience in 700 patients. *Chest* 1991;100:312-316.
[2] Tasdemir O, Vural KM, Karagoz H, Bayazit K. Coronary artery bypass grafting on the beating heart without the use of extracorporeal circulation: review of 2052 cases. *J Thorac Cardiovasc Surg* 1998;116:68-73.
[3] Ogus T, Ipek G, Isık O et al.. CABG on the beating heart without using pump oxgentor in high risk patients. *Turkish J Thorac Cardiovasc Surg* 1996;1:9-14.
[4] Subramanian VA, Sani G, Benetti FJ, Calafiore AM. Minimally invazive direct coronary bypass surgery: a multi-center report of preliminary clinical experience. *Circulation* 1995;92(Suppl I):645.

[5] Isik Ö, Daglar B, Kırali K, Balkanay M, Arbatlı H, Yakut C. Coronary bypass surgery via minithoracotomy on the beating heart. *Ann Thorac Surg* 1997;63 (Suppl):S57-60.

[6] Kırali K, Güler M, Dağlar B, et al. Videothoracoscopic internal mammary artery harvest for coronary bypass. *Asian Cardiovasc Thorac Ann* 1999;7:259-262.

[7] Baumgartner FJ, Gheissari A, Capouya ER, Panagiotides GP, Katouzian A, Yokoyama T. Technical aspects of total revascularization in off-pump coronary bypass via sternotomy approach. *Ann Thorac Surg* 1999;67:1653-1658.

[8] Buffolo E, Branco JN, Gerola LR et al.. Off-pump myocardial revascularization: critical analysis of 23 years' experience in 3866 patients. *Ann Thorac Surg* 2006;81:85-89.

[9] Kirali K, Rabus MB, Yakut N, et al. Early- and long-term comparison of the on- and off-pump bypass surgery in patients with left ventricular dysfunction. *Heart Surg Forum* 2002;5:177-181.

[10] Güler M, Kirali K, Toker ME, et al. Different CABG methods in patients with chronic obstructive pulmonary disease. *Ann Thorac Surg* 2001;71:152-157.

[11] Erentug V, Akıncı E, Kırali K, et al. Complete off-pump coronary revascularization in patients with dialysis-dependent renal disease. *Texas Heart Inst J* 2004;31:153-156.

[12] Marcheix B, Eynden FV, Demers P, Bouchard D, Cartier R. Influence of diabetes mellitus on long-term survival in systematic off-pump coronary artery bypass surgery. *Ann Thorac Surg* 2008;86:1181-1188.

[13] Kirali K, Mansuroğlu D, Kayalar N, Güzelmeriç F, Alp M, Yakut C. Markers of myocardial ischemia in the evaluation of the effect of left anterior descending coronary artery lesion and collateral circulation on myocardial injury in 1-vessel off-pump coronary bypass surgery. *Heart Surg Forum* 2003;6:143-148.

[14] Navia D, Vrancic M, Vaccarino G et al.. Total arterial off-pump coronary revascularization using bilateral internal thoracic arteries in triple-vessel disease: surgical technique and clinical outcomes. *Ann Thorac Surg* 2009;86:524-530.

[15] Toker ME, Ömeroğlu SN, Kırali K, Balkanay M, Yakut C. Using the bilateral internal mammary artery in the left or right coronary artery system: 5-year comparison of operation techniques and angiographic results. *Heart Surg Forum* 2005;8:345-350.

[16] Ömeroğlu SN, Kirali K, Güler M, et al. Midterm angiographic assessment of coronary artery bypass grafting without cardiopulmonary bypass. *Ann Thorac Surg* 2000;70:844-849.

[17] Angelini GD, Culiford L, Smith DK, et al. Effects of on- and off-pump coronary artery surgery on graft patency, survival, and healt-related quality of life: long-term follow-up up 2 randomized controlled trials. *J Thorac Cardiovasc Surg* 2009;137:295-303.

[18] Elevli G, Mataracı İ, Büyükbayrak F, Erkin A, Şişmanoğlu M, Kırali K. Complete revascularization with or without cardiopulmonary bypass using arterial grafts: The six-month angiographic results. *Turkish J Thorac Cardiovasc Surg* 2011;19:1-6.

[19] Clowes GH Jr, Neville WE, Hopkins A, Anzola J, Simeone FA. Factors contributing to success or failure in the use of a pump oxygenator for complete bypass of the heart and lung, experimental and clinical. *Surgery* 1954;36:557-579.

[20] Hoar PF, Hickey RF, Ullyot DJ. Systemic hypertension following myocardial revascularization: a method of treatment using epidural anesthesia. *J Thorac Cardiovasc Surg* 1976;71:859-864.

[21] El-Baz N, Goldin M. Continuous epidural infusion of morphine for pain relief after cardiac operations. *J Thorac Cardiovasc Surg* 1987;93:878-883.

[22] Karagöz H, Sönmez B, Bakkaloglu B, et al. Coronary artery bypass grafting in the conscious patient without endotracheal general anesthesia. *Ann Thorac Surg* 2000;70:91-96.

[23] Anderson MB, Kwong KF, Furst AJ, Salerno TA. Thoracic epidural anesthesia for coronary bypass via left anterior thoracotomy in the conscious patient. *Eur J Cardiothorac Surg* 2001;20:415-417.

[24] Zenati MA, Paiste J, Williams JP, Strindberg G, Dumouchel JP, Griffith BP. Minimally invasive coronary bypass without general endotracheal anesthesia. *Ann Thorac Surg* 2001;72:1380-1382.

[25] Vanek T, Straka Z, Brucek P, Widimsky P. Thoracic epidural anesthesia for off-pump coronary artery bypass without intubation. *Eur J Cardiothorac Surg* 2001;20:858-860.

[26] Aybek T, Dogan S, Neidhart G et al.. Coronary artery bypass grafting through complete sternotomy in conscious patients. *Heart Surg Forum* 2002;5:17-21.

[27] Souto GLL, Junior CSC, Souza JBS, et al. Coronary artery bypass in the ambulatory patient. *J Thorac Cardiovasc Surg* 2002;123:1008-1009.

[28] Chakravarthy M, Jawali V, Patil TA, Jayaprakash K, Shivananda NV. High thoracic epidural anesthesia as the sole anesthetic for performing multiple grafts in off-pump coronary artery bypass surgery. *J Cardiothorac Vasc Anesth* 2003;17:160-164.

[29] Paiste J, Bjerke RJ, Williams JP, Zenati MA, Nagy GE. Minimally invasive direct coronary artery bypass surgery under high thoracic epidural. *Anesth Analg* 2001;93:486-488

[30] Karagoz HY, Kurtoglu M, Ozerdem G, Bataloglu B, Korkmaz S, Bayazit K. Minimally invasive coronary artery bypass grafting: the rib cage lifting technique. *J Thorac Cardiovasc Surg* 1998;116:354-356.

[31] Kessler P, Neithard G, Bremerich DH et al.. High thoracic epidural anesthesia for coronary artery bypass grafting using two different surgical approaches in conscious patients. *Anesth Analg* 2002;95:791-797.

[32] Kırali K, Kayalar N, Koçak T, Yakut C. Reversed-J inferior sternotomy for awake coronary bypass. *Eur J Cardiothorac Surg* 2005;27:923-924.

[33] Watanabe G, Yamaguchi S, Tomiya S, Ohtake H. Awake subxyphoid minimally invasive direct coronary artery bypass grafting yielded minimum invasive cardiac surgery for high risk patients. *Interact Cardiovasc Thorac Surg* 2008;7:910-912.

[34] Lucchetti V, Moscariello C, Catapano D, Angelini GD. Coronary artery bypass grafting in the awake patient: combined thoracic epidural and lumbar subarachnoid block. *Eur J Cardiothorac Surg* 2004;26:658-659.

[35] Chakravarthy M, Jawali V, Manohar M et al.. Conscious off pump coronary artery bypass surgery-an audit of our first 151 cases. *Ann Thorac Cardiovasc Surg* 2005;11:93-97.

[36] Noiseux N, Prieto I, Bracco D, Basile F, Hemmerling T. Coronary artery bypass grafting in the awake patient combining high thoracic epidural and femoral nerve block: first series of 15 patients. *Br J Anaesth* 2008;100:184-189.

[37] Giglio MD, Amore AD, Zuffi A, Sokoli A. One-stage hybrid procedure: association between awake minimally invasive surgical revascularization and percutaneous coronary intervention. *Interact Cardiovasc Thorac Surg* 2009;9:551-553.

[38] Kırali K, Koçak T, Güzelmeriç F, Göksedef D, Kayalar N, Yakut C. Off-pump awake coronary revascularization using bilateral internal thoracic arteries. *Ann Thorac Surg* 2004;78:1598-1603.

[39] Kırali K. Composite bilateral internal thoracic artery grafts via standard sternotomy for lateral wall revascularization in conscious patients. *Heart Surg Forum* 2005;8:340-344.

[40] Chaney MA. Intrathecal and epidural anesthesia and analgesia for cardiac surgery. *Anesth Analg* 2006;102:45-64.

[41] Clemente A, Carli F. Thoracic epidural analgesia and the cardiovascular system. *Tech Reg Anesth Pain Manage* 2008;12:41-45.

[42] Yashiki N, Watanabe G, Tomita S, Nishida S, Yasuda T, Arai S. Thoracic epidural anesthesia for coronary bypass surgery affects autonomic neural function and arrhythmias. *Innovations* 2005;1:83-87.

[43] Niimi Y, Ichinose F, Saegusa H, Nakata Y, Morita S. Echocardiographic evaluation of global left ventricular function during high thoracic epidural anesthesia. *J Clin Anesth* 1997;9:118-124.

[44] Schmidt C, Hinder F, Aken HV, et al. The effect of high thoracic epidural anesthesia on systolic and diastolic left ventricular function in patients with coronary artery disease. *Anesth Analg* 2005;100:1561-1569.

[45] Gramling-Babb P. High thoracic epidural analgesia for relief of coronary ischemia syndrome without cardiac surgery. *Tech Reg Anesth Pain Manage* 2008;12:80-86.

[46] Hogan Q. Cardiovascular response to sympathetic block by regional anesthesia. *Reg Anesth* 1997;21:26-34.

[47] Groeben H. Epidural anesthesia and pulmonary function. *J Anesth* 2006;20:290-299.

[48] Hemmerling TM. Technical aspects of high thoracic epidural analgesia in cardiac surgery. *Tech Reg Anesth Pain Manage* 2008;12:46-53.

[49] Chakravarthy M, Nadiminti S, Krishnamurthy J, et al. Temporary neurologic deficits in patients undergoing cardiac surgery with thoracic epidural supplementation. *J Cardiothorac Vasc Anesth* 2004;18:512-520.

[50] Kırali K. Mini-T sternotomy for awake coronary revascularization with bilateral internal thoracic artery. *Interactive Cardiovasc Thorac Surg* 2004;3:S64-65.

[51] Cohn WE, Suen HC, Weintraub RM, Johnson RG. The "H" graft: an alternative approach for performing minimally invasive direct coronary artery bypass. *J Thorac Cardiovasc Surg* 1998;115:148-151.

[52] Kırali K, Yakut N, Güler M, et al. Radial artery in coronary bypass surgery: anatomical landsmarks and harvesting technique. *Turkish J Thorac Cardiovasc Surg* 1999;7:358-361.

[53] Kato Y, Matsumoto I, Tomita S, Watanabe G. A novel technique to prevent intra-operative pneumothorax in awake coronary artery bypass grafting: biomaterial neo-pleura. *Eur J Cardiothorac Surg* 2009;35:37-42

In: Off-Pump Coronary Artery Bypass Grafting
Editors: Shahzad G. Raja and Mohamed Amrani

ISBN: 978-1- 62081-549-6
© 2012 Nova Science Publishers, Inc.

*Chapter XIII*

# On-pump Beating-Heart Coronary Artery Bypass Grafting

*Ken Miyahara*
Division of Cardiovascular Surgery, Ichinomiya Municipal Hospital,
Ichinomiya, Aichi, Japan

## Abstract

Three operative procedures can be employed in isolated coronary artery bypass grafting (CABG): on-pump arrest CABG (conventional CABG), off-pump CABG (OPCAB), and on-pump beating-heart CABG. Conventional CABG, the standard technique applied in coronary artery surgery, has been used for over five decades and it is usually associated with complete revascularization and good graft patency rate. However, despite improvements in myocardial preservation techniques, the technique of aortic cross-clamping and cardioplegic arrest might induce myocardial and systemic organ damage, especially in extremely ill patients. Cardiopulmonary bypass (CPB) itself might induce a systemic inflammatory response, generate microemboli, and cause direct complications of the cannulation site. In the 1990s, to avoid the deleterious effects of CPB, aortic cross-clamping, and cardioplegic arrest, OPCAB was rediscovered with the advent of the stabilizer devices. While advances in the devices involved have made OPCAB safer, and it has been shown to be an effective technique in selected patients, controversy remains regarding graft patency, completeness of revascularization, incidence of recurrent or residual myocardial ischemia, need for reintervention, and long-term survival. Additionally, OPCAB is sometimes highly challenging and technically more demanding than conventional CABG, and it is associated with an acute conversion risk that causes death and serious complications in the hospital. Recent studies on myocardial revascularization using on-pump beating-heart CABG, a hybrid technique between conventional CABG and OPCAB, have shown this to be a reliable and effective method. Even in patients with severe left ventricular dysfunction or hemodynamic instability, such as acute myocardial infarction, CPB compensates for the hemodynamic instability by providing mechanical support to the systemic circulation, which enables optimal revascularization. The avoidance of cardioplegic arrest and the absence of reperfusion after cardioplegic arrest can eliminate intraoperative global myocardial ischemia, which might contribute to myocardial protection. By using CPB, on-pump beating-heart CABG results in the activation of inflammatory mediators whose effects are usually resolved within hours to days after surgery. This chapter focuses on the pros and cons of on-pump beating-heart CABG and provides an overview of the author's experience with this revascularization strategy.

## Introduction

For surgical treatment of coronary artery disease, on-pump arrest coronary artery bypass grafting (conventional CABG) has been performed for a long time. The technique of cardiopulmonary bypass (CPB), aortic cross-clamping, and cardioplegic arrest might induce myocardial and systemic organ damage, especially in patients who are extremely ill. Off-pump CABG (OPCAB) was rediscovered in the 1990s with the advent of the stabilizers and has been shown to be a safe and effective technique in selected patients. Controversy, however, remains as to the quality of anastomosis, and the procedure is associated with a potential acute conversion risk that causes death and serious complications in the hospital. On-pump beating-heart (OnP-BH) CABG is a hybrid technique combining conventional CABG and OPCAB, and recent studies using this technique have proved it to be a reliable and effective method, even in patients with severe left ventricular (LV) dysfunction or hemodynamic instability. The next sections describe this attractive technique and provide an overview of our own operative results.

## Historical Note

Experimentally, maintaining the heartbeat has been demonstrated to result in minimal myocardial edema and better LV function [1]. Clinically, Sweeney and Frazier [2] have demonstrated OnP-BH CABG to be an interesting trade-off, using biventricular assist devices and the β-blocker esmolol during coronary revascularization in severely ill patients. Perrault and colleagues [3] have described OnP-BH coronary operations as an acceptable trade-off between conventional CABG and OPCAB in high-risk patients with a low ejection fraction. They found that using CPB with the heart beating, without cross-clamping and cardioplegic arrest, is associated with less myocardial edema and ischemia. Since the work of Perrault, various studies have applied the OnP-BH technique for myocardial revascularization among both low- and high-risk patients [4–16].

## Surgical Technique

A standardized anesthetic protocol and pulmonary artery catheters are used in all patients. All operations are performed through a median sternotomy. Conduits are harvested and prepared, and the patients are heparinized with an initial dose of 300 IU/kg to achieve a target activated clotting time >450 s. The standard CPB circuit incorporates a roller pump and a hollow-fiber membrane oxygenator. The extracorporeal circuit is primed with 1,000 mL Hartmann solution, 150 mL mannitol, 20 mL sodium bicarbonate, and 4000 IU heparin.

The pericardium is opened, and epiaortic ultrasonographic scanning of the ascending aorta is performed to detect whether cannulation could be performed safely. CPB is established by means of aortic cannulation and insertion of a two-stage venous cannula through the right atrial appendage. The operation is then continued on the assisted beating heart. Distal anastomoses are constructed before proximal anastomoses. The left anterior descending coronary artery is revascularized first, followed by the circumflex and right coronary arteries.

Regional myocardial immobilization is achieved with a suction stabilizer (Octopus; Medtronic, Minneapolis, MN, USA; Guidant Acrobat; Guidant, Indianapolis, IN, USA), and an apical suction cardiac positioning device (Starfish; Medtronic) is used for revascularization of the circumflex and right coronary arteries to facilitate exposure. The CPB flow is fluctuates between 2.0–2.5 L/min/m$^2$ due to positioning of the heart and is maintained within this range. The systemic blood pressure is maintained at >60 mm Hg, the pulmonary arterial pressure and central venous pressure are kept appropriately, and the heart rate and electrocardiography are monitored carefully. The mixed venous oxygen saturation is maintained at >75%, the systemic temperature is kept between 36 and 37°C. Excessive decompression of the heart is avoided. LV venting is not needed [4]. During construction of the anastomoses, target vessel hemostasis is obtained with intravascular shunts (Clearview; Medtronic) or temporary occlusion of the proximal coronary artery (SaddleLoop vascular tape; Quest Medical, Allen, TX, USA). All distal anastomoses were made with running 7-0 polypropylene sutures, and the proximal anastomoses are created with 6-0 polypropylene sutures under a partial occlusion clamp or proximal anastomotic system (Enclose II; Novare Surgical Systems, Cupertino, CA, USA). A humidified carbon dioxide blower is used for better visualization. After weaning from CPB and decannulation, the heparin is reversed.

## Impact on Myocardial Enzyme Release

The impact of the three aforementioned myocardial revascularization strategies on myocardial enzyme release is shown in Figure 1. Data are for isolated primary elective double-vessel CABG performed between 2003 and 2009 at our institution. The postoperative maximum creatinine kinase myocardial band (CK-MB) values in the conventional CABG group were higher than those in the OnP-BH CABG group (32±15 *vs.* 23±11 IU/L, p<0.0001) and OPCAB group (32±15 *vs.* 21±12 IU/L, p=0.005), but the difference between the OnP-BH CABG and OPCAB groups (23±11 *vs.* 21±12 IU/L) was not statistically significant.

# CABG for Acute myocardial Infarction – Our Experience

Fibrinolytic therapy, percutaneous coronary intervention (PCI), or both is the preferred first-line therapy for acute myocardial infarction (AMI) [17]. CABG in the presence of or immediately after AMI is controversial because the mortality from emergency CABG for

AMI remains high [18-21]. However, we sometimes encounter selected patients requiring emergency surgical revascularization. Conventional CABG -the technique of aortic cross-clamping and cardioplegic arrest- might induce myocardial and systemic organ damage during this critical situation, which results in high mortality. The reasons for this poor result include both the patients' poor preoperative status, including cardiogenic shock [21] or organ failure, and myocardial damage after cardioplegic arrest.

To reduce the damaging effect of cardiac arrest and the mortality rate, we have adopted the technique of on-pump beating-heart (OnP-BH) CABG. We compared the clinical outcomes and laboratory data of patients undergoing conventional and OnP-BH CABG and evaluated the efficacy of the OnP-BH technique for the surgical treatment of AMI [5].

Between January 1999 and March 2005, 763 patients underwent isolated CABG at our institution. Of these patients, 61 (8%) underwent emergency operations for AMI (STEMI = ST-elevation myocardial infarction). We reviewed these 61 consecutive patients. In the first 23 patients, the conventional cardioplegic method was performed. In the most recent 38 patients, the OnP-BH procedure was used without cardioplegic arrest. The demographic and preoperative patient characteristics of the 2 groups were similar. No significant differences were observed between the groups in terms of age, sex, comorbidities, number of diseased vessels, AMI location, left main trunk lesion, shock, creatinine, and creatinine kinase myocardial band (CK-MB) values. The predicted mortality risk calculated by using EuroSCORE [22] was significantly higher in the OnP-BH CABG group than in the conventional CABG group (9.9 ± 1.6 vs. 9.0 ± 1.6, P = 0.048). The preoperative use of intra-aortic balloon pump (IABP) was also greater in the OnP-BH CABG group (78.9% vs. 43.5%, P = 0.005). These data mean that patients undergoing OnP-BH CABG were in more critical states than the patients undergoing conventional CABG. The time interval from the onset of AMI to CABG was similar (27.0 ± 22.0 vs. 18.3 ± 17.1 hours, P = 0.100).

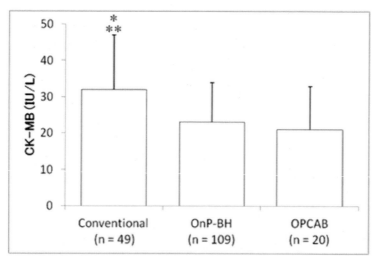

*p<0.0001 Conventional *vs.* OnP-BH, **p=0.005 Conventional *vs.* OPCAB. CK-MB (IU/L) = creatine phosphokinase myocardial band; Conventional = conventional CABG; OnP-BH = on-pump beating-heart CABG; OPCAB = off-pump CABG.

Figure 1. Postoperative maximum creatinine kinase myocardial band (CK-MB) values. Data are given as mean ± standard deviation.

## Table 1. Postoperative variables

| Postoperative variables | Conventional CABG (n=23) | On-pump beating CABG (n=38) | p value |
|---|---|---|---|
| max CK-MB* (mg/dL) | 188±359 | 106±86 | 0.256 |
| Duration of inotropic support* (days) | 5.2±4.3 | 6.1±4.1 | 0.476 |
| Duration of IABP use* (days) | 3.3±2.3 | 2.6±1.4 | 0.269 |
| Time to extubation* (hours) | 91.2±110.4 | 79.2±86.4 | 0.681 |
| Duration of ICU stay* (days) | 7.0±6.6 | 6.0±3.0 | 0.400 |
| Length of hospital stay* (days) | 31.8±19.3 | 29.8±21.0 | 0.715 |
| Graft patency (%) | 95.7 | 98.5 | 0.090 |
| Postoprative renal failure (Cre 2.0<) | 2 | 0 | 0.138 |
| Neurophysiologic complications | 0 | 0 | 1.000 |
| Hospital mortality (%) | 21.7 | 2.6 | 0.046 |

Cre, serum creatinine (mg/dL); IABP, intraaortic balloon pump; CK-MB, creatine phosphokinase myocardial band.
* Mean +/- standard deviation.

The diagnosis of AMI was based on clinical criteria, including electrocardiographic evidence (Q waves and ST-segment elevation) and characteristic increase in serum myocardial enzyme levels (creatine phosphokinase). Details are according to The Japan Adult Cardiovascular Surgery Database (JACVSD) (definitions are available online at http://www.jacvsd.umin.jp). All patients underwent emergency coronary angiography performed preoperatively by a cardiologist. Indications for emergency CABG included the following: patients with a contraindication for thrombolytic therapy, patients with coronary lesions unsuitable for primary PCI (including left main, complicated, and multiple lesions), and cardiogenic shock defined as a systolic blood pressure of less than 80 mm Hg with or without IABP and pressor support, as well as clinical signs of hypoperfusion. The criteria for preoperative insertion of an IABP were as follows: cardiogenic shock or refractory ventricular failure, hemodynamic instability with or without catecholamine, unstable refractory angina, intractable ventricular arrhythmia, and a critical left main stenosis (>70%).

The postoperative patient findings and early outcome data are presented in Table 1. The postoperative maximum CK-MB values in the conventional CABG group were higher than those in the OnP-BH CABG group (188 ± 359 vs. 106 ± 86 IU/L), but the difference was not statistically significant. The duration of inotropic support, duration of IABP use, time to extubation, duration of intensive care unit stay, and length of hospital stay were lower in the OnP-BH CABG group, but these differences did not reach significance. All surviving patients underwent early postoperative coronary angiography during their hospital stays. Graft patency in the OnP-BH CABG group was similar to that of the conventional CABG group (98.5% vs. 95.7%). Postoperative renal failure occurred in 2 patients in the conventional CABG group but in no patients in the OnP-BH CABG group (P = 0.138). These 2 patients required postoperative hemodialysis. No neurophysiologic complications developed in either group. Five hospital deaths occurred in the conventional CABG group (21.7%), whereas only 1 (2.6%) patient died in the OnP-BH CABG group. A significant reduction occurred in the observed mortality between the conventional and OnP-BH CABG groups (21.7% vs. 2.6%, P = 0.04), despite a higher predicted mortality risk calculated by using EuroSCORE (9.0 ± 1.6 vs. 9.6 ± 1.6, P = 0.048) and a greater use of a preoperative IABP (43.5% vs. 78.9%, P = 0.005). Three patients in the conventional CABG group required new insertion of an IABP, whereas no patients required this in the OnP-BH CABG group (P = 0.220).

# Comment

The technique of conventional CABG consists of CPB, aortic cross-clamping, and cardioplegic arrest. CPB itself might induce the systemic inflammatory response [6,7], generate microemboli [23], and cause direct complications of the cannulation site [24]. Many studies have been performed to investigate CPB-induced systemic inflammatory response. Wan et al. [6] demonstrated an isolated effect of CPB by comparing OnP-BH CABG and OPCAB, and reported significant elevation in the levels of interleukin (IL)-6, IL-8, and IL-10 and tumor necrosis factor-$\alpha$ during and immediately after the operations in the OnP-BH CABG group compared to the OPCAB group. No significant difference in clinical outcomes was observed between the two groups. Rastan and coworkers [7] performed a randomized study on patients with normal ventricular function. They examined coronary sinus blood and revealed that OnP-BH CABG causes more myocardial injury than OPCAB. Both these studies concluded that that the adverse effect of conventional CABG is due mainly to aortic cross-clamping and cardioplegic arrest, and not CPB. Conventional CABG offers a motionless and bloodless operative field, which is usually associated with complete revascularization and good graft patency rate.

However, despite improvements in myocardial preservation techniques and the use of cardiac-assist devices such as an IABP, morbidity and mortality are high, especially in very ill patients [18-20].

Resurgence of OPCAB was brought about by the advent of the stabilizers. OPCAB does not require CPB, aortic cross-clamping, or cardioplegic arrest. Advances in devices such as apical suction cardiac positioning devices have rendered it safer to revascularize the circumflex and right coronary arteries. Intravascular shunts facilitate the anastomoses and maintain coronary flow. OPCAB seems to be an ideal procedure, which is thought to eliminate the drawbacks of conventional CABG. Several studies [25-35] including randomized controlled studies [28,29,31,34] and propensity score analyses [30,35] have compared OPCAB and conventional CABG, revealing that the former is safe in selected patients and that it has a short-to-long-term cardiac outcome comparable or superior to that of conventional CABG. Note, however, that some of these studies excluded emergency patients with AMI, left main coronary artery stenosis, reoperation, or major left ventricular hypertrophy or dilatation, which has limited the results.

Over the past decade, controversy has persisted regarding graft patency [26,29,36], completeness of revascularization [30,33,36], incidence of recurrent or residual myocardial ischemia [26,29], and need for reintervention [26,33] following OPCAB. OPCAB is not always associated with complete revascularization, and less complete revascularization and poor graft patency are suspected to be the main causes of a higher incidence of repeat revascularization as compared to conventional CABG. Moreover, OPCAB is sometimes highly challenging and technically more demanding than conventional CABG. Outcomes may thus have been influenced by the surgeon's experience [36]. Puskus [31], who has performed >2500 OPCAB procedures himself, has commented that occasionally, he still encounters something that is new or different. Something unexpected can always occur during an operation, and not everyone is able to reproduce excellent results. Even with the leading experts for OPCAB in Japan, early graft patency without stenosis is inferior to that of with on-pump CABG [34].

OPCAB is associated with an acute conversion risk that causes death and serious complications in the hospital [37-42], which is its most serious drawback. Even recently, a conversion rate of 2.1–12.4% has been reported [28,31,32,36]. In 2008, 1.9% of patients in Japan were converted from OPCAB to on-pump bypass in isolated, primary CABG, and their hospital mortality reached 7.4% [37], which means that when we select OPCAB, 0.14% of patients will die from conversion. This is not negligible. We should not stick to OPCAB when the hemodynamic state is unstable or appears to be worsening. The conversion risks are difficult to quantify precisely [40], although suggested predictors of conversion have included previous CABG, congestive heart failure, a surgeon with insufficient experience, a low ejection fraction, and recent myocardial infarction [38,41,43].

OnP-BH CABG is a novel hybrid technique combining conventional CABG and OPCAB, and advances in OPCAB devices have made it easier to execute. OnP-BH CABG is an attractive technique that maintains a beating heart with the aid of CPB but without aortic cross-clamping or cardioplegic arrest. The avoidance of cardioplegic arrest can eliminate intraoperative global myocardial ischemia, which might contribute to myocardial protection [3]. The beating heart can preserve native coronary blood flow, which might reduce myocardial injury [7]. Another advantage of OnP-BH surgery is that it allows optimal exposure of the coronary arteries [44]. This avoids extreme upward retraction of the heart, especially during revascularization of the circumflex branches, which might contribute to better myocardial protection [44]. For these reasons, this technique may have the potential to compensate partially for the drawbacks of OPCAB. Darwazah et al. [8] have found that the number of grafts performed per patient was significantly higher among patients who underwent OnP-BH CABG compared to those who had OPCAB. As to the number of grafts performed, conflicting results have been obtained, including in our own studies. Some studies have been in favor of OPCAB or conventional bypass over OnP-BH [4,5,7], while others have been in favor of OnP-BH [8,9]. The technique enables even high-risk patients to avoid serious manipulation and allows subsequent complete revascularization [8,10,11].

We do not believe that OPCAB should be used in all patients with AMI. An appropriate circulatory support system should be applied to improve their hemodynamic status and compensate for visceral organ perfusion because most of the patients are hemodynamically unstable and have poor perfusion of their visceral organs. CPB has a preventive role when cardiac arrest or severe hemodynamic alterations occur during surgical intervention [21]. Vassiliades and associates [41] have suggested considering the OnP-BH technique to prevent catastrophic sudden hemodynamic collapse in CABG. Ferrari et al. [13] strongly believe that OnP-BH can lead to acceptable results and that it remains an attractive alternative to conventional CABG and OPCAB. The greatest benefits are the reduction of hemodynamic instability caused by surgical manipulations, absence of global myocardial ischemia, and absence of reperfusion after cardioplegic arrest. CPB can unload the heart and guarantee adequate organ perfusion [7]. We, however, have found no difference in the incidence of renal failure, although OnP-BH CABG seems to cause significantly less renal dysfunction [12]. Since our published study [5], we have treated another 45 patients with AMI (STEMI) and have applied this technique consistently [45]. The results have been excellent, with an overall hospital mortality of 2.2%. The only patient who died had a left main trunk infarction and required percutaneous cardiopulmonary support preoperatively.

Since 2008, in the annual report of the Japanese Association for Thoracic Surgery, OnP-BH CABG has been added to the questionnaire about isolated CABG procedures, in addition to the other two techniques. This means that OnP-BH CABG has become recognized as an independent procedure for isolated CABG. According to the most recent report [37], the proportion of OnP-BH CABG was 10.1%, whereas those of OPCAB and on-pump arrest were 63.2% and 26.7%, respectively. The proportion of OPCAB being performed in Japan is extremely high at over 60% since 2004, as compared to 20% in the United States [31]. Different from other institutes in Japan, adoption of OPCAB is lower in our institute.

A few reports have criticized OnP-BH CABG. Pegg et al. [14] compared OnP-BH CABG to conventional CABG for patients with impaired ventricular function. They estimated ventricular geometry by cardiac magnetic resonance imaging and biochemical markers. They demonstrated that the area under the curve for troponin was higher in OnP-BH CABG than conventional CABG, and that the incidence of new irreversible myocardial injury was significantly higher in OnP-BH CABG than in conventional CABG. Their patients had impaired ventricular function but were not hemodynamically unstable because they were all tolerant of magnetic resonance before surgery. They speculated that the most likely mechanism was inadequate coronary perfusion to distal myocardial territories in patients with severe proximal coronary disease.

Before our methodology for OnP-BH CABG was standardized, we applied LV venting during OnP-BH CABG as well as conventional CABG, as described by our colleague Mizutani [4]. Low cardiac output developed in several cases after bypass grafting. We speculate that excessive decompression of the heart caused a reduction in coronary flow. We have since abandoned LV venting.

One drawback of OnP-BH CABG is the cost increase related to perfusion and disposable devices. Another disadvantage is that it requires manipulation of the ascending aorta for inflow cannula insertion, which might cause atheromatous macroemboli [45]. Femoral cannulation must be considered when atheromatous changes of the ascending aorta exist. We have had one experience of femoral inflow in a patient with AMI.

## Our Strategy for Isolated CABG

As we presented at the 63th Annual Scientific Meeting of the Japanese Association for Thoracic Surgery in 2010, hospital mortality in a recent consecutive series of 482 isolated CABG procedures at our hospital was only 0.2%. The proportion of OnP-BH CABG was 85% (OPCAB and conventional CABG were 11% and 4%, respectively). We have been using OnP-BH CABG for patients with hemodynamic instability or LV dysfunction, as well as in elective surgical patients. During OnP-BH CABG, we have had no experience of hemodynamic collapse or conversion to conventional CABG. At present, conventional CABG is not considered as a procedure for isolated CABG. In fact, no conventional CABG has been performed at our institute since December 2006.

In order to choose the most appropriate surgical strategy we consider hemodynamic status, LV function, elective or emergency surgery, coronary artery anatomy, presence of left main trunk lesion, AMI, and calcification or atheromatous changes of the ascending aorta. If the patients are hemodynamically stable and LV function is good, we can choose OPCAB or OnP-BH CABG according to the surgeon's preference and the demands of the particular situation. In other cases, OnP-BH CABG is considered first, except in patients with aortic problems. Even in such cases, however, femoral or subclavian arterial cannulation can be considered if OnP-BH CABG is necessary.

## Conclusion

OnP-BH CABG is a hybrid technique combining conventional CABG and OPCAB. Even in patients with severe LV dysfunction or hemodynamic instability such as AMI, CPB compensates for hemodynamic instability and provides mechanical support to the systemic circulation, which enables one to perform optimal revascularization. The avoidance of cardioplegic arrest and the absence of reperfusion after cardioplegic arrest can eliminate intraoperative global myocardial ischemia, which might contribute to myocardial protection.

## References

[1] Mehlhorn U, Allen SJ, Adams DL, Davis KL, Gogola GR, Warters RD. Cardiac surgical conditions induced by beta-blockade: effect on myocardial fluid balance. *Ann Thorac Surg* 1996;62:143-150.

[2] Sweeney MS, Frazier OH. Device-supported myocardial revascularization: safe help for sick hearts. *Ann Thorac Surg* 1992;54:1065-1070.

[3] Perrault LP, Menasche P, Peynet J, Faris B, Bel A, de Chaumaray T, Gatecel C, Touchot B, Bloch G, Moalic JM. On-pump, beating-heart coronary artery operations in high-risk patients: an acceptable trade-off? *Ann Thorac Surg* 1997;64:1368-1373.

[4] Mizutani S, Matsuura A, Miyahara K, Eda T, Kawamura A, Yoshioka T, Yoshida K. On-pump beating-heart coronary artery bypass: A propensity matched analysis. *Ann Thorac Surg* 2007;83:1368-1373.

[5] Miyahara K, Matsuura A, Takemura H, Saito S, Sawaki S, Yoshioka T, Ito H. On-pump beating-heart coronary artery bypass grafting after acute myocardial infarction has lower mortality and morbidity. *J Thorac Cardiovasc Surg* 2008;135:521-526.

[6] Wan IY, Arifi AA, Wan S, Yip JH, Sihoe AD, Thung KH, Wong EM, Yim AP. Beating heart revascularization with without cardiopulmonary bypass: evaluation of inflammatory response in a prospective randomized study. *J Thorac Cardiovasc Surg* 2004;127:1624-1631.

[7] Rastan AJ, Bittner HB, Gummert JF, Wather T, Schewick CV, Girdauskas E, Mohr FW. On-pump beating heart versus off-pump coronary artery bypass surgery—evidence of pump-induced myocardial injury. *Eur J Cardiothorac Surg* 2005;27:1057-1064.

[8] Darwazah AK, Bader V, Isleem I, Helwa K. Myocardial revascularization using on-pump beating heart among patients with left ventricular dysfunction. *J Cardiothoracic Surg* 2010;5:109.

[9] Prifti E, Bonacchi M, Giunti G, Proietti P, Leacche M, Salica A, Sani G, Brancaccio G. Does on-pump/beating-heart coronary artery bypass grafting offer better outcome in end-stage coronary artery disease patients? *J Card Surg* 2000;15:403-410.

[10] Gulcan O, Turkoz R, Turkoz A, Caliskan E, Sezgin AT. On-pump/beating-heart myocardial protection for isolated or combined coronary artery bypass grafting in patients with severe left ventricular dysfunction: assessment of myocardial function and clinical outcome. *Heart Surg Forum* 2005;8:E178-E182.

[11] Munos E, Calderon J, Pillois X, Lafitte S, Ouattara A, Labrousse L, Roques X, Barandon L. Beating-heart coronary artery bypass surgery with the help of mini extracorporeal circulation for very high-risk patients. *Perfusion* 2011;26:123-131.

[12] Prifti E, Bonacchi M, Frati G, Giunti G, Proietti P, Leacche M, Massetti M, Babatasi G, Sani G. Beating heart myocardial revascularization on extracorporeal circulation in patients with end-stage coronary artery disease. *Cardiovasc Surg* 2001;9:608-614.

[13] Ferrari E, Stalder N, von Segesser LK. On-pump beating heart coronary surgery for high risk patients requiring emergency multiple coronary artery bypass grafting. *J Cardiothorac Surg* 2008, 3:38.

[14] Pegg TJ, Selvanayegam JB, Francis JM, Karamitsos TD, Maunsell Z, Yu LM, Neubauer S, Taggart DP. Randomized Trial of on-pump Beating heart and conventional cardioplegic arrest in Coronary artery Bypass Surgery patients with impaired left ventricular Function using cardiac Magnetic Resonance Imaging and Biochemical Markers. *Circulation* 2008;118:2130-2138.

[15] Folliguet TA, Philippe F, Larrazet F, Dibie A, Czitrom D, Le Bret E, Bachet J, Laborde F. Beating heart revascularization with minimal extracorporeal circulation in patients with a poor ejection fraction. *Heart Surg Forum* 2002;6:19-23.

[16] Edgerton JR, Herbert MA, Jones KK, Prince SL, Acuff T, Carter D, Dewey T, Magee M, Mack M. On-Pump Beating Heart Surgery Offers an Alternative for Unstable Patients Undergoing Coronary Artery Bypass Grafting. *Heart Surg Forum* 2004;7:8-15.

[17] Eagle KA, Guyton RA, Davidoff R, Edwards FH, Ewy GA, Gardner TJ, Hart JC, Herrmann HC, Hillis LD, Hutter AM Jr, Lytle BW, Marlow RA, Nugent WC, Orszulak TA; American College of Cardiology; American Heart Association. ACC/AHA 2004 guideline update for coronary artery bypass graft surgery: a report of the American College of Cardiology/American Heart Association Task Force on Practice Guidelines (Committee to Update the 1999 Guidelines for Coronary Artery Bypass Graft Surgery). *Circulation* 2004;110:e340-437.

[18] Wasvary H, Shannon F, Bassett J, O'Neill W. Timing of coronary artery bypass grafting after acute myocardial infarction. *Am Surg* 1997;63:710-715.

[19] Kaul TK, Fields BL, Riggins SL, Dacumos GC, Wyatt DA, Jones CR. Coronary artery bypass grafting within 30 days of an acute myocardial infarction. *Ann Thorac Surg* 1995;59:1169-1176.

[20] Quigley RL, Milano CA, Smith LR, White WD, Rankin JS, Glower DD. Prognosis and management of anterolateral myocardial infarction in patients with severe left main disease and cardiogenic shock. The left main shock syndrome. *Circulation* 1993;88(suppl):II65-I170.

[21] Yamagishi I, Sakurada T, Abe T. Emergency coronary artery bypass grafting after acute myocardial infarction. What influences early postoperative mortality? *Ann Thorac Cardiovasc Surg* 1998;4:28-33.

[22] Nashef SA, Roques F, Michel P, Gaducheau E, Lemeshow S, Salamon R. European System for Cardiac Operative Risk Evaluation (EuroSCORE). *Eur J Cardiothorac Surg* 1999;16:9-13.

[23] Diegeler A, Hirsch R, Schneider F, Schilling LO, Falk V, Rauch T, Mohr FW. Neuromonitoring and neurocognitive outcome in off-pump versus conventional coronary bypass operation. *Ann Thorac Surg* 2000;69:1162–1166.

[24] Hartman GS, Yao FS, Bruefach M 3rd, Barbut D, Peterson JC, Purcell MH, Charlson ME, Gold JP, Thomas SJ, Szatrowski TP. Severity of aortic atheromatous disease diagnosed by transesophageal echocardiography predicts stroke and other outcomes associated coronary artery surgery: a prospective study. *Anesth Analg* 1996;83:701-708.

[25] Bull DA, Neumayer LA, Stringham JC, Meldrum P, Affleck DG, Karwande SV. Coronary artery bypass grafting with cardiopulmonary bypass versus off-pump cardiopulmonary bypass grafting: does eliminating the pump reduce morbidity and cost? *Ann Thorac Surg* 2001;71:170-175.

[26] Gundry SR, Romano MA, Shattuck OH, Razzouk AJ, Bailey LL. Seven-year follow-up of coronary artery bypasses performed with and without cardiopulmonary bypass. *J Thorac Cardiovasc Surg* 1998;115:1273-1278.

[27] Mack M, Bachand D, Acuff T, Edgerton J, Prince S, Dewey T, Magee M. Improved outcomes in coronary artery bypass grafting with beating-heart techniques. *J Thorac Cardiovasc Surg* 2002;124:598-607.

[28] van Dijk D, Nierich AP, Jansen EW, Nathoe HM, Suyker WJ, Diephuis JC, van Boven WJ, Borst C, Buskens E, Grobbee DE, Robles De Medina EO, de Jaegere PP; Octopus Study Group. Early outcome after off-pump versus on-pump coronary bypass surgery: results from a randomized study. *Circulation* 2001;104:1761-1766.

[29] Khan NE, De Souza A, Mister R, Flather M, Clague J, Davies S, Collins P, Wang D, Sigwart U, Pepper J. A randomized comparison of off-pump and on-pump multivessel coronary-artery bypass surgery. *N Engl J Med* 2004;350:21-28.

[30] Sabik JF, Gillinov AM, Blackstone EH, Vacha C, Houghtaling PL, Navia J, Smedira NG, McCarthy PM, Cosgrove DM, Lytle BW. Does off-pump coronary surgery reduce morbidity and mortality? *J Thorac Cardiovasc Surg* 2002;124:698-707.

[31] Puskas JD, Williams WH, O'Donnell R, Patterson RE, Sigman SR, Smith AS, Baio KT, Kilgo PD, Guyton RA. Off-pump and on-pump coronary artery bypass grafting are associated with similar graft patency, myocardial ischemia, and freedom from reintervention: long-term follow-up of a randomized trial. *Ann Thorac Surg* 2011;91:1836-1842; discussion 1842-1843.

[32] Landoni G, Pappalardo F, Crescenzi G, Aletti G, Marchetti C, Poli D, Franco A, Rosica C, Zangrillo A. The outcome of patients requiring emergency conversion from off-pump to on-pump coronary artery bypass grafting. *Eur J Anaesthesiol* 2007;24:317-322.

[33] Attaran S, Shaw M, Bond L, Pullan MD, Fabri BM. Does off-pump coronary artery revascularization improve the long-term survival in patients with ventricular dysfunction? *Interact Cardiovasc Thorac Surg* 2010;11:442-446.

[34] Kobayashi J, Tashiro T, Ochi M, Yaku H, Watanabe G, Satoh T, Tagusari O, Nakajima H, Kitamura S; Japanese Off-Pump Coronary Revascularization Investigation (JOCRI)

Study Group. Early outcome of a randomized comparison of off-pump and on-pump multiple arterial coronary revascularization. *Circulation* 2005;112:Suppl:I338-I343.

[35] Kuss O, von Salviati B, Börgermann J. Off-pump versus on-pump coronary artery bypass grafting: a systematic review and meta-analysis of propensity score analyses. *J Thorac Cardiovasc Surg* 2010;140:829-835.

[36] Shroyer AL, Grover FL, Hattler B, Collins JF, McDonald GO, Kozora E, Lucke JC, Baltz JH, Novitzky D; Veterans Affairs Randomized On/Off Bypass (ROOBY) Study Group. On-pump versus off-pump coronary-artery bypass surgery. *N Engl J Med* 2009;361:1827-1837.

[37] Sakata R, Fujii Y, Kuwano H. Thoracic and cardiovascular surgery in Japan during 2008. Annual report by the Japanese Association for Thoracic Surgery. *Gen Thorac Cardiovasc Surg* 2010;58:356-383.

[38] Edgerton JR, Dewey TM, Magee MJ, Herbert MA, Prince SL, Jones KK, Mack MJ. Conversion in off-pump coronary artery bypass grafting: an analysis of predictors and outcomes. *Ann Thorac Surg* 2003;76:1138-1143.

[39] Légaré JF, Buth KJ, Hirsch GM. Conversion to on pump from OPCAB is associated with increased mortality: results from a randomized controlled trial. *Eur J Cardiothorac Surg* 2005;27:296-301.

[40] Reeves BC, Ascione R, Caputo M, Angelini GD. Morbidity and mortality following acute conversion from off-pump to on-pump coronary surgery. *Eur J Cardiothorac Surg* 2006;29:941-947.

[41] Vassiliades TA Jr, Nielsen JL, Lonquist JL. Hemodynamic collapse during off-pump coronary artery bypass grafting. *Ann Thorac Surg* 2002;73:1874-1879.

[42] Ashraf O. Is off-pump therapy really the right choice in urgent coronary grafting? *J Thorac Cardiovasc Surg* 2006;132:211-212.

[43] Soltoski P, Salerno T, Levinsky L, Schmid S, Hasnain S, Diesfeld T, Huang C, Akhter M, Alnoweiser O, Bergsland J. Conversion to cardiopulmonary bypass in off-pump coronary artery bypass grafting: its effect on outcome. *J Card Surg* 1998;13:328-334.

[44] Borowski A, Korb H. Myocardial infarction in coronary bypass surgery using on-pump, beating heart technique with pressure- and volume-controlled coronary perfusion. *J Card Surg* 2002;17:272-278.

[45] Varatharajah K, Rosenfeldt FL. Changes in noninfarcted myocardium explain benefits of on-pump beating-heart coronary artery bypass grafting for acute myocardial infarction. *J Thorac Cardiovasc Surg* 2009;137:1575-1576.

In: Off-Pump Coronary Artery Bypass Grafting
Editors: Shahzad G. Raja and Mohamed Amrani

ISBN: 978-1-62081-549-6
© 2012 Nova Science Publishers, Inc.

*Chapter XIV*

# Anesthesia for Off-pump Coronary Artery Bypass Grafting

*Daniel Bainbridge*
Department of Anesthesia & Perioperative Medicine, Schulich School of Medicine,
University of Western Ontario, London, Ontario, Canada

## Abstract

Off-pump coronary artery bypass (OPCAB) surgery presents unique challenges to the anesthesiologist and the ability to understand both the procedure and its effects on the heart is crucial to being able to provide optimal anesthetic care to the patient and allow for early extubation and rapid recovery after the surgery is completed. OPCAB surgery requires the heart to be positioned in a manner which contributes to hemodynamic instability. In addition, the heart may become ischemic during the procedure because of compromised blood flow through the coronary artery being bypassed. This chapter will highlight the differences between conventional heart surgery and OPCAB surgery. It will focus on the diagnosis and management of hemodynamic changes and ischemia occurring during the procedure. Special mention will be made of techniques to prevent hypothermia, bleeding and rhythm disturbances during OPCAB surgery. In addition to OPCAB surgery, a section will discuss the special OPCAB technique of robotic surgery with or without hybrid revascularization, with special emphasis on techniques for lung isolation and the use of bivalirudin as an alternate anticoagulant. Finally the recovery of OPCAB patients will be reviewed with emphasis on early extubation through the avoidance of common complications such as hypothermia, hemodynamic instability and bleeding.

## Introduction

Anesthesia for off pump coronary artery bypass (OPCAB) grafting at its core is similar to anesthesia for any other cardiac surgical procedure, with the goals of maintaining the patient in an anesthetized state, maintaining stable vital signs by monitoring and treating changes in blood pressure or heart rate, and to provide excellent surgical operating conditions. It relies on close communication between the anesthesiologist and surgeon so that hemodynamic changes can be anticipated. This is crucial as OPCAB surgery presents some very unique challenges for the anesthesiologist, such as maintaining hemodynamic stability with a displaced, ischemic heart which makes providing anesthesia for such cases demanding.

The primary considerations for OPCAB surgery is the maintenance of hemodynamic stability, especially during the suturing of the distal anastomosis. During this time the heart is restrained and ischemia may occur. Monitoring and treating hemodynamic changes while preventing rhythm disturbances, and maintaining normothermia in the presence of an open chest can be difficult. The primary goal is to allow for the rapid recovery of the patient after surgery and thus minimize delays in discharge from both the intensive care unit (ICU) and the hospital.

OPCAB surgery has been likened to fixing a car engine while it is still running, as it provides unique challenges for both surgeon and anesthesiologist. Careful communication and a team approach are essential. This chapter will discuss in detail some of these unique challenges. In addition to conventional OPCAB surgery brief mention will be made of the anesthetic considerations in hybrid robotic procedures.

## Anesthesia for OPCAB Surgery

Anesthetic management of OPCAB patients is similar to conventional heart surgery. An arterial line and central line are placed for monitoring purposes. Five lead electrocardiogram (ECG), pulse oximetry and non invasive blood pressure cuff are all placed for monitoring before during and after surgery. General anesthesia is induced in the usual fashion typically employing a balanced approach using hypnotics (benzodiazepine or propofol), narcotics, and muscle relaxants. A single lumen endotracheal tube is inserted, although robotic procedures require lung isolation and so double lumen tubes are used in these cases. Anesthesia is maintained through the use of inhaled agents and intermittent boluses of narcotics and muscle relaxants as needed. Transesophageal echocardiography is frequently employed as an additional ischemic monitor. Pulmonary artery catheters may be used to monitor pulmonary pressures during the procedure or as a cardiac output monitor during heart displacement usually at the discretion of the anesthesiologist.

The remainder of the anesthetic differs sharply from conventional bypass surgery and these differences will be outlined and discussed in the following section [1].

## Pain Control

Regional analgesic techniques may be employed in OPCAB patients as the risks of epidural hematoma [2,3], which has stirred controversy in conventional CABG surgery, are theoretically reduced in OPCAB surgery owing to the avoidance of cardiopulmonary bypass (CPB). Popular techniques include thoracic epidural analgesia, or intrathecal morphine. Both are usually performed prior to induction to decrease the risk of nerve injury. While pain from OPCAB surgery is the same as from conventional techniques, there is sometimes a patient expectation that recovery will be faster and pain reduced by choosing 'less invasive' techniques. The benefit from regional anesthesia for OPCAB surgery are mainly seen in reductions in pain scores [4], although there may be improvements in pulmonary function [5,6] and reductions in perioperative arrhythmias [7]. However the risk/benefit profile of regional anesthesia has not been fully quantified and many centers employ similar post operative analgesic regimens to conventional heart surgery. There are now numerous reports of performing 'awake' OPCAB using thoracic epidural anesthesia. The benefit of performing the surgery awake (usually with sedation and sometimes non-invasive ventilation) is not clear [8,9]. Overall, there are too few studies with too few patients to adequately quantify the risks and benefits of regional anesthesia for OPCAB surgery. There is currently no evidence for benefit in awake OPCAB surgery.

## Hemodynamic Considerations

OPCAB surgery is associated with significant and rapid hemodynamic changes owing to the positioning of the heart and the use of stabilization devices to permit performance of the distal anastomosis. Also, vessel occlusion, required to perform the distal anastomosis, may induce ischemia which further impairs hemodynamic stability and may induce not only hypotension but arrhythmias.

The two different immobilization device groups: those which suspend the heart (Octopus, Medtronic) and those which compress the heart (CoroNeo retractors, CoroNeo Inc, Montreal) produce different hemodynamic changes. In addition, the use of intracoronary shunts, and location of the target vessel (left anterior descending [LAD], circumflex or right coronary artery), induce different degrees of hemodynamic compromise (Table 1). The degree of hemodynamic change has been extensively studied [10-17]. Consistently OPCAB is associated with reductions in systemic pressures, and increases in pulmonary and central venous pressures and a decrease in cardiac output. This is a result of reductions in ventricular compliance especially on the right side of the heart. The smaller chamber sizes can be seen on transesophageal echocardiography (TEE). Most studies which examined the hemodynamic effects of heart positioning placed patients in Trendelenberg position, and employed inotropes, accounting for the consistent decrease in MAP of only 1-15%. This intervention may have underestimated the full effect of heart positioning on hemodynamic changes.

As seen in Table 1, the greatest hemodynamic changes are typically seen during grafting of the circumflex coronary artery, as the heart is twisted and displaced laterally putting the greatest pressure on the right ventricle. Grafting of the left anterior descending and right coronary artery (posterior descending artery) resulted in the least amount of hemodynamic compromise. Again evidence for impaired ventricular compliance, especially on the right side, is supported by studies in which hemodynamic changes have been reversed by the use of right heart assist devices. The right ventricle is sensitive to externally applied forces owing to its thin wall and low internal pressures. Interestingly, patients with poor ejection fractions appear to tolerate heart positioning as well as patientswith normal ejection fractions [18], which again supports RV impairment as the main mechanism of the hemodynamic changes [19].

Table 1. Degree of hemodynamic compromise during grafting of the three target territories

**LAD Anastomosis**

|   | BP | PAP | PCWP | CVP | CO |
|---|---|---|---|---|---|
| Suction | ↓ 5% | ↑ 30% | ↑ 30% | ↑ 20% | ↓ 5% |
| Compression | ↓ 7% | ↑ 20% | ↑ 5% | ↔ | ↓ 10% |

**Circumflex**

|   | BP | PAP | PCWP | CVP | CO |
|---|---|---|---|---|---|
| Suction | ↓ 5% | ↔ | ↑ 40% | ↑ 30% | ↓ 15% |
| Compression | ↓ 10% | ↑ 15% | 13 | 18 | ↓ 15% |

**Posterior Descending Anastomosis**

|   | BP | PAP | PCWP | CVP | CO |
|---|---|---|---|---|---|
| Suction | ↔ | ↑ 5% | ↑ 30% | ↑ 40% | ↓ 5% |
| Compression | ↓ 10% | ↑ 10% | ↑ 10% | ↑ 10% | ↓ 10% |

BP- Systemic blood pressure, PAP- Pulomonary artery pressure, PCWP- Pulmonary capillary wedge pressure, CVP-central venous pressure, CO- cardiac output.

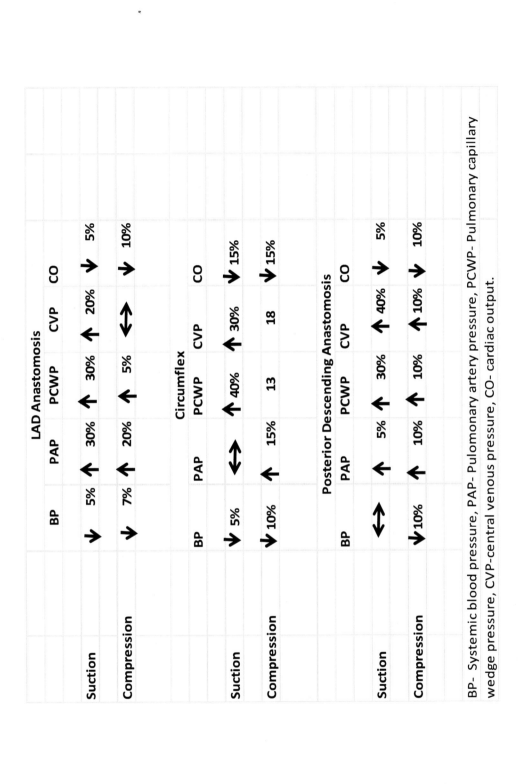

BP- Systemic blood pressure, PAP- Pulmonary artery pressure, PCWP- Pulmonary capillary wedge pressure, CVP-central venous pressure, CO- cardiac output.

The hemodynamic changes that occur with displacement and stabilization of the heart often occur within seconds and stabilize after 5 minutes, so that late hemodynamic changes as a result of positioning tend not to occur [14] If hemodynamic changes persist or are unresponsive to treatment, ischemia may be the cause and careful examination of the heart on TEE and ST segments on ECG should be made.

## Management of Hemodynamic Changes

One of the keys to management of hemodynamic changes as a result of positioning is to communicate with the surgeon and anticipate heart displacement. If the patient does not tolerate the change then the heart can be returned to its resting position and inotropes or volume given to increase the blood pressure before attempting to reposition the heart. Patience and persistence is often rewarded in OPCAB surgery. Other options for the treatment of hemodynamic changes should consist of increasing venous return to the heart and increasing systemic vascular resistance to maintain arterial pressures. Venous return can be increased quickly by the use of the Trendelenberg position (20-30° head down). Volume loading using 500-1000 ml of crystalloid or colloid, with target CVP's of 10-12 in the supine patient can also be used. An additional advantage of the Trendelenberg position is that it can improve surgical exposure during the grafting of the posterior descending artery. If these measures are insufficient to maintain MAP's within 10-20% of baseline then the addition of inotropes/vasopressors may be tried. Levophed is commonly used as it can increase systemic vascular resistance while maintaining cardiac output. However, phenylephrine, epinephrine or dopamine can be used. Usually this is sufficient to maintain hemodynamic stability (Table 2). During this time monitoring of cardiac output either directly (pulmonary artery catheter or TEE) or indirectly with urine output should be undertaken to ensure adequate tissue perfusion. Serial arterial blood gases are often also helpful to ensure that the serum lactate is not increasing.

If hemodynamic deterioration persists after positioning, then a cause must be sought. Ischemia is the most likely cause and can reduce cardiac contractility. New onset ST segment changes or new onset wall motion abnormalities on TEE should raise the suspicion of ischemia. This may be treated by inserting a shunt into the vessel being grafted if a shunt was not previously placed or by attempting to improve blood flow and reduce myocardial oxygen consumption by increasing MAP and lowering heart rate. Nitroglycerin may also be beneficial (Table 3).

If hemodynamic deterioration persists then an incision in the right pericardium/pleura will allow the right heart to 'herniate' slightly into the right chest cavity, alleviating compression on the right heart and allowing an increase in filling.

## Assist Devices for Hemodynamic Support

While the main goal of OPCAB surgery is to avoid conventional CPB, the use of right heart assist devices has been explored as a 'bridge' or hybrid technique between conventional cardiac surgery and pure OPCAB techniques. Right heart bypass does not require an oxygenator, avoids cannulation of the aorta (and therefore cerebral emboli) and should support the right heart, which is the main ventricle affected by positioning during OPCAB. Several studies have examined the use of right heart support devices during OPCAB and shown minimal hemodynamic changes with positioning with these devices [20-24].

Intra-aortic balloon pumps (IABP) have also been inserted in patients undergoing OPCAB surgery in order to either reduce hemodynamic changes or reduce ischemic episodes during OPCAB surgery [25-27]. IABP devices are commonly used in patients with left main disease as a method of reducing ischemia during grafting. Some investigators have also placed the devices in patients with poor ejection fractions. These devices are usually placed prior to positioning for OPCAB surgery, in anticipation of hemodynamic or ischemic changes, however they may be considered if recurrent instability occurs despite multiple attempts at positioning the heart, or to treat refractory ischemia.

**Table 2. Management of intraoperative hypotension during off-pump coronary artery bypass grafting**

| Treatment of Hypotension |
|---|
| Trendelenberg Position |
| Volume loading 4-5 ml/kg |
| Inotropes |
|    Levophed |
|    Dopamine |
|    Epinephrine |
|    Phenylephrine |
| Rule out ischemia |
| Rule out mitral regurgitation |

**Table 3. Management of intraoperative ischemia during off-pump coronary artery bypass grafting**

| Management of Ischemia |
|---|
| Increase Oxygen Supply |
|    Increase blood pressure (increase preload) |
|    Insert coronary shunt |
|    Coronary vasodilators |
|    Treat anemia |
| Reduce Oxygen Demand |
|    Decrease heart rate (treat tachycardia) |
|    Decrease contractility |
| Consider IABP |

IABP = intra-aortic balloon pump.

## Monitoring

Routine monitoring is similar in OPCAB surgery as conventional bypass surgery. A comprehensive pre- and post operative TEE examination should be performed in any patient who has a TEE inserted. Although the aorta is spared cannulation, examination of the aorta for plaque using TEE is important as OPCAB surgery does not preclude, and in fact makes possible, a no touch aortic technique using either all arterial grafts or sequential grafting. This should be considered in patients with significant plaque in the ascending aorta or in patients who have heavily calcified or 'porcelain' aortas. Intermittent examination of the heart should also be performed during the procedure. While transgastric images are often lost during cardiac positioning, the long axis transesophageal images are maintained and information about wall motion function (for ischemia monitoring) and global LV and RV function (to estimate cardiac output) are easily obtained.

The main concern in OPCAB surgery is cardiac ischemia, especially during positioning and distal anastomosis therefore the main goal of intraoperative monitoring is to detect ischemic changes early before they become hemodynamically significant and to look for the possible causes of hemodynamic instability which fails to adequately respond to either fluid loading or inotropes.

Ischemia monitoring, as in conventional bypass, is done using the ECG and TEE.

Neither ECG nor TEE is 100% specific for ischemia during OPCAB surgery and heart positioning with a stabilizer can lead to false positives [28]. Usually, some degree of new onset ST segment elevation or depression occurs during positioning and anastomosis. The ECG axes and voltages may also change during cardiac manipulation which may make ST segment interpretation difficult.

On TEE, wall motion abnormalities are induced by the stabilizer itself. In addition to false positives, false negatives are also possible as positioning may result in areas of myocardium which are poorly visualized on TEE and the elevation of the heart out of the chest may reduce voltages on the ECG to such an extent that interpretation is not possible. Ischemia should be suspected if new and persistent ST segment elevation occurs, or if new persistent wall motion abnormalities occur.

Another common cause of hemodynamic instability during OPCAB surgery is new or worsening mitral regurgitation which may be evident on TEE and can be secondary to either positioning itself (resulting in the distortion of the valve) or ischemia of one of the papillary muscles resulting in restricted leaflet motion [29,30].

This is often suspected when positioning results in a greater decrease in blood pressure than expected or a dramatic rise in pulmonary pressures. It is always wise to examine the mitral valve following any cardiac position change.

If the cause of the mitral regurgitation is secondary to cardiac positioning then often small changes in the heart/stabilizer position can result in dramatic decreases in the amount of MR. However, if the MR is caused by ischemia, then this needs to be aggressively treated, as the hemodynamic changes caused by the MR may dramatically worsen the ischemia and further exacerbate instability which may require conversion to CPB.

## Arrhythmias

Bradycardia often occurs during RCA grafting a result of ischemia to the SA or AV nodes. It seems to occur most frequently during anastomosis of a low grade lesion (<70% occlusion) likely because low grade lesions rarely have collateral circulation. Bradycardia is readily apparent on ECG, is easy to anticipate, based on lesion anatomy and site of grafting, and is easily treatable with ventricular pacing. Many surgeons will place pacemaker leads prior to distal RCA grafting to minimize hemodynamic compromise if heart block should occur.

Tachyarrythmias including atrial fibrillation and ventricular tachycardia may also occur due to either directly mechanical stimulation or induced by ischemia. Again ischemia should be aggressively treated. The use of amiodarone, magnesium or the treatment of low serum potassium levels may reduce the frequency or rate of tachyarrythmias in the irritable heart. External or internal defibrillator paddles should be immediately available if the rhythm becomes unstable.

## Conversion to Conventional Bypass Grafting

One of the most feared complications of OPCAB surgery is rapid decompensation requiring emergency cardiopulmonary bypass. Patients who are emergently converted to CPB have more complications and a worse outcome than either patients who successfully undergo either OPCAB or conventional bypass surgery Studies suggest that compared to OPCAB surgery, mortality rates are increased 2-6 times [31,32]. The causes for the increased mortality are unclear and may be related to patient or procedural factors. For this reason both surgeon and anesthesiologists should be ready to emergently convert to conventional bypass surgery. This decision should be made in a timely and controlled fashion whenever possible to reduce the insult caused by hypotension or ischemia. Blood gas analysis should be performed soon after initiation of CPB and any abnormalities corrected. Finally, weaning from bypass may be more difficult owing to stunned myocardium and this should be anticipated before coming off.

## Anticoagulation Management

Management of anticoagulation during OPCAB surgery is varied, and very little consensus exists on optimum strategies, which reflects a paucity of evidence in the current literature [33]. Heparin is the most common anticoagulant used during OPCAB surgery although, patients with for example heparin-induced thrombocytopenia and thrombosis (HITT) are often selected to undergo OPCAB surgery so that heparin can be avoided and in these cases bivalirudin is often the most frequent alternative [34,35]. The ideal activated clotting time (ACT) target when using heparin is also varied, with some institutions using half dose heparin with target ACTs in the 250 second range to full dose heparin with targets over 400 seconds. The main advantage of lowering the heparin dose is the theoretical reduction in bleeding post-operatively. The advantage of using high dose heparin is the ability to convert to on pump bypass immediately, if needed.

Literature from cardiac catheterization procedures suggests, in the absence of clopidogrel or glycoprotein IIb/IIIa inhibitors, that a target ACT of 375 seconds results in the greatest benefit from ischemic complications [36,37]. However, with the use of clopidogrel and/or glycoprotein IIb/IIIa inhibitors the degree of anticoagulation over 200 seconds had little impact on ischemic events and resulted in greater bleeding [38]. The former trials involved primarily balloon angioplasty, while the later trials involved primarily stenting. Based on the available information it can be inferred that for OPCAB an ACT in the range of 300-400 seconds should be targeted in patients who have had clopidogrel/aspirin stopped for 3-5 days. While patients still taking anti-platelet agents may toleratelower target ACTs.

While there has been concern that patients become hypercoagulable following OPCAB surgery there is no evidence for this [39]. In addition, incomplete protamine reversal can lead to increased blood loss and so complete reversal of heparin with protamine should be the aim, with the return of ACTs to baseline [40].

## Temperature Management

One often overlooked aspect of anesthesia for OPCAB surgery is maintenance of normothermia. Hypothermia can contribute to reductions in blood pressure and cardiac output making the maintenance of hemodynamic changes more complex. It may also contribute to a coagulopathy, which will increase blood loss. It impairs cognitive and respiratory function and so may prolong recovery from anesthesia and delay extubation and discharge from the ICU. Hypothermia is caused by many factors including a cold room/operating table, an exposed patient with an open chest, the use of cold intravenous (iv) fluids and the use of cold irrigation solutions. Maintaining normothermia in OPCAB patients is made more challenging by the need to keep at least one leg, both groins and the chest exposed which limits patient access and the ability to place forced air warming blankets. Typically a fluid warmer is used to ensure iv fluids are over $35^{\circ}C$ [41]. This is especially important if volume boluses are used. The use of a forced air warming blanket or more frequently two, one over the head and one over the lower body/undraped leg, aid in maintaining normothermia. Novel techniques and devices have also been shown to be effective [42-44]. Finally, if these fail then increasing the temperature of the room or the use of full body forced air warmers in ICU may be necessary to quickly rewarm the patient.

## Blood Conservation

One consistent advantage of OPCAB surgery over conventional bypass grafting is the reductions in blood product utilization. This is likely the result of avoiding CPB which causes hemodilution and greater blood loss. However, techniques can be employed to further limit blood loss during OPCAB surgery and these include the use of cell savers and antifibrinolytics.

Cell saver can be used throughout surgery to collect and process shed blood in the surgical field. It may be most beneficial on small patients, those with anemia, and those with known preexisting bleeding disorders (eg. preoperative clopidogrel use). Unlike conventional bypass, where cardiotomy suction can be used instead of cell saver, there is no disadvantage to using cell saver during surgery, however, if large quantities of blood are processed fresh frozen plasma may be required to replace lost coagulation factors discarded during cell saver blood processing [45-47].

Antifibrinolytics can be used for OPCAB surgery, although there has been concern that there use will result in an increase in thrombotic events, current trials do not support this [48,49]. Tranexamic acid has been shown to effectively reduce chest tube loss and transfusion rates in patients undergoing OPCAB surgery [48]. Most trials used a 1 gram loading dose followed by 200-400 mg/h as an infusion. The overall effect was a 50% reduction in chest tube drainage, the effect being consistent with or without the use of cell salvage devices.

## Robotic Surgery and Hybrid Procedures

### Anesthetic Considerations

There are two primary differences between robotic surgery with or without hybrid revascularization and conventional OPCAB surgery. The first is the use of one lung anesthesia and the second is the use of bivalirudin and clopidogrel as anticoagulants in hybrid surgery instead of heparin [50].

### One Lung Anesthesia

While one lung anesthesia (OLA) is easy to institute, there are some particular considerations during robotic or robotic hybrid procedures compared to thoracic surgery. There are three potential techniques to isolate lung ventilation. Double lumen tubes (DLT) are the gold standard for OLA and work well in robotic procedures. They are the most frequently used device, with a left sided DLT being placed in most patients. Following lung isolation CPAP of 10-13 cm $H_2O$ is created in the left pleura to permit access to the left internal mammary artery. This often aids lung collapse and shunts blood to the ventilated lung. In addition, ultra fast track management is possible with robotic procedures so the patient can be extubated in the operating room which avoids the need to replace the double lumen tube with a single lumen tube for long term ventilation in the ICU. If the patient is not a candidate for ultra fast track management (bleeding, hypothermia, hemodynamic instability), the tube should be exchanged for a single lumen endotracheal tube as it is better tolerated for ventilatory weaning. Univent tubes or bronchial blockers may also be used to provide OLA and offer an alternative to DLT. As the left lung needs to be blocked, Univent tubes may be difficult to place. The bronchial blocker can be guided using fiberoptic bronchscopy, so it is easier to place but more expensive Both alternatives do not require the tube to be exchanged following surgery and so are better suited to patients who may require ICU ventilation.

Pulmonary artery pressures should be monitored during OLA as increases may be dramatic owing to one lung anesthesia and the tension pneumothorax created in the left hemithorax. Elevated PA pressures are one of the main reasons for conversions to sternotomy during this procedure. Management of pulmonary hypertension includes the use of nitroglycerin, deepening anesthesia, milrinone, and avoiding hypoxemia and acidosis. Reducing intrathoracic insufflation pressures may also help.

# Anticoagulation

For hybrid cases in which a stent is deployed the lack of anti-platelet agents has led to a concern over the use of heparin as sole anticoagulant during stent deployment. Studies using bivalirudin suggest it is as effective as heparin plus glycoprotein IIb/IIIa inhibitors and so bivalirudin has been used as sole anticoagulant during both robotic OPCAB internal mammary artery to left anterior descending artery anastomosis and for subsequent stent deployment. Bivalirudin is a 20 amino acid synthetic peptide direct thrombin inhibitor. Bivalirudin is active against both unbound and clot bound thrombin which may be why it is more efficacious in coronary stent insertions. The binding of bivalirudin to thrombin is reversible and has a half life of 30 minutes. Elimination is through kidney filtration, however no dosage adjustment is necessary in patients with a creatinine clearance greater than 60 ml/min. Another method of elimination is the degradation of bivalirudin by thrombin, so blood, isolated in a cardiotomy reservoir for example, will eventually show clot formation. The dose of bivalirudin is 1.75 mg/kg bolus followed by a continuous infusion of bivalirudin at 0.75 mg/kg/hr. An ACT should be done every 15-20 minutes during the infusion. The bivalirudin infusion is started prior to the occlusion of the internal mammary artery and continued until stent deployment, to minimize the risk of acute graft or stent thrombosis. Bivalirudin has been used successfully as an anticoagulant during OPCAB surgery. Several trials have investigated the safety and efficacy of bivalirudin use during OPCAB surgery. The largest of these trials, the EVOLUTION-OFF study enrolled a total of 156 patients [34]. There was no difference in the clinical endpoints but there was a statistically significant increase in incidence of stroke in the heparin arm. A smaller study in 100 patients showed no difference in bleeding rates or other clinical outcomes in those who received heparin compared to those who did not [35]. The primary limitation in the use of bivalirudin is that ACT measurements may not correlate to the degree of anticoagulation [51].

The use of bivalirudin in percutaneous coronary procedures has gained widespread acceptance following the publication of several trials which suggest the superiority of bivalirudin over heparin. The largest of these was the REPLACE-2 trial which compared bivalirudin with provisional GPIIb/IIIa inhibitors (7% of patients received GPIIb/IIIa) versus heparin and GPIIb/IIIa inhibitors in 6010 patients undergoing PCI. While the study showed the non-inferiority of bivalirudin for important clinical events, the bivalirudin group also had less bleeding and was more cost effective [52].

In addition to the use of bivalirudin during bypass, patients also receive clopidogrel 300 mg per NG tube after stent deployment. Clopidogrel reduces stent thrombosis following PCI.

A meta-analysis of trials comparing aspirin alone vs aspirin and ticlopidine demonstrated an OR of 0.23 ( 95% CI 0.11–0.49, $P=0.0001$) for death or myocardial infarction following stenting favoring the use of ticlopidine [53]. The benefits of clopidogrel occur early after stenting, within two hours, suggesting that early administration is beneficial [54]. However, there is a recognized risk of major bleeding with the use of multiple antiplatelett agents therefore the initiation of clopidogrel should be delayed until several hours after surgery [55].

## Early Extubation and fast Track Management

OPCAB surgical patients are often ideal candidates for fast track programs and can be rapidly extubated following surgery. Some centers have even proposed an ultrafast track program in which OPCAB patients are extubated immediately after the surgical procedure, within the operating room [56-58]. The common factors that prevent early extubation include ongoing bleeding, hemodynamic instability, worsening metabolic acidosis, and hypothermia.

Bleeding issues are usually minor, as CPB is avoided, and most studies suggest blood loss is lower with OPCAB surgery [59]. A repeat ACT should be checked to ensure adequate reversal of heparin. The chest should be explored to ensure there are no bleeding sites. If bleeding is brisk then coagulation studies (INR, PTT, platelet count) should be sent. The patient's temperature should be checked as a coagulopathy secondary to hypothermia is also common. Hemodynamic instability occurs post surgery due either to ongoing ischemia, myocardial stunning or hypovolemia. Repeat TEE assessment with the heart in anatomical position can often help with diagnosing the cause of instability. Ensuring the patient is not anemic or acidotic is also important. If acidosis is present then signs of poor cardiac output should be elicited and the causes treated. Sometimes epinephrine infusions themselves will contribute to a metabolic acidosis and this drug should be discontinued if it is felt to be the cause. Patients with temperatures less than $36°C$ should remain intubated as hypothermia can impair both mentation and respiration both directly and through its effect on anesthetic drug clearance. It is best to take these patients directly to the ICU or recovery area intubated and rewarm them using full body forced air warmers. When the temperature rises above $36°C$ they can be extubated.

The management of these patients upon arrival in the ICU is essentially the same as for conventional bypass patients. Routine blood tests and chest X-Ray are performed on admission. The patient is monitored during their stay and extubated and eventually discharged as they meet criteria. OPCAB patients often require more fluid in the ICU owing to the lack of pump prime and mediastinal salvage that occurs in conventional bypass cases.

The use of ultra fast track approach has resulted in some institutions bypassing ICU entirely and sending patients to a recovery room and then up to the general ward. This approach should be individualized to the patient and the disposition determined at the end of the procedure with the ability to transfer to an ICU bed if complications arise.

## Conclusion

Anesthesia for OPCAB surgery is challenging to the anesthesiologist and requires an in depth understanding of the procedure and the complications associated with heart positioning. While the number of OPCAB cases being performed has fluctuated over the last 10 years it appears that there are certainly patients that benefit from such approaches. Hence, OPCAB surgery offers a useful alternative approach to revascularization in these patients. At the same time as the surgical procedures becomes less invasive the anesthetic required is becoming ever more demanding.

# References

[1] Bainbridge D, Cheng DC. Minimally invasive direct coronary artery bypass and off-pump coronary artery bypass surgery: anesthetic considerations. *Anesthesiol Clin* 2008;26:437-52.

[2] Rosen DA, Hawkinberry DW, 2nd, Rosen KR, Gustafson RA, Hogg JP, Broadman LM. An epidural hematoma in an adolescent patient after cardiac surgery. *Anesth Analg* 2004; 98:966-9.

[3] Ho AM, Chung DC, Joynt GM. Neuraxial blockade and hematoma in cardiac surgery: estimating the risk of a rare adverse event that has not (yet) occurred. *Chest* 2000;117:551-5.

[4] Caputo M, Alwair H, Rogers CA, et al. Thoracic epidural anesthesia improves early outcomes in patients undergoing off-pump coronary artery bypass surgery: a prospective, randomized, controlled trial. *Anesthesiology* 2011;114:380-90.

[5] Mehta Y, Vats M, Sharma M, Arora R, Trehan N. Thoracic epidural analgesia for off-pump coronary artery bypass surgery in patients with chronic obstructive pulmonary disease. *Ann Card Anaesth* 2010; 13: 224-30.

[6] Suryaprakash S, Chakravarthy M, Gautam M, et al. Effect of thoracic epidural anesthesia on oxygen delivery and utilization in cardiac surgical patients scheduled to undergo off-pump coronary artery bypass surgery: A prospective study. *Ann Card Anaesth* 2010;14:192-6.

[7] Bakhtiary F, Therapidis P, Dzemali O, et al. Impact of high thoracic epidural anesthesia on incidence of perioperative atrial fibrillation in off-pump coronary bypass grafting: a prospective randomized study. *J Thorac Cardiovasc Surg* 2007;134:460-4.

[8] Watanabe G, Tomita S, Yamaguchi S, Yashiki N. Awake coronary artery bypass grafting under thoracic epidural anesthesia: great impact on off-pump coronary revascularization and fast-track recovery. *Eur J Cardiothorac Surg* 2011;40788-93.

[9] Noiseux N, Prieto I, Bracco D, Basile F, Hemmerling T. Coronary artery bypass grafting in the awake patient combining high thoracic epidural and femoral nerve block: first series of 15 patients. *Br J Anaesth* 2008;100:184-9.

[10] Kwak YL, Oh YJ, Jung SM, Yoo KJ, Lee JH, Hong YW. Change in right ventricular function during off-pump coronary artery bypass graft surgery. *Eur J Cardiothorac Surg* 2004;25:572-7.

[11] Watters MP, Ascione R, Ryder IG, Ciulli F, Pitsis AA, Angelini GD. Haemodynamic changes during beating heart coronary surgery with the 'Bristol Technique'. *Eur J Cardiothorac Surg* 2001;19:34-40.

[12] Mueller XM, Chassot PG, Zhou J, et al. Hemodynamics optimization during off-pump coronary artery bypass: the 'no compression' technique. *Eur J Cardiothorac Surg* 2002;22:249-54.

[13] Do QB, Goyer C, Chavanon O, Couture P, Denault A, Cartier R. Hemodynamic changes during off-pump CABG surgery. *Eur J Cardiothorac Surg* 2002;21:385-90.

[14] Shinn HK, Oh YJ, Kim SH, Lee JH, Lee CS, Kwak YL. Evaluation of serial haemodynamic changes during coronary artery anastomoses in patients undergoing off-pump coronary artery bypass graft surgery: initial experiences using two deep pericardial stay sutures and octopus tissue stabilizer. *Eur J Cardiothorac Surg* 2004;25:978-84.

[15] Nierich AP, Diephuis J, Jansen EW, Borst C, Knape JT. Heart displacement during off-pump CABG: how well is it tolerated? *Ann Thorac Surg* 2000;70:466-72.

[16] Eldrup N, Rasmussen NH, Yndgaard S, Bigler D, Berthelsen PG. Impact of off-pump coronary artery surgery on myocardial performance and beta-adrenoceptor function. *J Cardiothorac Vasc Anesth* 2001;15:428-32.

[17] Mathison M, Edgerton JR, Horswell JL, Akin JJ, Mack MJ. Analysis of hemodynamic changes during beating heart surgical procedures. *Ann Thorac Surg* 2000;70:1355-60.

[18] Fiore G, Latrofa ME, Tunzi P, et al. Hemodynamics in off-pump surgery: normal versus compromised preoperative left ventricular function. *Eur J Cardiothorac Surg* 2005;27:488-93.

[19] Couture P, Denault A, Limoges P, Sheridan P, Babin D, Cartier R. Mechanisms of hemodynamic changes during off-pump coronary artery bypass surgery. *Can J Anaesth* 2002;49:835-49.

[20] Sharony R, Autschbach R, Porat E, et al. Right heart support during off-pump coronary artery bypass surgery--a multi-center study. *Heart Surg Forum* 2002;5:13-6.

[21] Livi U, Gelsomino S, Da Col P, et al. The A-Med right heart support for off-pump coronary artery bypass grafting. *Ital Heart J* 2001;2:502-6.

[22] Mathison M, Buffolo E, Jatene AD, Jatene FB, Reichenspurner H, Matheny RG, Shennib H, Akin JJ, Mack MJ: Right heart circulatory support facilities coronary artery bypass without cardiopulmonary bypass. *Ann Thorac Surg* 2000;70:1083-5.

[23] Lundell DC, Crouch JD. A miniature right heart support system improves cardiac output and stroke volume during beating heart posterior/lateral coronary artery bypass grafting. *Heart Surg Forum* 2003;6:302-6.

[24] Lima LE, Jatene F, Buffolo E, et al. A multicenter initial clinical experience with right heart support and beating heart coronary surgery. *Heart Surg Forum* 2001;4:60-4.

[25] Vohra HA, Dimitri WR. Elective intraaortic balloon counterpulsation in high-risk off-pump coronary artery bypass grafting. *J Card Surg* 2006;21:1-5.

[26] Vohra HA, Briffa NP. Routine preoperative insertion of IABP in high-risk off-pump coronary artery bypass grafting. *Heart Surg Forum* 2005;8:E94-5.

[27] Kim KB, Lim C, Ahn H, Yang JK. Intraaortic balloon pump therapy facilitates posterior vessel off-pump coronary artery bypass grafting in high-risk patients. *Ann Thorac Surg* 2001;71:1964-8.

[28] Shiga T, Terajima K, Matsumura J, et al. Local cardiac wall stabilization influences the reproducibility of regional wall motion during off-pump coronary artery pass surgery. *J Clin Monit Comput* 2000;16:25-31.

[29] George SJ, Al-Ruzzeh S, Amrani M. Mitral annulus distortion during beating heart surgery: a potential cause for hemodynamic disturbance--a three-dimensional echocardiography reconstruction study. *Ann Thorac Surg* 2002;73:1424-30.

[30] Kinjo S, Tokumine J, Sugahara K, et al. Unexpected hemodynamic deterioration and mitral regurgitation due to a tissue stabilizer during left anterior descending coronary anastomosis in off-pump coronary artery bypass graft surgery. *Ann Thorac Cardiovasc Surg* 2005;11:324-8.

[31] Patel NC, Patel NU, Loulmet DF, McCabe JC, Subramanian VA. Emergency conversion to cardiopulmonary bypass during attempted off-pump revascularization results in increased morbidity and mortality. *J Thorac Cardiovasc Surg* 2004;128:655-61.

[32] Landoni G, Pappalardo F, Crescenzi G, Aletti G, Marchetti C, Poli D, Franco A, Rosica C, Zangrillo A: The outcome of patients requiring emergency conversion from off-pump to on-pump coronary artery bypass grafting. *Eur J Anaesthesiol* 2007;24:317-22.

[33] Englberger L, Streich M, Tevaearai H, Carrel TP. Different anticoagulation strategies in off-pump coronary artery bypass operations: a European survey. *Interact Cardiovasc Thorac Surg* 2008;7:378-82.

[34] Smedira NG, Dyke CM, Koster A, et al. Anticoagulation with bivalirudin for off-pump coronary artery bypass grafting: the results of the EVOLUTION-OFF study. *J Thorac Cardiovasc Surg* 2006;131:686-92.

[35] Merry AF, Raudkivi PJ, Middleton NG, et al. Bivalirudin versus heparin and protamine in off-pump coronary artery bypass surgery. *Ann Thorac Surg* 2004;77:925-31.

[36] Montalescot G, Cohen M, Salette G, et al. Impact of anticoagulation levels on outcomes in patients undergoing elective percutaneous coronary intervention: insights from the STEEPLE trial. *Eur Heart J* 2008;29:462-71.

[37] Chew DP, Bhatt DL, Lincoff AM, et al. Defining the optimal activated clotting time during percutaneous coronary intervention: aggregate results from 6 randomized, controlled trials. *Circulation* 2001;103:961-6.

[38] Brener SJ, Moliterno DJ, Lincoff AM, et al. Relationship between activated clotting time and ischemic or hemorrhagic complications: analysis of 4 recent randomized clinical trials of percutaneous coronary intervention. *Circulation* 2004;110:994-8.

[39] Tanaka KA, Thourani VH, Williams WH, et al. Heparin anticoagulation in patients undergoing off-pump and on-pump coronary bypass surgery. *J Anesth* 2007;21:297-303.

[40] Gatti G, Pugliese P. Heparin reversal in off-pump coronary artery bypass surgery: complete, partial, or no reversal? *Cardiovasc Surg* 2002;10:245-50.

[41] Jeong SM, Hahm KD, Jeong YB, Yang HS, Choi IC. Warming of intravenous fluids prevents hypothermia during off-pump coronary artery bypass graft surgery. *J Cardiothorac Vasc Anesth* 2008;22:67-70.

[42] Calcaterra D, Ricci M, Lombardi P, Katariya K, Panos A, Salerno TA. Reduction of postoperative hypothermia with a new warming device: a prospective randomized study in off-pump coronary artery surgery. *J Cardiovasc Surg (Torino)* 2009;50:813-7.

[43] Engelen S, Berghmans J, Borms S, Suy-Verburg M, Himpe D. Resistive heating during off-pump coronary bypass surgery. *Acta Anaesthesiol Belg* 2007;58:27-31.

[44] Kim JY, Shinn H, Oh YJ, Hong YW, Kwak HJ, Kwak YL. The effect of skin surface warming during anesthesia preparation on preventing redistribution hypothermia in the early operative period of off-pump coronary artery bypass surgery. *Eur J Cardiothorac Surg* 2006;29:343-7.

[45] Damgaard S, Steinbruchel DA. Autotransfusion with cell saver for off-pump coronary artery bypass surgery: a randomized trial. *Scand Cardiovasc J* 2006;40:194-8.

[46] Niranjan G, Asimakopoulos G, Karagounis A, et al. Effects of cell saver autologous blood transfusion on blood loss and homologous blood transfusion requirements in patients undergoing cardiac surgery on- versus off-cardiopulmonary bypass: a randomised trial. *Eur J Cardiothorac Surg* 2006;30:271-7.

[47] Ysasi A, Trujillo MJ, Tuesta ID, Llorens R, Herreros E. [Cell saver devices in coronary revascularization surgery without extracorporeal circulation reduce transfusion requirements]. *Rev Esp Anestesiol Reanim* 2006;53:465-70.

[48] Adler Ma SC, Brindle W, Burton G, et al. Tranexamic acid is associated with less blood transfusion in off-pump coronary artery bypass graft surgery: a systematic review and meta-analysis. *J Cardiothorac Vasc Anesth* 2011;25:26-35.

[49] Wang G, Xie G, Jiang T, et al. Tranexamic acid reduces blood loss after off-pump coronary surgery: a prospective, randomized, double-blind, placebo-controlled study. *Anesth Analg* 2011 Jul. [Epub ahead of print]

[50] Bainbridge D, Dobkowski W. Hybrid coronary artery bypass grafting. *Anesthesiol Clin* 2008;26:453-63.

[51] Jones PM, Bainbridge D, Dobkowski W, et al. Comparison of MAX-ACT and K-ACT values when using bivalirudin anticoagulation during minimally invasive hybrid off-pump coronary artery bypass graft surgery. *J Cardiothorac Vasc Anesth* 2011;25:415-8.

[52] Lincoff AM, Bittl JA, Harrington RA, et al. Bivalirudin and provisional glycoprotein IIb/IIIa blockade compared with heparin and planned glycoprotein IIb/IIIa blockade during percutaneous coronary intervention: REPLACE-2 randomized trial. *JAMA* 2003;289:853-63.

[53] Mehta SR, Yusuf S. The Clopidogrel in Unstable angina to prevent Recurrent Events (CURE) trial programme; rationale, design and baseline characteristics including a meta-analysis of the effects of thienopyridines in vascular disease. *Eur Heart J* 2000;21:2033-41.

[54] Yusuf S, Zhao F, Mehta SR, et al. Effects of clopidogrel in addition to aspirin in patients with acute coronary syndromes without ST-segment elevation. *N Engl J Med* 2001;345:494-502.

[55] Kiai B, McClure S, Stewart P, et al. Simultaneous integrated coronary artery revascularization with long term angiographic follow-up. *J Thorac Cardiovasc Surg* 2008:136:702-8.

[56] Borracci RA, Dayan R, Rubio M, Axelrud G, Ochoa G, Rodriguez LD. [Operating room extubation (ultra fast-track anesthesia) in patients undergoing on-pump and off-pump cardiac surgery]. *Arch Cardiol Mex* 2006;76:383-9.

[57] Straka Z, Brucek P, Vanek T, Votava J, Widimsky P. Routine immediate extubation for off-pump coronary artery bypass grafting without thoracic epidural analgesia. *Ann Thorac Surg* 2002;74:1544-7.

[58] Djaiani GN, Ali M, Heinrich L, et al. Ultra-fast-track anesthetic technique facilitates operating room extubation in patients undergoing off-pump coronary revascularization surgery. *J Cardiothorac Vasc Anesth* 2001;15:152-7.

[59] Cheng DC, Bainbridge D, Martin JE, Novick RJ. Does off-pump coronary artery bypass reduce mortality, morbidity, and resource utilization when compared with

conventional coronary artery bypass? a meta-analysis of randomized trials. *Anesthesiology* 2005;102:188-203.

In: Off-Pump Coronary Artery Bypass Grafting
Editors: Shahzad G. Raja and Mohamed Amrani
ISBN: 978-1- 62081-549-6
© 2012 Nova Science Publishers, Inc.

*Chapter XV*

# Verification of Graft Patency in Off-pump Coronary Artery Bypass Grafting

### *Ramanan Umakanthan, Marzia Leacche, Christopher R. Byrne and John G. Byrne*

Vanderbilt Heart & Vascular Institute, Department of Cardiac Surgery, Vanderbilt University Medical Center, Nashville, Tennessee, US

## Abstract

Off-pump coronary artery bypass (OPCAB) surgery is becoming an increasingly popular and frequently utilized therapeutic modality. OPCAB circumvents the requirements for cardiopulmonary bypass and its associated risks while still affording the opportunity for optimal coronary revascularization. There is relatively limited information, however, detailing the postoperative long term patency of the grafts. As with conventional on-pump coronary artery bypass grafting (CABG), long term outcomes, such as survival, freedom from angina, and quality of life, depend on graft patency and completeness of revascularization. In conventional on-pump CABG, approximately 20% to 30% of all grafts are no longer patent at 12 months. In addition, 3% to 12% of grafts fail immediately or in the early postoperative period. As OPCAB surgery is technically more demanding compared to standard on-pump CABG, there is a potential risk of lower patency of the grafts. The long-term outcomes of CABG, whether it be on-pump or off-pump, is dependent upon the assessment of graft patency in the intra-operative or immediate postoperative period, so that any graft defects can be detected and addressed immediately. Three major techniques have been utilized for the verification of graft patency in OPCAB. These techniques are transit time flow measurement, intra-operative fluorescent imaging, and less commonly, coronary angiography. Although intra-operative coronary angiography is considered the "gold standard" for the assessment of graft patency, it is not available in the operating rooms of most institutions as it requires specially designed "hybrid operating rooms". Each of these techniques, however, have their own respective advantages and disadvantages and have contributed beneficially in varying degrees to the verification of graft patency in off-pump coronary artery bypass surgery. This chapter provides a comprehensive account of pros and cons and results of the various techniques used for assessment of graft patency in OPCAB grafting.

# Introduction

Coronary artery bypass grafting (CABG) is still one of the most common surgical procedures performed in the United States each year. In appropriately selected patients with coronary artery disease (CAD), it results in increased survival, relief of angina, restored physical activity, and improved quality of life [1,2]. However, conventional on-pump CABG uses cardioplegic arrest and cardiopulmonary bypass (CPB) and raises the concerns of whether the associated complications related to CPB may hinder an otherwise successful procedure. Hence, interest in off-pump coronary artery bypass (OPCAB) surgery stems from the fact that it presents surgeons with the option of coronary revascularization without the potential risks of extracorporeal support. Widespread utilization of this technique, nevertheless, remains sporadic. This can be attributed to the fact that much of the literature reporting outcomes of the technique is relatively inconclusive as to the overall benefit of this technique and questions still linger regarding its ultimate benefits.

One of the major questions regarding OPCAB is how its graft patency rates compare to standard on-pump CABG. In a meta-analysis of 5 randomized trials by Parolari et al. [3], the data on 675 patients who had undergone OPCAB or standard CABG and follow-up coronary angiography 3 to 12 months after surgery were analyzed. The meta-analysis found the risk of graft occlusion in OPCAB to be increased approximately 1.51 times compared to standard CABG (odds ratio, 1.51; 95% confidence intervals, 1.15 to 1.99; $p = 0.003$).

The anastomosis of left internal mammary artery (LIMA) to the left anterior descending artery (LAD) is considered the "gold standard" graft in CABG surgery, due to its excellent patency rates [1,2]. Early patency of LIMA to LAD grafts is almost 100% followed by long-term patency of 92%-99% at 1 year, 90%-95% at 10 years [4-8]. Saphenous vein grafts (SVG), however, have much poorer patency rates. One year SVG failure rates are approximately 26% (range 7-30%) [4,8-10], and only about 50%-60% of SVG remain patent at 10 years after CABG surgery [4,11-15].

Vein graft failure within the first month after surgery is cause by acute thrombosis of the vein graft, between one to twelve months after surgery is caused by neo-intimal hyperplasia, and after twelve months is caused by progression of atherosclerosis. Thus, early graft thrombosis can have devastating consequences [16-18]. Graft thrombosis usually results from technical reasons, such as small target vessel size resulting in poor distal runoff, anastomotic occlusion, size mismatch between the graft and the target vessel creating turbulent flow, and a disruption of the endothelial layer due to mechanical trauma and manual distention.

As OPCAB is a technically more challenging procedure than conventional on-pump CABG, graft thrombosis caused by technical errors could be more prominent, therefore there is a need for intra-operative graft patency assessment.

Intraoperative graft patency has usually been assessed indirectly by utilizing the following parameters: absence of new ischemic electrocardiographic changes, absence of new wall-motion abnormalities in the area of the bypass on a trans-esophageal echocardiogram, good distal runoff on manual palpation, and absence of signs of hemodynamic instability. The tradeoff, however, in following this logic is that these methods are valuable only if significant myocardial ischemia develops. Some patients, however, develop "silent ischemia" depending on the size of the vessel grafted, diffusiveness of disease and presence of collaterals.

A variety of different techniques have been developed for intra-operative verification of graft patency. These techniques are coronary angiography [19-21], intra-operative fluorescent imaging (IFI) [22], and transit-time-flow measurements (TTFM) [23,24]. Although other techniques such as electromagnetic flowmetry [25], Doppler ultrasound velocity measurements [26,27], thermal coronary angiography [28], and epicardial color Doppler scanning [29] have also been attempted, these have failed to reliably detect occluded grafts.

# Current Verification Techniques Used to Assess Graft Patency in OPCAB

## Transit Time Flow Measurement

Transit time flow measurement (TTFM) [30] is the most commonly used method to assess grafts patency. It utilizes a flow probe that has two ultrasonic transducers and a fixed acoustic reflector. With the transducers and the reflector held perpendicularly to the graft axis, the transducer transmits an ultrasound signal which travels upstream and downstream from the direction of the blood flow through the reflector. Due to the fact that the ultrasound signal travels faster if transmitted in the same direction of the flow, the difference in time span between the two signals is calculated and defined as the transit time. The transit time is proportional to the actual flow. Hence, calculating the transit time for signal propagation between the two transducers paves the foundation for this technique. The measurements obtained are then expressed as the mean graft flow (MGF), the diastolic flow index, which is the percentage of total flow occurring in diastole, and the pulsatility index (PI), which is an estimate of the resistance to graft flow. When the MGF is greater than 30 ml/min, the graft is considered patent, while an MGF of less than 5 ml/min is indicative of graft occlusion. Further analysis is required if a MGF between 5 and 30 ml/min is obtained. In such cases, a diastolic flow-index greater than 50% of the MGF and a pulsatility index under 5 indicate graft patency [30].

## Intraoperative Fluorescence Imaging

Intraoperative fluorescence imaging (IFI) is another established technique that has been utilized to analyze graft patency [31]. This procedure is based on the fluorescent properties of the plasma protein binding dye indocyanine green (ICG). Delivered through a central venous catheter during OPCAB, ICG subsequently binds to proteins within the plasma and fluoresces when illuminated with a near-infrared laser beam. Molecules of ICG generally absorb light at a wavelength of 806 nm and fluoresce at a wavelength of 830 nm. The source of illumination is situated approximately 30 cm above the heart and designed to analyze a surface area of 7.5 cm x 7.5 cm, with 1 to 2 cm of soft tissue penetration. Deeper soft tissue penetration is not recommended in order to minimize the potential risks of thermal injury to myocardial tissue. A charge-coupled device (CCD) video camera, mounted over the operating field, is used to capture the fluorescing radiation and depict the movement of the ICG dye through the graft, the coronary-artery lumen, the perfusion territory, and the coronary veins. Each graft requires a few minutes for imaging [31].

## Coronary Angiography

Coronary angiography is another technique that can be used for verification of graft patency and is very reliable. It is commonly referred to as the "gold standard" for verification of graft patency [28]. However, it is not available in the majority of the operating rooms (ORs) in most institutions as rather stringent demands and requirements have to be met for its successful implementation. Specifically designed state-of-art "hybrid ORs" are required in order to allow for intraoperative angiography during coronary procedures. Hence, it is less common than TTFM and IFI. We have, however, found this technique to be a very valuable resource for intraoperative graft assessment [1,32] due to the successful implementation of one the first hybrid ORs in the US at the Vanderbilt Heart and Vascular Institute in 2005. The technique is relatively straightforward. Prior to administration of heparin for the surgical procedure, a femoral sheath is inserted into the left or right femoral artery using the Seldinger technique. After the surgery is completed, coronary angiography is performed to verify graft patency. This is done by injecting the iso-osmolar contrast medium iodixanol (Visipaque™) into the sheath and utilizing fluoroscopy to visualize the real time images as the contrast progresses along its path. If a defect in graft patency is detected, surgical or percutaneous graft revisions can be performed in the same intraoperative setting. Repeat angiography can then be performed to ensure the grafts are now patent before chest closure. At the end of the procedure, the heparin is reversed with Protamine, the sheath removed, and a Syvek Patch® (Marine Polymer Technologies, Danvers, MA) applied, in addition to 12 minutes of manual compression on the groin. Coronary angiography is contraindicated in patients with advanced vascular disease. This is defined as grade 4-5 atheromatous disease in the descending thoracic aorta which is detected on transesophageal echocardiogram as this could pose challenges to vascular access. This technique is also contraindicated in patients with a pre-operative serum creatinine over 2.0 mg/dL in order to minimize the risk of renal complications from contrast exposure.

# Advantages and Disadvantages of the Respective Techniques

## Transit Time Flow Measurement

The use of TTFM is beneficial because it is noninvasive, simple, quick, reproducible, and representative of flow within the graft. However, graft assessment by TTFM has the potential shortcoming of being affected by dynamic variables such as blood pressure, heart rate, graft diameter, and flow competition [33]. It is also difficult to interpret anastomotic quality as a single function of mean graft flow [33]. This technique does not provide specific details about grafts. Based on the flow data provided by TTFM, it is only possible to detect the patency of a graft. This technique is not capable of identifying whether poor graft flow represents an anastomotic problem, a conduit problem, or a disease in the target coronary artery. The location of an obstruction is also hard to ascertain using TTFM [34] and this method is capable of detecting graft failures in only about 1%-8% of grafts [40-49]. As this technique does not provide a visual image of the graft, it is generally limited in scope when compared to IFI and coronary angiography.

## Intraoperative Fluorescence Imaging

Using IFI has several advantages. The procedure is minimally invasive, with no need for arterial puncture, and also avoids ionizing radiation. Adverse reactions are very uncommon, although there have been a few allergic reactions reported [22,50]. This techniques provides semi-quantitative estimates of flow with real-time images [22,50].

***This technique, however, is only semi-quantitative and does not allow for an exact measure of graft flow. The technique also allows for precise definition of anastomotic quality in only about 75% of grafts.*** Imaging can only occur when the chest is open and pedicled internal thoracic artery conduits are less well visualized than skeletonized ones. Finally, tissue penetration is very limited, making it difficult to obtain accurate imaging of intra-myocardial arterial segments [33].

Hence, while IFI appears to have distinct advantages over TTFM, it still has limitations to the imaging it can provide when compared to coronary angiography.

## Coronary Angiography

Coronary angiography is regarded as the "gold standard" in graft assessment because it can identify the patency of grafts more accurately than the other two verification methods. In a previous study which compared diagnostic capabilities of coronary angiography, TTFM and IFI [49], it was shown that IFI was able to correctly detect 83% of abnormal/occluded grafts out of 100% of abnormal/occluded grafts identified by coronary angiography, while TTFM was able to detect only 25% of abnormal/occluded grafts [49]. In addition, IFI correctly detected 87% of grafts that had non-occlusive lesions, while TTFM didn't identify these abnormalities [43].

This technique allows for timely graft revision by surgical intervention. It also provides for direct feedback for quality control and technical improvement when implementing a technically demanding surgical procedure, such as OPCAB [51].

Using coronary angiography does have a few challenges. Advanced vascular disease or impaired renal function may preclude the technique as previously stated. The use of intra-operative coronary angiography ideally requires the use of a hybrid OR which integrates cardiac surgical OR capabilities with that of endovascular imaging and therapy. While this ultimately implies that graft verification and revision can be performed in one interventional setting, the construction of a hybrid OR can prove to be a tedious and challenging process.

Effective design of the hybrid OR is a long complex process that requires a multi-disciplinary team approach. A multi-disciplinary team approach and learning curve will be required from all the teams involved such as cardiology, cardiac surgery, anesthesiology, support staff and the OR nursing staff.

Also the spatial dimensions required of a hybrid OR should optimally be between approximately 750-900 feet [35] with a minimum floor-to-ceiling height of 10 feet, so that it can accommodate floor or ceiling mounted C-arms for 3D rotational angiography [35,36].

Equipment within the hybrid OR has to be optimally situated such that it does not cause potential conflicts among the teams involved regarding spatial constraints. A specially designed operating table has to be utilized such that it is ideally set up with the imaging and monitoring equipment in the hybrid OR. As it is crucial all teams involved have unrestricted access to the imaging and monitoring systems in the hybrid OR, at least four ceiling-mounted flat screens that display imaging and monitoring information should be placed in the four quadrants of the room, without interfering with the OR lights

Radio-protective precautions are another important factor to consider. The hybrid OR requires lead-lined walls of 2 to 3 mm thickness and OR staff will be required to wear lead aprons during procedures. As infection risk could be higher, due to the larger number of personnel and equipment, a laminar air-flow ceiling and very careful adherence to sterile techniques are prudent. In addition as the angiograms are performed with the X-ray camera moving in the vicinity of an open chest, special precaution should be given to sterile draping. At our institution, we practice triple sterile draping of the open wound and double draping of the camera.

Finally, the financial expenditure required to build a hybrid OR can vary between 2 to 4 million dollars depending on the specific needs and resources required. Certain institutions, particularly smaller ones, may not have the necessary resources to build a hybrid OR. Therefore the practicality and feasibility of such an endeavor have to be carefully considered.

Hence, while intra-operative angiography is clearly superior to TTFM and IFI in its ability to verify graft patency, all of the aforementioned factors must be carefully taken into account by individual institutions before considering it implementation.

# Results of the Respective Techniques Used for Graft Assessment in OPCAB

There have been several studies [31-33,42,45,51-56] that have used TTFM, IFI, and coronary angiography for the verification of graft patency in OPCAB procedures. The results of these studies have been summarized in detail in Table 1. The results of these studies are discussed next.

## Transit Time Flow Measurement

Transit time flow measurement has been found to be reasonably effective in detecting highly stenotic coronary anastomoses. A prospective study performed by Kim et al. [33] indicates that it is a reliable intra-operative tool to predict graft flow impairment in OPCAB. Five variables (flow pattern, mean flow, pulsatility index, insufficiency ratio, and fast Fourier transformation ratio) were measured and compared between 103 normal and 14 abnormal (occluded or competitive) grafts. The researchers were able to predict graft flow complications with sensitivity of 96.2% and specificity of 76.9% after their criteria for abnormal grafts were applied [33].

**Table 1. Graft Patency Verification Techniques Used in Studies**

| First Author | Year | Citation Number | # of Patients | # of grafts | When imaging was performed | Interventions performed (Grafts or Patients as indicated) |
|---|---|---|---|---|---|---|
| **TTFM** | | | | | | |
| Kim | 2005 | 33 | 58 | 117 | Intra-operative | N/A |
| D'Ancona | 2000 | 42 | 409 | 1145 | Intra-operative | 37/1145 (3%) grafts revised & 33/409 (8%) patients had revision |
| Schmitz | 2003 | 45 | 201 OPCAB/ 695 CABG | 295 OPCAB/ 1952 CABG | Intra-operative | N/A |
| **IFI** | | | | | | |
| Waseda | 2009 | 31 | 137 | 507 | Intra-operative | 6/507 (1%) grafts revised |
| Reuthebuch | 2004 | 52 | 38 | 124 (107 analyzed) | Intra-operative | 4/107 (4%) analyzed grafts revised |
| Takahashi | 2004 | 53 | 72 | 290 | Intra-operative | 4/290 (1%) grafts revised |
| **Coronary Angiogram** | | | | | | |
| Kim | 2010 | 51 | 1345 | 2998 | Postoperative 0 to 3 days | 35/1345 (3%) patients had revision |
| Bonatti | 2003 | 54 | 23 | 33 | Intra-operative | 14/23 (61%) grafts revised (2 revisions, 1 additional graft placed & 11 intraluminal injection with nitroglycerine) |
| Zehr | 2000 | 55 | 50 | 144 | Imme-diate postoperative | 7/50 (14%) patients had revision |
| Wiklund | 2000 | 56 | 84 | 113 | Postoperative 0 to 5 days | 3/84 (4%) patients had revision |
| Hoff | 2011 | 32 | 56 (43 underwent completion angiography) | 65 (48 underwent completion angiography) | Intra-operative | 4/48 (8%) analyzed grafts revised |

D'Ancona et al. [42] also found TTFM to be a reasonable tool to monitor the effectiveness of OPCAB in a prospective study they performed. The authors routinely used TTFM in the OPCAB procedures after 1996 and after three years determined it to be a helpful measurement technique. TTFM enabled surgeons to detect stenoses causing a 50% or greater narrowing of the anastomoses. As a result of TTFM findings, 3% (37/1145) of the grafts underwent revision. However, they did find that TTFM was not effective in determining less than critical stenoses that were found through angiography after operation [42].

In a retrospective study by Schmitz et al. [45] comparing CABG and OPCAB, results of TTFM were compared in 695 patients who underwent on-pump CABG with 201 patients who had OPCAB. Flow measurements were lower in OPCAB patients for all grafts performed. In particular, mean LIMA to LAD graft flows for OPCAB vs. CABG were 27.22 $\pm$ 15.55 mL/min vs. 40.25 $\pm$22.92 mL/min ($p$ < 0.001). Also, mean SVG to LAD graft flows for OPCAB vs. CABG were 37.79 $\pm$ 34.79 mL/min vs. 59.93 $\pm$ 33.00 mL/min ($p$ = 0.025). These findings however did not lead to increased myocardial damage as postoperative cardiac enzymes (CK-MB and troponin I) were significantly lower in OPCAB patients. In particular, median troponin I values for OPCAB vs. CABG were 1.2 (range 0.9 to 2.3) ug/L vs. 7.8 (range 7.0 to 8.3) ug/L. The authors noted that this marked decrease in troponin I values does suggest myocardial benefit in OPCAB although the TTFM values are markedly lower. Hence they concluded that although TTFM flows may help detect graft failure from technical errors, TTFM measurements should be correlated simultaneously with clinical parameters (eg. electrocardiogram, transesophageal echocardiogram, hemodynamic data), particularly in OPCAB.

### Intraoperative Fluorescence Imaging

Intra-operative fluorescence imaging has also been found to be helpful in detecting graft failure in OPCAB and more effective than TTFM. In a prospective study by Waseda et al. [31], patients undergoing OPCAB received IFI analysis, intra-operative TTFM, and postoperative angiography. IFI was initially attempted in a total of 507 grafts in 137 patients undergoing OPCAB. Due to hemodynamic instability and/or anatomical position of the grafts, acquisition of images was not possible in 37 grafts. Ninety one grafts were classified as only partially analyzable, thereby rendering the remaining 379 grafts amenable to analysis. However, 14 patients declined coronary angiography. As a result, 289 grafts from 116 patients were available for full comparison of IFI with TTFM and coronary angiography. Six grafts (1%) with acceptable TTFM results were diagnosed with graft failure by IFI, which required grafts revision. The patency of these revised grafts was confirmed by postoperative angiography. In contrast, 21 grafts with unsatisfactory TTFM results were deemed acceptable by IFI and postoperative angiography showed that 20 of the grafts were patent. Thus the IFI system provided good correlation with coronary angiography. They did agree that coronary angiography was still capable of identify more graft failure than IFI.

In another prospective study performed by Reuthebuch et al. [52], an ICG based imaging system was used to analyze OPCAB procedures. There were a total of 38 patients in the study, and 107 of 124 grafts were analyzed. According to the authors, the system was easy to handle and there were no adverse reactions to the ICG. It was determined that 4/107 (4%) of the analyzed grafts needed revision. In this study, the authors stated the images were of such high quality that they were almost equivalent to angiography, but without the need for catheter insertion and radiography. The course of the coronary arteries, which may be otherwise difficult to locate in obese patients, could be located using this imaging system. The researchers concluded that an ICG- based imaging system is safe and simple to use and has clinical utility in the assessment of graft patency in OPCAB [52].

A similar ICG based imaging system was also described in a prospective study by Takahashi et al. [53]. Good-quality images were obtained in 290 grafts of 72 OPCAB cases. Four grafts (1%) were revised because of defects detected by this system. The authors concluded that this was a useful technique for intra-operative graft verification and serves as a safety net because OPCAB is a technically difficult procedure [53].

## Coronary Angiography

The effectiveness of coronary angiography in OPCAB has been studied several times. In a prospective study performed by Kim et al. [51], authors examined 1345 patients who had undergone OPCAB. Patients underwent OPCAB without (group I, n= 234) or with (group II, n= 1111) intra-operative TTFM. Early postoperative angiography was performed in 95% of the patients at 1.6 +/- 1.2 postoperative days. A total of 33/1345 (3%) grafts were revised. The authors determined, however, that although TTFM did help decrease the incidence of reoperation, there were still 1.8% of patients who required reoperation on the basis of early angiography findings despite intra-operative TTFM-guided revision [51].

In another prospective study by Bonatti et al. [54], 33 grafts were evaluated via intra-operative angiography in 23 patients who underwent beating heart surgery. Fourteen (61%) revisions were performed due to graft stenosis in 2 grafts requiring surgical revision, 1 patient requiring an additional bypass graft due to angiography findings, and vasospasm in 11 patients requiring injection of nitroglycerin. All patients were free of angina 6 months after surgery. The authors concluded that intra-operative angiography may improve the results of OPCAB coronary surgery [54].

Some studies, however, have stated that the role of angiography in OPCAB is not very clearly delineated. In a study performed by Zehr et al. [55], 50 OPCAB patients had immediate post-operative coronary angiography. Angiographic graft patency was 90% each for the internal thoracic grafts (n=51), radial artery grafts (n=17), and saphenous vein graft (n=76). Seven (14%) patients returned to the OR as result of catheterization findings. All graft defects were discovered in the absence of hemodynamic instability or electrocardiogram changes. Despite promptly discovering and rectifying defects, the authors stated that in hospital mortality was still 1/50 (2%), while 1/50 (2%) patients required permanent pacemakers, and 1/50 (2%) patients required reoperation for bleeding. The authors concluded that the interpretation of immediate post-operative angiography is difficult because of significant spasms in native vessels and grafts immediately after surgery. Therefore, the value of immediate postoperative coronary angiogram for long-term patency is not clear [55].

Similar conclusions were also drawn from a study performed by Wiklund et al. [56]. Eighty four patients receiving 113 grafts were examined. An angiogram was performed on these patients within 5 days after surgery. Grafts were graded in the following manner: grade A (unimpaired run-off), grade B1 (<50% stenosis), grade B2 (>50% stenosis), and grade O (occlusion). Patients with B2 stenosis had a follow up angiogram 4-30 months after surgery. Overall graft patency was 96 %. Three (4%) patients required revision. The 14 patients that had B1 stenosis did not have any clinical signs of ischemia. Eight of the 12 patients that had B2 stenosis according to the immediate postoperative angiography had a normal angiogram at their re-angiography. The authors determined that since a majority of the stenoses visualized immediately after surgery were not present in later angiographies, interpretation of the angiogram is an unreliable tool immediately after the procedure [57].

In a study performed at our institution by Hoff et al. [32], 56 patients underwent minimally invasive OPCAB through a left thoracotomy. Forty three patients underwent completion angiography in which 48 grafts were analyzed. Four (8%) of the analyzed grafts required intervention after the initial surgery. Three of the grafts required stent placement because the grafts had anastomotic stenoses. The other finding led to the placement of an additional vein graft. A patient who did not undergo completion angiogram after surgery had myocardial infarction and thus required a stent for anastomotic stenosis. Hence, it is our experience that completion angiography definitely helps detect graft defects in a timely fashion and could substantially aid graft patency and clinical outcomes [32].

## Conclusion

There are a variety of techniques that are available for the verification of graft patency in OPCAB. As we have observed, each technique has their respective advantages and disadvantages. Also, some techniques, such as coronary angiography, which have a high degree of accuracy, may not be available at certain institutions. Nevertheless, each of these techniques has proven to be of varying degrees of benefit in verification of graft patency in different studies (Table 1) with coronary angiography leading to the highest percentage of intervention.

While OPCAB procedure has accrued a substantial amount of popularity over the last several years, future randomized control trials will be required to assess the full extent of its benefits and how its graft patency compares to that of conventional CABG.

## References

[1] Byrne JG, Leacche M, Vaughan DE, Zhao DX. Hybrid cardiovascular procedures. *JACC Cardiovasc Interv* 2008;1:459–468.

[2] Schmitto JD, Rajab TK, Cohn LH. Prevalence and variability of internal mammary graft use in contemporary multivessel coronary artery bypass graft. *Curr Opin Cardiol* 2010;25:609–612.

[3] Parolari A, Alamanni F, Polvani G, et al. Meta-analysis of randomized trials comparing off-pump with on-pump coronary artery bypass graft patency. *Ann Thorac Surg* 2005;80:2121-5.

[4] Alexander JH, Hafley G, Harrington RA, et al. Efficacy and safety of edifoligide, an E2F transcription factor decoy, for prevention of vein graft failure following coronary artery bypass graft surgery: PREVENT IV: A randomized controlled trial. *JAMA* 2005;294:2446–2454.

[5] Kim KB, Cho KR, Jeong DS. Midterm angiographic follow-up after off-pump coronary artery bypass: Serial comparison using early, 1-year, and 5-year postoperative angiograms. *J Thorac Cardiovasc Surg* 2008;135:300–307.

[6] Hayward PA, Buxton BF. Contemporary coronary graft patency: 5-Year observational data from a randomized trial of conduits. *Ann Thorac Surg* 2007;84:795–799.

[7] Tatoulis J, Buxton BF, Fuller JA. Patencies of 2127 arterial to coronary conduits over 15 years. *Ann Thorac Surg* 2004;77:93–101.

[8] Magee MJ, Alexander JH, Hafley G, et al. Coronary artery bypass graft failure after on-pump and off-pump coronary artery bypass: findings from PREVENT IV. *Ann Thorac Surg.* 2008;85:494-9.

[9] Puskas JD, Williams WH, Mahoney EM, et al. Off-pump vs. conventional coronary artery bypass grafting: Early and 1-year graft patency, cost, and quality-of-life outcomes: A randomized trial. *JAMA* 2004;291:1841–1849.

[10] Barner HB. Operative treatment of coronary atherosclerosis. *Ann Thorac Surg* 2008;85:1473–1482.

[11] Goldman S, Zadina K, Moritz T, et al. Long-term patency of saphenous vein and left internal mammary artery grafts after coronary artery bypass surgery: results from a Department of Veterans Affairs Cooperative Study. *J Am Coll Cardiol* 2004;44:2149–56.

[12] Desai ND, Cohen EA, Naylor CD, et al. A randomized comparison of radial-artery and saphenous-vein coronary bypass grafts. *N Engl J Med* 2004;351:2302–9.

[13] Widimsky P, Straka Z, Stros P, et al. One-year coronary bypass graft patency: A randomized comparison between off-pump and on-pump surgery angiographic results of the PRAGUE-4 trial. *Circulation* 2004;110:3418–3423.

[14] Straka Z, Widimsky P, Jirasek K, et al. Off-pump versus on-pump coronary surgery: Final results from a prospective randomized study PRAGUE-4. *Ann Thorac Surg* 2004;77:789–793.

[15] Kim KB, Lim C, Lee C, et al. Off-pump coronary artery bypass may decrease the patency of saphenous vein grafts. *Ann Thorac Surg* 2001;72:S1033–S1037.

[16] Bourassa MG. Fate of venous grafts: the past, the present and the future. *J Am Coll Cardiol* 1991;17:1081-1083.

[17] Fitzgibbon GM, Kafka HP, Leach AJ, Keon WJ, Hooper GD, Burton JR. Coronary bypass graft fate and patient outcome: angiographic follow-up of 5,065 grafts related to survival and reoperation in 1,388 patients during 25 years. *J Am Coll Cardiol* 1996;28:616-626.

[18] Bryan AJ, Angelini GD. The biology of saphenous vein graft occlusion: etiology and strategies for prevention. *Curr Opin Cardiol* 1994;9:641-649.

[19] Elbeery JR, Brown PM, Chitwood WR Jr. Intraoperative MIDCABG arteriography via the left radial artery: a comparison with Doppler ultrasound for assessment of graft patency. *Ann Thorac Surg* 1998;66:51-55.

[20] Hol PK, Lingaas PS, Lundblad R, et al. Intraoperative angiography leads to graft revision in coronary artery bypass surgery. *Ann Thorac Surg* 2004;78:502-505.

[21] Zhao DX, Leacche M, Balaguer JM, et al. Routine intraoperative completion angiography after coronary artery bypass grafting and 1-stop hybrid revascularization results from a fully integrated hybrid *catheterization laboratory/operating room. J Am Coll Cardiol* 2009;20;53:232-241.

[22] Taggart DP, Choudhary B, Anastasiadis K, Abu-Omar Y, Balacumaraswami L, Pigott DW. Preliminary experience with a novel intraoperative fluorescence imaging

technique to evaluate the patency of bypass grafts in total arterial revascularization. *Ann Thorac Surg* 2003;75:870-873.

[23] Canver CC, Dame NA. Ultrasonic assessment of internal thoracic artery graft flow in the revascularized heart. Ann Thorac Surg 1994;58:135-8.

[24] Walpoth BH, Bosshard A, Genyk I, et al., Transit-time flow measurement for detection of early graft failure during myocardial revascularization, Ann Thorac Surg 1998;**6**:1097-1100.

[25] Louagie YA, Haxhe JP, Buche M, et al. Intraoperative electromagnetic flowmeter measurements in coronary artery bypass grafts, Ann Thorac Surg 1994;**57**:357–364.

[26] Segadal L, Matre K, Engedal H, et al. Estimation of flow in aortocoronary grafts with a pulsed ultrasound Doppler meter, Thorac Cardiovasc Surg. 1982;**30**:265–268.

[27] Laustsen J, Pedersen EM, Terp K, et al. Validation of a new transit time ultrasound flowmeter in man. Eur J VascEndovasc Surg 1996;**12**:91–96.

[28] Falk V, Walther T, Philippi A, et al. Thermal coronary angiography for intraoperative patency control of arterial and saphenous vein coronary artery bypass grafts: results in 370 patients. *J Card Surg* 1995;10:147-160.

[29] Haverstad R, Vitale N, Tjomsland O, et al. Intraoperative color Doppler ultrasound assessment of LIMA-to-LAD anastomoses in off-pump coronary artery bypass grafting, Ann Thorac Surg 2002;**74**:S1390–S1394.

[30] Laustsen J, Pedersen EM, Terp K, et al. Validation of a new transit time ultrasound flowmeter in man. Eur J VascEndovasc Surg 1996;**12**:91–96.

[31] Waseda K, Ako J, Hasegawa T, et al. Intraoperative fluorescence imaging system for on-site assessment of off-pump coronary artery bypass graft. *J Am Coll Cardiol Img* 2009;2:604-612.

[32] Hoff SJ, Ball SK, Leacche M, et al. Results of completion arteriography after minimally invasive off-pump coronary artery bypass. *Ann Thorac Surg* 2011;91:31-6.

[33] Kim KB, Kang CH, Lim C. Prediction of graft flow impairment by intraoperative transit time flow measurement in off-pump coronary artery bypass using arterial grafts. *Ann Thorac Surg* 2005;80:594-8.

[34] Leacche M, Balaguer JM, Byrne JG. Intraoperative graft assessment. *Semin Thorac Cardiovasc Surg* 2009l;21:207-12.

[35] Kpodonu J, Raney A. The cardiovascular hybrid room a key component for hybrid interventions and image guided surgery in the emerging specialty of cardiovascular hybrid surgery. *Interact Cardiovasc Thorac Surg* 2009;9:688-692.

[36] Nollert G, Wich S. Planning a cardiovascular hybrid operating room: the technical point of view. *Heart Surg Forum* 2009;12:E125-E130.

[37] Umakanthan R, Leacche M, Petracek MR, et al. Safety of minimally invasive mitral valve surgery without aortic cross-clamp. *Ann Thorac Surg* 2008;85:1544-9.

[38] Umakanthan R, Leacche M, Petracek MR, et al. Combined PCI and minimally invasive heart valve surgery for high risk patients. *Current Treatment Options in Cardiovascular Medicine* 2009;11:492-498.

[39] Byrne JG, Leacche M, Unic D, et al. Staged initial percutaneous coronary intervention followed by valve surgery ("hybrid approach") for patients with complex coronary and valve disease. *J Am Coll Cardiol* 2005;45:14-18.

[40] Herman C, Sullivan JA, Buth K, et al. Intraoperative graft flow measurements during coronary artery bypass surgery predict in-hospital outcomes. *Interact Cardiovasc Thorac Surg* 2008;7:582-585.

[41] Balacumaraswami L, Abu-Omar Y, Choudhary B, et al. A comparison of transit-time flowmetry and intraoperative fluorescence imaging for assessing coronary artery bypass graft patency. *J Thorac Cardiovasc Surg* 2005;130:315-320.

[42] D'Ancona G, Karamanoukian HL, Ricci M, et al. Graft revision after transit time flow measurement in off-pump coronary artery bypass grafting. *Eur J CardiothoracSurg 2000*;17:287-293.

[43] Jakobsen HL, Kjaergard HK. Severe impairment of graft flow without electrocardiographic changes during coronary artery bypass grafting. *Scand Cardiovasc J* 1999;33:157-159.

[44] Hirotani T, Kameda T, Shirota S, et al. An evaluation of the intraoperative transit time measurements of coronary bypass flow. *Eur J CardiothoracSurg* 2001;19:848-852.

[45] Schmitz C, Ashraf O, Schiller W, et al. Transit time flow measurement in on-pump and off-pump coronary artery surgery. *J Thorac Cardiovasc Surg* 2003;126:645-650.

[46] Kjaergard HK, Irmukhamedov A, Christensen JB, et al. Flow in coronary bypass conduits on-pump and off-pump. *Ann Thorac Surg* 2004;78:2054-2056.

[47] Hassanein W, Albert AA, Arnrich B, et al. Intraoperative transit time flow measurement: off-pump versus on-pump coronary artery bypass. *Ann Thorac Surg* 2005;80:2155-2161.

[48] Tokuda Y, Song MH, Ueda Y, et al. Predicting early coronary artery bypass graft failure by intraoperative transit time flow measurement. *Ann Thorac Surg* 2007; 84:1928-1933.

[49] Desai ND, Miwa S, Kodama D, et al. A randomized comparison of intraoperative indocyanine green angiography and transit-time flow measurement to detect technical errors in coronary bypass grafts. *J Thorac Cardiovasc Surg* 2006;132:585-594.

[50] Speich R, Saesseli B, Hoffmann U, Neftel KA, Reichen J. Anaphylactoid reactions after indocyanine-green administration. *Ann Intern Med* 1988;109:345-346.

[51] Kim KB, Kim JS, Kang HJ, et al. Ten-year experience with off-pump coronary artery bypass grafting: lessons learned from early postoperative angiography. *J Thorac Cardiovasc* Surg 2010;139:256-62.

[52] Reuthebuch O, Häussler A, Genoni M, et al. Novadaq SPY: intraoperative quality assessment in off-pump coronary artery bypass grafting. *Chest* 2004;125:418-24.

[53] Takahashi M, Ishikawa T, Higashidani K, Katoh H. SPY: an innovative intra-operative imaging system to evaluate graft patency during off-pump coronary artery bypass grafting. *Interact Cardiovasc Thorac Surg* 2004;3:479-83.

[54] Bonatti J, Danzmayr M, Schachner T, Friedrich G. Intraoperative angiography for quality control in MIDCAB and OPCAB. *Eur J Cardiothorac Surg* 2003;24:647-9.

[55] Zehr KJ, Handa N, Bonilla LF, Abel MD, Holmes DR Jr. Pitfalls and results of immediate angiography after off-pump coronary artery bypass grafting. *Heart Surg Forum* 2000;3:293-9.

[56] Wiklund L, Johansson M, Brandrup-Wognsen G, Bugge M, Rådberg G, Berglin E. Difficulties in the interpretation of coronary angiogram early after coronary artery bypass surgery on the beating heart. *Eur J Cardiothorac Surg* 2000;17:46-51.

[57] Hol PK, Fosse E, Mork BE, et al. Graft control by transit time flow measurement and intraoperative angiography in coronary artery bypass surgery. *Heart Surg Forum* 2001;4:254-257.

*Chapter XVI*

# Atrial Pacing for Off-pump Coronary Artery Bypass Grafting

*Vassilios S. Gulielmos, Emmanouela G. Dalamanga and Pavlos G. Papoulidis*
Department of Cardiac Surgery, Euromedica - Geniki Kliniki Thessaloniki, Thessaloniki, Greece

## Abstract

Atrial pacing is one of the adjuncts for facilitating off-pump coronary artery bypass surgery. Atrial pacing is commenced prior to displacing the heart and assists in achieving stable hemodynamics. It is proven that atrial pacing increases blood pressure, cardiac output, cardiac index and decreases left ventricular end-diastolic pressure, stroke volume and central venous pressure. Use of atrial pacing assists in decreasing the size of heart leading to better tolerance while tilting the heart for exposure of back wall vessels. Even when mitral regurgitation is apparent, atrial pacing either decreases mitral incompetence or does not allow further increase. This chapter provides an overview of the benefits of atrial pacing particularly as the described maneuver is used routinely at authors' institution with virtual elimination of hemodynamic deterioration and conversion to cardiopulmonary bypass.

## Introduction

Off-pump coronary artery bypass (OPCAB) surgery is considered to be the most modern technique for more than a decade now, even though it was initiated in the mid sixties by Kolessov. The reason for this is probably the fact that coronary artery bypass grafting (CABG) on cardiopulmonary bypass (CPB) became a routine procedure after Favaloro presented a large series using extracorporal circulation and standardizing the technique validating the safety and reproducibility of conventional CABG on CPB.

Adoption of conventional CABG resulted in apparent abandonment of beating heart CABG. However, in many developing countries such as in South America and Asia, off-pump procedures thrived for decades due to financial and economic constraints. OPCAB surgery saw resurgence once Cornelius Borst developed a system for safe and reproducible beating heart bypass surgery [1]. The advantages of this technique compared to the CPB procedures became obvious [2-5] within a short span of time, however even after 2 decades following rediscovery it has not been universally adopted.

Compromising hemodynamics, while tilting the heart for exposure of back wall coronaries, is one of the main reasons for hesitance to adopt it. In order to maintain hemodynamic stability a hand full of maneuvers were proposed, such as right rotation of the patient, Trendelenburg position [6], the "Lima stitch" and use of additional devices such as X-pose or Star-fish. In the present chapter we will discuss the use and benefits of "temporary atrial pacing" for maintaining stable hemodynamics during OPCAB surgery.

## Procedure and Explanation

Prior to commencing grafting temporary epicardial atrial pacemaker wires are attached to the right atrium and atrial pacing started at a rate of 90 beats per minute. The positive hemodynamic effect becomes immediately apparent in terms of increasing systolic blood pressure, diastolic blood pressure and mean blood pressure. In parallel, the decrease of left atrial pressure is also evident more than the decrease of central venous pressure (CVP). Left atrial pressure (LAP) is directly measured at our institution, using a catheter positioned intraoperatively through the right upper pulmonary vein into the left atrium, instead of using the indirect information from a pulmonary artery (Swan-Ganz) catheter. A study performed in Dresden in year 2000 to prove the positive effects of atrial pacing also revealed immediate increase of cardiac output (CO) and cardiac index (CI) with statistical significance even in a very small group of patients due to the great difference [7].

It is indeed feasible to pace most patients up to 90 beats per minute, because majority of them arrive in the operating room with normal heart rate or bradycardia due to being on beta blockers. Following induction of general anaesthesia, the negative chronotropic effects of beta blockers become more apparent and pulse decreases down to even 50 beats per minute.

The rationale for pacing at a rate of 90 beats per minute is evidence-based. Already in the 70s Sowton [8] showed that human heart achieves its maximum performance in different situations at different rates. At rest the best performance is around 90 beats per minute with both CO and CI achieving their maximum levels. It is no wonder then why blood pressure also rises offering to the surgical team a better initial hemodynamic situation. This phenomenon gains more importance while tilting the heart for exposing back wall vessels of the left ventricle.

During grafting on the circumflex territory for stabilizing the target site, the heart is pressed against the right aspects of pericardium, which means that left ventricular geometry is easily deformed especially in a ventricle with low EF. As a result the performance of the left ventricle is further decreased with possible deterioration of hemodynamics leading to conversion to CPB. It is also well known that conversion to CPB during off-pump procedures is a great intraoperative risk factor for increased mortality [9], meaning thereby that any maneuver helping to avoid use of CPB is most important.

The law of LaPlace shows that the stress being exercised to the chamber wall is proportional to the size of the chamber radius (Figure 1). With increasing size of the radius, wall stress also increases independently from the hydrostatic pressure within the left ventricle. The longer the radius of the ventricle the higher the stress force exercised to the interior wall of the left ventricle.

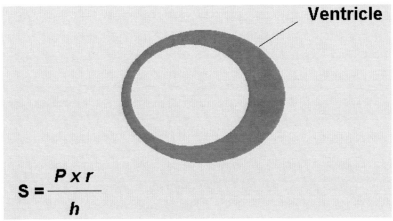

S = Wall Stress
P = Pressure
r = Radius
h = Wall Thickness

Figure 1. Law of LaPlace: When pressure or radius increase, wall stress increases.

Atrial pacing clearly decreases stroke volume as well as the radius of the left ventricular chamber [7] (Figure 1). Resultant wall stress reduction improves the contracting condition of the left ventricle and the beneficial results become evident when the heart is displaced, for gaining access to the posterior aspects of the heart.

In case of mild to moderate mitral valve incompetence, particularly in the setting of low left ventricular ejection fraction, Trendelenburg maneuver increases mitral regurgitation. The mechanism on most occasions is the following: Trendelenburg maneuver → increase of ventricular and atrial load → atrial and ventricular dilatation → increased mitral valve incompetence → further increasing volume load → ventricular dilation ect. leading to ventricular decompensation and necessity for CPB. Atrial pacing interferes and breaks this circulus vitiosus by reducing the radius of the left ventricle thus stabilising the hemodynamic condition of the patient. The correction of electrical atrial-ventricular interval additionally leads to competence of the mitral valve, resulting in better tolerance of cardiac displacement and enucleation.

At our institution we routinely use this maneuver not only in our first time OPCAB procedures but also in redo cases with functioning LIMA-graft as well as in valve surgery when hemodynamic support is needed. The maneuver helps to almost completely eliminate hemodynamic deterioration and reduces the need for conversion to extracorporeal circulation during OPCAB procedures to practically zero.

## Conclusion

Over the past two decades several tips, tricks and tools have been devised to maintain stable hemodynamic situation during OPCAB surgery. Apart from right rotation of the patient, Trendelenburg maneuver, intra-coronary shunts and "Lima stitch", temporary atrial pacing has emerged as a useful adjunct to avoid deterioration of hemodynamics during beating heart operations. The better performance of the left ventricle with higher blood pressure, lower LAP, lower CVP, higher CO and CI, leads to decreased left ventricular wall stress through reduction of the chamber radius. All these improvements lead to achievement of hemodynamic stability, following displacement of the heart for access to vessels on the back of the heart, and eliminate conversion to CPB. The extended use of all the tricks and tools including routine atrial pacing will allow wider acceptance of off-pump procedures.

## References

[1]  Borst C, Jansen EW, Tulleken CA, et al. Coronary artery bypass grafting without cardiopulmonary bypass and without interruption of native coronary flow using a novel anastomosis site restraining device ("Octopus"). *J Am Coll Cardiol* 1996; 27:1356-1364.

[2]  Ascione R, Lloyd CT, Underwood MJ, Gomes WJ, Angelini GD. On-pump versus off-pump coronary revascularization: evaluation of renal function. *Ann Thorac Surg* 1999;68:493-498.

[3]  Strüber M, Cremer JT, Gohrbandt B, et al. Humane cytokine responses to coronary artery bypass grafting with and without cardiopulmonary bypass. *Ann Thorac Surg* 1999;68:1330-1335.

[4]  Trehan N, Mishra M, Sharma OP, Mishra A, Kasliwal RR. Further reduction in stroke after off-pump coronary artery bypass grafting: a 10-year experience. *Ann Thorac Surg* 2001;72:1026-1032.

[5]  Wan S, Izzat MB, Lee TW, Wan IYP, Tang NLS, Yim APC. Avoiding cardiopulmonary bypass in multivessel CABG reduces cytokine response and myocardial injury. *Ann Thorac Surg* 1999;68:52-57.

[6]  Gründeman PF, Borst C, Verlaan CW, Meijburg H, Mouës CM, Jansen EW. Exposure of circumflex branches in the tilted, beating porcine heart: echocardiographic evidence of right ventricular deformation and the effect of right or left heart bypass. *J Thorac Cardiovasc Surg* 1999;118:316-23.

[7]  Gulielmos V, Kappert U, Eller M, Sahre H, Alexiou K, Georgi C, Nicolai J, Hartmann N. Improving hemodynamics by atrial pacing during off-pump bypass surgery. *Heart Surg Forum 2003*;6:E179-82.

[8]  Sowton E. Hemodynamic studies in patients with artificial pacemakers. *Brit Heart J* 1964;26:737-746.

[9]  Soltoski P, Salerno T, Levinsky L, et al. Conversion to cardiopulmonary bypass in off-pump coronary artery bypass grafting: its effect on outcome. *J Card Surg* 1998;13:328-34.

# Index

### #

20th century, 26, 65, 109, 175

### A

Abraham, 161
access, vii, 13, 30, 37, 108, 111, 112, 137, 138, 139, 144, 147, 150, 151, 155, 160, 166, 171, 181, 182, 189, 191, 199, 201, 204, 232, 233, 257, 258
accounting, 57, 191, 225
acetylcholine, 56, 58
acid, 9, 184, 203, 233, 239
acidity, 91
acidosis, 234, 235
AD, 50, 158, 208, 219, 237
adhesions, 3, 8, 9, 18, 26, 125, 131, 144, 145, 151, 155, 166
adipose, 187, 203
adipose tissue, 187, 203
adjustment, 234
administrative support, 134
adrenaline, 7
adrenoceptors, 68, 178
advancement(s), 81, 105, 171
adventitia, 80, 177
adverse effects, xi, 26, 173, 176
adverse event, 108, 236
age, 8, 21, 96, 97, 110, 115, 117, 132, 147, 155, 171, 214
aggressiveness, 165
Air Force, 4
airways, 177
albumin, 90, 91
ALT, 154
alters, 69
American Heart Association, 220
amino, 234
amino acid, 234
amputation, 1
analgesia, xi, 173, 174, 175, 176, 179, 182, 183, 186, 191, 202, 209, 224, 236, 239
analgesic, 181, 224
anatomy, 12, 15, 55, 56, 69, 103, 105, 125, 127, 135, 165, 186, 187, 188, 204, 218, 231
anemia, 229, 233
anesthesiologist, xi, xii, 30, 42, 173, 182, 185, 223, 224, 235
anesthetics, 1, 186, 187, 199
aneurysm, 18, 155, 187
anger, 5
angina, xiii, 3, 5, 6, 7, 8, 9, 10, 11, 13, 15, 16, 18, 20, 21, 24, 31, 50, 108, 110, 115, 118, 130, 132, 155, 156, 161, 171, 179, 186, 215, 239
angiogram, 17, 76, 111, 116, 165, 171
angiography, xiii, 3, 12, 13, 14, 15, 16, 19, 20, 21, 22, 23, 27, 67, 76, 77, 112, 116, 130, 133, 139, 155, 156, 170, 171, 215
angioplasty, x, 22, 107, 109, 118, 171
angiotensin II, 56, 69
angiotensin receptor antagonist, 68, 72
anticoagulant, x, xiii, 121, 187, 223, 231, 234
anticoagulation, 99, 140, 183, 194, 231, 232, 234, 238, 239
antispasmodics, 72
anxiety, 185, 186
aorta, 5, 10, 11, 12, 13, 14, 15, 16, 22, 26, 38, 40, 46, 47, 54, 66, 70, 90, 92, 97, 98, 99, 100, 101, 104, 122, 124, 144, 145, 146, 148, 149, 150, 151, 153, 157, 160, 164, 190, 191, 200, 203, 204, 213, 218, 229, 230
aortic regurgitation, 188
aortic valve, 3, 125, 137
APC, 71, 72, 258
apex, 11, 30, 40, 41, 48, 49, 50, 101, 111, 113, 201

Argentina, 17, 23, 28
arginine, 56
arrest, xii, 17, 23, 105, 122, 137, 144, 146, 168, 211, 212, 214, 216, 217, 218, 219, 220
arrhythmia, xi, 173, 205, 215
arrhythmias, 96, 166, 225
arterial blood gas, 228
arteries, viii, xi, 5, 7, 10, 12, 13, 15, 16, 22, 27, 28, 30, 40, 54, 55, 56, 57, 58, 59, 60, 61, 62, 63, 67, 68, 69, 70, 71, 72, 73, 75, 77, 96, 102, 103, 110, 111, 124, 125, 167, 173, 178, 187, 207, 209
arteriography, 11, 15
arteriosclerosis, 69
asbestos, 9
Asia, 256
aspiration, 177, 191, 203, 205
assessment, xiii, 33, 70, 72, 77, 78, 87, 89, 98, 111, 116, 124, 133, 156, 161, 202, 207, 220, 235
assimilation, 97
asthma, 125
asymptomatic, 7, 8, 11, 26, 170
atelectasis, 114, 177, 180
atherosclerosis, 24, 31, 58, 59, 60, 61, 62, 90, 97, 101, 105, 125, 132, 146, 147, 148, 153, 178
atherosclerotic plaque, 77, 188
atmosphere, 197
atrial fibrillation, 30, 116, 154, 179, 231, 236
atrial septal defect, 27
atrioventricular block, 187
atrium, 178
attachment, 193
attitudes, 97
audit, 208
authorities, 11
autonomic nervous system, 177
autopsy, 2, 3, 5, 22
avoidance, x, xi, xii, xiii, 1, 77, 85, 97, 123, 143, 145, 147, 148, 167, 173, 174, 175, 180, 186, 211, 217, 219, 223, 224

## B

bacteria, 4
balloon angioplasty, 117, 164, 232
barotrauma, 177
barriers, 187
base, 11, 99, 101
basophils, 56
beating heart totally endoscopic coronary artery bypass grafting (BHTECAB), x, 121, 122
beef, 9
beneficial effect, 189

benefits, ix, x, xiii, 16, 22, 78, 95, 103, 106, 122, 123, 125, 137, 160, 165, 174, 185, 217, 222, 225, 235, 255, 256
benign, 20, 21
benzodiazepine, 224
beta blocker, 256
bicarbonate, 182, 213
*Bilateral*, 10, 204
biological behavior, viii, 53, 60
bleeding, xiii, 10, 29, 78, 88, 102, 103, 116, 127, 130, 131, 132, 133, 149, 150, 159, 167, 169, 171, 184, 187, 202, 223, 232, 233, 234, 235
blood clot, 18
blood flow, xiii, 8, 9, 10, 13, 23, 24, 26, 27, 29, 30, 39, 56, 59, 61, 100, 146, 176, 178, 179, 180, 183, 186, 187, 199, 217, 223, 228
blood pressure, xiii, 39, 40, 98, 103, 148, 151, 167, 169, 178, 181, 213, 224, 228, 229, 230, 232, 255, 256, 258
blood supply, 2, 6, 8, 12, 55, 59, 119
blood transfusion(s), 4, 23, 137, 147, 164, 239
blood vessels, 8, 22, 56, 69, 77
bone, 5, 9
bradycardia, xi, 46, 64, 100, 173, 178, 179, 184, 187, 256
bradykinin, 55, 58
brain, 126
brass, 3
Brazil, 23, 25, 28
breathing, 191, 192, 193, 194, 200, 202
Britain, 8
bronchopneumonia, 2
bronchospasm, 184
brothers, 6

## C

cadaver, 7, 14, 134
calcification, 103, 111, 127, 129, 132, 134, 188, 218
calcium, 19, 58, 63, 64, 65, 71, 72, 89
calcium channel blocker, 89
caliber, 28
campaigns, 1
candidates, 28, 96, 110, 114, 165, 166, 188, 235
carbon, 1, 17, 167, 182, 202, 205, 213
carbon dioxide, 1, 17, 167, 182, 202, 205, 213
cardiac arrest, 2, 4, 13, 28, 32, 214, 217
cardiac arrhythmia, 179
cardiac catheterization, 5, 164, 232
cardiac operations, 5, 175, 176, 208
cardiac output, xiii, 3, 38, 40, 47, 98, 126, 178, 179, 201, 218, 224, 225, 228, 230, 232, 235, 237, 255, 256

cardiac surgery, vii, 1, 4, 5, 26, 27, 29, 90, 98, 105, 119, 122, 123, 124, 132, 136, 139, 164, 169, 174, 175, 176, 181, 184, 185, 208, 209, 228, 236, 239
cardiac tamponade, 2, 4
cardiogenic shock, 21, 22, 96, 110, 214, 215, 220
cardiologist, 22, 64, 132, 165, 168, 215
cardiomyopathy, 110, 155
cardioplegia, 19, 144, 145, 146, 159
cardiovascular system, 176, 209
carotid bruit, 96
carotid duplex, 96
carotid endarterectomy, 96, 187
cartilage, 167, 168, 193, 197
cascades, 147
catheter, 3, 5, 13, 22, 38, 39, 72, 97, 98, 100, 111, 155, 164, 165, 166, 169, 170, 171, 181, 183, 191, 228, 256
causation, 26
CBP, 164
cellulitis, 84
cerebrovascular complications, 117
cerebrovascular disease, 77
challenges, ix, xii, 30, 77, 95, 96, 97, 125, 130, 144, 145, 157, 165, 206, 223, 224
channel blocker, 19, 89
chemical, 3, 9
CHF, 187
Chicago, 6
China, 53
chloroform, 2
choline, 13
chronic obstructive pulmonary disease, 110, 125, 166, 180, 187, 204, 207, 236
chylothorax, 90
circulation, x, xii, 3, 5, 8, 9, 11, 15, 23, 24, 38, 50, 69, 89, 91, 131, 139, 143, 168, 174, 175, 186, 188, 206, 207, 211, 219, 220, 231, 239, 255, 257
City, 12, 16, 75, 128
classification, viii, 53, 60, 61, 62, 68, 72
clinical application, 27, 175
clinical trials, 65, 238
closure, 15, 27, 87, 105, 129, 151, 170, 203, 205
$CO_2$, 30, 81, 82, 85, 86, 87, 88, 102, 149
coagulopathy, 98, 232, 235
coarctation, 13
coherence, 77, 92, 93
collaboration, xi, 173
collateral, 8, 9, 11, 12, 15, 24, 89, 103, 122, 168, 169, 186, 188, 207, 231
collateralization, 101
coma, 184
commercial, 79, 136
communication, 182, 185, 186, 224

communication skills, 185
community, 77, 125, 136
compensation, 136, 140
competition, 82, 136, 178
compilation, vii
complement, 147
complexity, 17, 76, 136, 144
compliance, 182, 225
complications, vii, viii, ix, xii, xiii, 12, 15, 18, 27, 75, 78, 84, 85, 95, 96, 108, 109, 114, 116, 126, 164, 167, 168, 169, 170, 171, 174, 177, 179, 180, 184, 186, 192, 206, 211, 212, 215, 216, 217, 223, 231, 232, 235, 238
compression, viii, 2, 29, 37, 40, 41, 43, 46, 47, 48, 99, 102, 228, 236
computed tomography, 139, 144
computer, 29, 140, 141
conductance, 55, 60, 63
conduction, 126, 179, 183
conductivity, 178
congenital heart disease, 6
congestive heart failure, 20, 43, 86, 110, 130, 187, 217
congress, 13, 17
connective tissue, 88
consensus, 170, 231
consent, 130
conservation, 148
construction, 27, 30, 171, 213
consumption, 180
contingency, 98
contour, 111
controlled studies, 216
controlled trials, ix, 95, 105, 147, 159, 207, 238
controversial, 110, 213
controversies, x, xi, 21, 122, 143, 144, 163
conversion rate, 115, 217
conversion to cardiopulmonary bypass, xiii, 130, 149, 238, 255
conviction, 96
cooling, 97
coordination, 82
COPD, 43, 111, 115
coronary angioplasty, xi, 108, 163, 169
Coronary artery bypass grafting (CABG), viii, 75, 242
coronary artery disease, xi, 6, 7, 11, 19, 20, 21, 26, 30, 104, 105, 108, 137, 140, 144, 145, 160, 164, 165, 173, 176, 179, 183, 209, 212, 219, 220
coronary bypass surgery, xi, 21, 32, 50, 54, 76, 91, 118, 159, 169, 173, 190, 206, 207, 209, 221, 222, 238
coronary heart disease, 31, 179

coronary thrombosis, 3, 26
correlation, 174
cosmetic, 164, 190, 193
cost, 84, 135, 140, 147, 174, 176, 186, 191, 218, 221, 234
cost effectiveness, 174, 191
cost saving, 147
cotton, 9
cough, 180, 185, 186, 194, 199, 202, 204
cough reflex, 204
coughing, 204
counterbalance, 176
covering, 118, 191, 192
CPB, xii, 38, 46, 49, 108, 109, 110, 111, 114, 115, 123, 144, 146, 147, 148, 149, 152, 153, 155, 156, 161, 164, 165, 166, 167, 168, 169, 174, 176, 211, 212, 213, 216, 217, 219, 224, 228, 230, 231, 232, 235, 255, 256, 257, 258
creatine, 214, 215
creatine phosphokinase, 214, 215
creatinine, 213, 214, 215, 234
CRF, 58
critical analysis, 207
critical state, 214
CT, 32, 66, 77, 105, 124, 125, 133, 258
CT scan, 125
CV, 219
cycles, 102
cytokines, 147

## D

danger, 2
data analysis, 20
data set, 136
database, 76, 158
death rate, 76
deaths, 2, 4, 12, 28, 170, 171
decreased myocardial ischemia, xi, 173
deep venous thrombosis, 86
defects, xiii, 205
defibrillation, 4, 5, 126, 149
defibrillator, 98, 111, 115, 126, 231
deficiency, 110
deficit, 11, 181
deformation, 38, 44, 46, 258
degradation, 234
dehiscence, 84
delirium, 186
dentist, 2
depression, 19, 21, 184, 194, 230
depth, ix, 95, 96, 126, 235
dermatome, 185

desiccation, 87
detectable, 48
developing countries, 256
diabetes, 57, 76, 86, 110, 175, 207
diabetic patients, 105
dialysis, 207
diaphragm, 41, 46, 99, 127, 151, 152, 182, 184, 194, 204
diastolic blood pressure, 256
diastolic pressure, xiii, 17, 40, 255
diffusion, 199
dilation, 89, 90, 91, 257
direct measure, 180
disability, 11
disabled patients, 21
discomfort, 174, 176, 185, 186, 199, 200, 201, 202, 204
discrimination, 182
diseases, 57, 126
dislocation, 192
displacement, 30, 38, 39, 40, 41, 43, 46, 48, 98, 99, 100, 101, 103, 167, 191, 193, 200, 224, 228, 237, 257, 258
disposition, 235
distress, 202, 204, 205
distribution, 41, 59, 68, 165, 171
doctors, 16
dogs, 8, 9, 14, 22, 27, 28, 30, 129
dominance, 22
donors, 12
dopamine, 228
dorsal aorta, 59
dosage, 190, 234
drainage, 127, 152, 191, 202, 205, 206, 233
drug reactions, 177
drugs, 65, 184
durability, 203
dyspnea, 199, 204

## E

echocardiogram, 42, 87, 124
edema, 48, 84, 177, 212
editors, vii
education, 140
efferent nerve, 178
elderly population, 24
electrocardiogram, 3, 17, 38, 111, 181, 224
electrocautery, 93, 190, 194, 195
electrodes, 3
electrolyte, 91
emboli, 87, 104, 145, 229
embolism, 85, 87, 92

embolization, 87, 145
embolus, 5, 18
embryology, 56, 59
emergency, 15, 17, 23, 110, 111, 125, 169, 183, 213, 214, 215, 216, 218, 220, 221, 231, 238
employment, 20, 125
empyema, 125
endocarditis, 4, 6
endocardium, 180, 183
endoscope, 79, 80, 82, 126
endothelial NO synthase, 58
endothelium, 54, 55, 56, 58, 66, 68, 77, 90, 91, 178
endotracheal intubation, xi, 150, 173, 174, 179, 180, 182, 205
energy, 77
England, 3, 4
enlargement, 188
environment, 4, 135
enzyme, 213, 215
epicardium, 8, 9, 11, 113, 129, 136, 178
epidural hematoma, 181, 184, 185, 224, 236
epinephrine, 176, 177, 228, 235
equipment, 3, 42, 136
esophagus, 46, 47, 100
ETA, 57, 69
etiology, 38, 39, 40, 69, 126
Europe, 2, 79
evidence, vii, 9, 39, 44, 56, 60, 66, 87, 89, 106, 144, 146, 147, 156, 159, 161, 164, 215, 219, 225, 231, 232, 256, 258
evolution, vii, ix, x, 1, 2, 3, 47, 75, 77, 143
examinations, 96
excision, 14, 18
excitability, 178
exclusion, 131, 132, 165
exercise, 20, 21, 178
exercise performance, 21
exertion, 8
expertise, 30, 110
exposure, viii, xiii, 29, 30, 32, 33, 40, 41, 45, 46, 47, 48, 49, 50, 98, 99, 100, 101, 102, 103, 104, 111, 123, 128, 136, 149, 151, 152, 167, 191, 192, 200, 204, 213, 217, 228, 255, 256
extraction, 2

## F

factor analysis, 119
false negative, 230
false positive, 230
fantasy, 1
fascia, 88, 104, 127, 190, 195, 197

fat, 8, 9, 11, 26, 49, 88, 99, 102, 111, 112, 113, 118, 127, 134, 135, 150, 193
fear, 206
fiber(s), 177, 213
fibrillation, 131, 179
fibrin, 87, 99, 203
fibrinolytic, xi, 173, 176, 179
fibrosis, 125
filtration, 234
financial, 256
fires, 129
first generation, 122
fish, 10, 256
fixation, 38, 49
fluid, 38, 39, 79, 86, 98, 219, 230, 232, 235
fluid balance, 219
fluorescence, 156
Foley catheter, 181
Food and Drug Administration, 24, 122
force, 257
formaldehyde, 9
formation, 77, 85, 99, 118, 234
fractures, 29
fragility, 87
France, 3
freedom, x, xiii, 110, 117, 121, 122, 123, 132, 221
fresh frozen plasma, 233
friendship, 11

## G

ganglion, 7, 177
gastroparesis, 152
general anaesthesia, 256
general anesthesia, xi, 170, 173, 174, 175, 176, 177, 180, 181, 182, 185, 186, 189, 190, 192, 203, 204, 205, 206, 208
general practitioner, vii
geometry, 41, 44, 101, 218, 256
Georgia, 95
Germany, 107
glasses, 28
glue, 203
graft technique, 11, 190, 193, 197, 201
gravity, 41, 201
Greece, 4, 255
growth, 69, 96
growth factor, 69
guidance, 131
guidelines, 70, 106, 125

## H

hair, 97
harvesting, viii, xii, 63, 64, 70, 75, 76, 77, 79, 84, 86, 87, 91, 92, 93, 99, 112, 123, 127, 129, 134, 151, 155, 173, 183, 191, 192, 193, 194, 195, 196, 199, 203, 209
HE, 31, 63, 64, 118
healing, 2
health, 18
heart attack, 26
heart block, 231
heart disease, 19, 54
heart failure, 2, 5, 7, 8, 9, 100, 131
heart rate, 38, 64, 126, 174, 178, 179, 183, 186, 205, 213, 224, 228, 229, 256
heat loss, 181
hematoma, 47, 84, 154, 184, 194, 236
hematomas, 85, 89
hemodialysis, 215
hemodynamic deterioration, xi, xiii, 46, 48, 173, 228, 238, 255, 257
hemodynamic instability, viii, xii, xiii, 37, 149, 185, 211, 215, 217, 218, 219, 223, 230
hemorrhage, 99, 187
hemostasis, 104, 113, 129, 147, 149, 191, 192, 213
herniate, 46, 228
high risk patients, 22, 24, 125, 175, 176, 206, 208, 220
histamine, 56
histology, 7, 67
history, vii, 1, 7, 13, 25, 26, 30, 65, 86, 96, 124, 147
HIV, 138
HM, 32, 221
hormones, 176, 177
hospital death, 110, 215
hospitalization, xi, 163, 170
host, 38
human, 9, 10, 14, 16, 22, 30, 39, 40, 56, 57, 58, 61, 65, 66, 68, 69, 70, 71, 72, 92, 126, 256
human immunodeficiency virus, 126
human skin, 9
human subjects, 39
Hunter, 5
hybrid, ix, x, xi, xii, xiii, 26, 105, 107, 110, 117, 121, 123, 125, 130, 132, 133, 137, 138, 139, 155, 163, 164, 165, 168, 171, 176, 208, 211, 212, 217, 219, 223, 224, 228, 233, 234, 239
hyperactivity, 184
hyperplasia, 87
hypertension, 19, 115, 175, 177, 207
hyperthermia, 177
hyperthyroidism, 7
hypertrophy, 130, 216
hyperventilation, 202
hypotension, 38, 41, 47, 91, 98, 149, 177, 180, 184, 225, 229, 231
hypothermia, xiii, 177, 223, 233, 235, 238
hypothesis, 55
hypovolemia, 180, 183, 235
hypoxemia, 180, 234
hypoxia, 126, 177, 194, 204, 205
hysterectomy, 2

## I

iatrogenic, 46, 110, 203
ID, 239
ideal, vii, xi, 28, 29, 30, 78, 82, 110, 163, 165, 171, 189, 216, 231, 235
identification, 77, 127, 167, 168
IEA, 55, 56, 57, 58, 59, 61, 62
IL-8, 216
IMA, 45, 54, 55, 56, 57, 58, 59, 60, 61, 62, 63, 64, 65, 69, 71, 109, 112, 123, 124, 129, 134, 175, 176, 183, 186, 190, 191, 192, 193, 194, 201, 203
image(s), 12, 13, 77, 127, 136, 156, 230
imagination, 5
immobilization, 40, 112, 213, 225
immune response, 179
implants, 11, 12, 13
improved ventricular function, avoidance, xi, 173
improvements, vii, xii, 1, 17, 20, 21, 169, 211, 216, 225, 258
impulses, 3
in vitro, 57, 69, 70
incidence, x, xii, 29, 30, 58, 59, 60, 62, 78, 87, 93, 108, 110, 143, 144, 156, 169, 179, 211, 216, 217, 218, 234, 236
induction, 224, 256
industry, 29, 76, 78, 137
infarction, 6, 10, 13, 15, 17, 18, 19, 20, 76, 78, 116, 145, 205, 217, 222
infection, 3, 4, 89, 167, 184
inferior vena cava, 38, 100, 149
inferiority, 234
inflammation, 147, 159
inflammatory disease, 125
inflammatory mediators, xii, 29, 212
inflation, 113, 177
informed consent, 185
infrared spectroscopy, 138
inhibition, 69, 76, 140, 179
inhibitor, 71, 234
initiation, 103, 178, 231, 235
injure, 192

injury(s), 4, 17, 23, 32, 41, 47, 48, 51, 77, 84, 85, 86, 87, 88, 89, 90, 93, 102, 106, 114, 126, 127, 131, 139, 145, 147, 149, 159, 177, 180, 191, 192, 194, 205, 207, 216, 217, 218, 219, 224, 258
innominate, 9, 99
insertion, 125, 129, 175, 181, 183, 187, 204, 213, 215, 218, 237
institutions, vii, xiii, 153, 171, 231, 235
insulin, 110, 115
integrity, xi, 89, 163, 167, 193
intensive care unit, 11, 30, 114, 147, 174, 186, 191, 205, 215, 224
interference, 39, 77, 102, 183
intervention, viii, ix, xi, 14, 53, 60, 62, 105, 107, 108, 116, 118, 132, 136, 138, 153, 163, 164, 165, 166, 169, 170, 171, 172, 182, 208, 213, 225, 238, 239
intima, 103
intoxication, 204
intra-aortic balloon pump, 19, 21, 43, 104, 152, 154, 214, 229
intracerebral hemorrhage, 116
intravenous fluids, 149, 181, 238
intravenously, 87, 179, 183, 202
iodine, 9
iron, 9
irradiation, 148, 166
irrigation, 232
irritability, 182, 202, 204
ischemia, x, xii, xiii, 10, 23, 41, 42, 43, 50, 89, 100, 102, 103, 110, 112, 143, 145, 151, 166, 168, 169, 171, 176, 183, 195, 205, 209, 212, 223, 224, 225, 228, 229, 230, 231, 235
isolation, xiii, 134, 223, 224, 233
isotonic solution, 64, 65
Israel, 14
issues, 42, 78, 98, 104, 170, 235
iteration, 123

## J

Japan, 211, 215, 216, 217, 218, 222
jejunum, 8

## K

$K^+$, 57, 65
kidney, 12, 234
knees, 86
kyphosis, 125

## L

laceration, 2
lack of confidence, 16
laparoscopic surgery, 140
laparotomy, 41, 100, 148, 161, 194
L-arginine, 69
laryngoscope, 79
larynx, 4
lead, x, 10, 23, 27, 46, 47, 87, 89, 90, 97, 98, 100, 121, 122, 123, 136, 180, 217, 224, 230, 232, 258
leakage, 39, 155
learning, ix, x, 29, 92, 97, 105, 107, 108, 114, 117, 121, 130, 132, 134, 135, 136, 137, 191, 194, 206
left atrium, 3, 40, 100, 256
left internal mammary artery (LIMA), ix, 26, 107, 108, 127, 145, 149, 197, 242
left ventricle, 2, 4, 11, 12, 18, 24, 40, 99, 108, 136, 149, 188, 200, 256, 257, 258
left ventricular end-diastolic pressure, xiii, 40, 255
legs, 126
lesions, ix, 19, 21, 22, 28, 30, 99, 105, 107, 108, 109, 130, 164, 165, 166, 169, 170, 171, 186, 188, 215, 231
leukocytes, 48
lifetime, 27
ligament, 190
light, 3, 77, 109
liver, 152
living beating heart, vii, 1
local anesthesia, 181, 182
local anesthetic, 10, 179, 182, 190, 191, 192, 199
low risk, 135
lumen, 11, 15, 54, 64, 150, 178, 224, 233
lung disease, 166
lymphedema, 86

## M

magnesium, 231
magnetic resonance, 218
magnetic resonance imaging, 218
magnitude, 57
majority, 19, 29, 78, 108, 181, 256
malignancy, 110
man, 2, 5, 7, 8, 18, 26
management, vii, xiii, 1, 4, 17, 19, 42, 43, 63, 76, 97, 98, 103, 114, 130, 132, 138, 220, 223, 224, 228, 233, 235
manipulation, ix, x, 29, 77, 85, 87, 95, 98, 101, 129, 143, 145, 167, 189, 205, 217, 218, 230
mannitol, 213

## Index

mapping, 86
Maryland, 121
mast cells, 56
materials, 22, 26
matter, 13
MB, 118, 139, 207, 208, 213, 214, 215, 258
mean arterial pressure, 39, 40, 149
measurement(s), xiii, 3, 72, 156, 161, 181, 234
mechanical ventilation, xi, 173, 174, 175, 179, 180, 183, 187, 191, 194, 203
mechanical ventilator, 182
median, 12, 23, 76, 99, 102, 115, 123, 144, 147, 151, 152, 153, 154, 165, 174, 175, 181, 182, 185, 189, 190, 191, 192, 194, 195, 197, 204, 205, 212
mediastinitis, 148
mediastinum, 4, 99, 104, 124, 167
medical, 2, 3, 4, 17, 18, 19, 20, 21, 22, 29, 76, 114, 117
medicine, 3, 92
mellitus, 175, 207
mentor, 30
messenger RNA, 55, 68
meta-analysis, 78, 116, 118, 222, 234, 239, 240
metabolic acidosis, 235
metabolites, 178
metabolizing, 178
methodology, 218
Mexico, 12
microscope, 16
microscopy, 77
migration, 181
military, 4
miniature, 129, 136, 237
miniaturization, 105
Minimally invasive direct coronary artery bypass (MIDCAB), ix, 107, 108
Minneapolis, 99, 101, 102, 103, 152, 213
mitochondria, 23
mitral insufficiency, 41
mitral regurgitation, xiii, 100, 188, 229, 230, 238, 255, 257
mitral stenosis, 5
mitral valve, 41, 135, 139, 140, 188, 230, 257
mixing, 46
models, 29, 48, 140
modifications, 63, 126
Moon, 92
morbidity, ix, xi, 12, 29, 38, 105, 106, 107, 108, 130, 143, 144, 146, 147, 152, 156, 159, 161, 163, 164, 174, 176, 216, 219, 221, 238, 239
morphine, 208, 224
mortality rate, 4, 16, 20, 116, 153, 164, 169, 214, 231

mortality risk, 214, 215
Moses, 118
MR, 68, 69, 106, 138, 140, 230
muscarinic receptor, 56, 178
muscle relaxant, 224
muscles, 26, 179, 180, 182, 193, 204, 230
music, 186
myocardial infarction, xii, 3, 6, 9, 10, 13, 15, 17, 18, 19, 21, 22, 26, 28, 29, 76, 78, 96, 104, 110, 116, 125, 130, 133, 145, 152, 153, 154, 158, 165, 168, 169, 171, 179, 187, 211, 213, 214, 217, 219, 220, 222, 234
myocardial ischemia, xi, xii, 6, 26, 42, 100, 131, 146, 147, 173, 177, 178, 180, 185, 205, 207, 211, 216, 217, 219, 221
myocardial necrosis, 29, 48
myocardial revascularization, vii, xi, xii, 1, 10, 11, 12, 16, 23, 25, 26, 27, 28, 29, 30, 31, 32, 49, 50, 54, 66, 67, 109, 119, 122, 147, 155, 156, 159, 163, 164, 206, 207, 211, 212, 213, 219, 220, 252
myocardium, x, 6, 8, 9, 10, 11, 16, 24, 26, 28, 47, 48, 103, 108, 109, 121, 128, 136, 146, 165, 175, 177, 179, 180, 222, 230, 231

## N

narcotics, 176, 224
nasogastric tube, 152, 182
nasopharynx, 186
nausea, 177
necrosis, 12
negotiating, 137
nerve, 7, 8, 9, 41, 46, 56, 85, 89, 90, 93, 113, 127, 146, 149, 150, 151, 184, 199, 203, 208, 224, 236
nervous system, 179
Netherlands, 45
neural function, 209
neuropathy, 177
neuropeptides, 56
neurotoxicity, 184
New England, 78, 92
nitrates, 19, 20, 21
nitric oxide, 2, 54, 55, 61, 66, 68, 69, 72, 178
nitric oxide synthase, 55, 68
nitrous oxide, 1
Nobel Prize, 3, 25, 26
nodes, 231
noncalcified, 110
norepinephrine, 56, 57, 176, 177, 178
North America, 20
Norway, 2
nurses, vii, 134
nutrition, 10

## O

obesity, 110, 111, 125, 166
obstruction, 5, 8, 11, 14, 15, 16, 18, 39, 40
occlusion, 6, 8, 9, 13, 14, 17, 19, 23, 26, 27, 31, 33, 54, 57, 62, 77, 89, 99, 100, 101, 102, 103, 104, 110, 111, 112, 113, 115, 116, 123, 125, 132, 133, 146, 151, 153, 156, 168, 170, 188, 213, 225, 231, 234
octopus, 32, 43, 237
oesophageal, 11
off-pump coronary artery bypass (OPCAB), vii, 25, 37, 96, 160, 174, 242
OH, 79, 97, 99, 219, 221
oil, 3
omentum, 8, 11, 26, 151
operations, vii, viii, x, 1, 4, 8, 11, 12, 14, 16, 18, 23, 25, 43, 44, 75, 89, 115, 122, 123, 134, 135, 137, 144, 152, 155, 164, 174, 187, 194, 212, 214, 216, 219, 238, 258
optimization, 236
organ(s), xii, 55, 56, 59, 61, 65, 96, 140, 147, 152, 211, 212, 214, 217
ostium, 14
outpatient, xi, 173
ox, 19
oxygen, 9, 10, 40, 42, 174, 176, 177, 179, 180, 182, 186, 203, 205, 213, 228, 236
oxygen consumption, 179, 180, 228

## P

pacing, xiii, 43, 47, 50, 98, 100, 102, 104, 111, 231, 255, 256, 257, 258
pain, xi, 1, 5, 6, 7, 9, 11, 17, 20, 78, 84, 85, 114, 119, 163, 167, 168, 174, 176, 180, 182, 184, 185, 186, 190, 191, 192, 193, 202, 205, 208, 224
pain tolerance, 191
pallor, 5
palpation, 146
parallel, 12, 48, 111, 193, 203, 256
paralysis, 182, 184, 204
parathyroid, 7
parathyroid glands, 7
paresis, 184
paresthesias, 89
patent ductus arteriosus, 4
pathology, 109, 187, 188
pathophysiology, 8
pectoralis major, 8
pelvis, 150
penetrance, 136
penicillin, 4
peptide, 56, 69, 234
percutaneous coronary intervention (PCI), ix, 107, 108, 213
perforation, 4
perfusion, 7, 11, 16, 26, 27, 48, 100, 103, 130, 131, 138, 139, 145, 146, 166, 176, 179, 180, 183, 188, 217, 218, 222
pericardial sac, 8, 30
pericarditis, 9
pericardium, 4, 8, 9, 18, 41, 46, 47, 48, 49, 99, 100, 101, 112, 113, 127, 136, 144, 145, 146, 149, 150, 151, 152, 191, 192, 193, 194, 199, 200, 201, 203, 213, 228, 256
peripheral vascular disease, 86, 96, 110, 159
peritoneal cavity, 81
peritoneum, 151
permission, 2, 5, 60, 91
permit, 18, 151, 225, 233
perseverance, 109
pH, 64, 65, 90, 91
pharmacological intervention, viii, 53, 60, 62
pharmacology, 56
Philadelphia, 14
physical activity, 21
physical health, 132
physical properties, 178
physicians, 7, 8, 78, 137, 170
physics, 3
Physiological, 59
physiology, 56
pigs, 38, 39, 136
placebo, 239
plaque, 230
platelet count, 235
platform, 2, 83, 99, 101
pleura, 146, 190, 192, 194, 195, 202, 205, 209, 228, 233
pleural cavity, 113, 191, 193
pleural effusion, 116, 125
pleural spaces, 99
pleuritis, 125
plexus, 7
PM, 66, 119, 159, 221, 239
pneumonectomy, 96
pneumonia, 177
pneumothorax, xii, 167, 174, 190, 193, 194, 195, 197, 202, 204, 205, 209, 234
policy, 20
polypropylene, 112, 149, 151, 152, 199, 213
polyvinyl chloride, 22
population, x, 76, 78, 115, 117, 121, 122, 137, 152
potassium, 19, 56, 57, 71, 231

potential benefits, 176
preparation, 70, 72, 73, 78, 86, 90, 92, 97, 113, 238
preservation, xi, xii, 23, 63, 70, 77, 126, 163, 173, 211, 216
pressure gradient, 87
prevention, 71, 87
principles, 14, 27, 47, 101, 104, 126
probe, 38, 40, 181
progressive atherosclerotic disease, x, 143
project, 158
prophylactic, 130
prostate cancer, 140
prostatectomy, 140
prosthesis, 11
protection, x, xii, 65, 84, 103, 104, 108, 122, 126, 143, 145, 146, 147, 212, 217, 219, 220
prototypes, 29
PTFE, 48
PTT, 235
publishing, 27
pulmonary artery pressure, 102
pulmonary capillary wedge pressure, 180
pulmonary edema, 125
pulmonary function test, 124
pulmonary hypertension, 166, 234
pumps, 229

# Q

quality of life, xii, xiii, 20, 108, 119, 126, 137, 144, 174, 207
questionnaire, 217

# R

radiation, 125
radius, 257, 258
RE, 221
reactivity, 56, 57, 59, 60, 61, 62, 69, 180
reading, 60
real time, 29, 77, 136
reality, 136
reasoning, 6
receptors, 57, 58, 69, 178
recognition, 19, 96, 97, 153
recommendations, 87
reconstruction, 12, 15, 50, 237
recovery, x, xi, xii, 2, 3, 4, 14, 107, 114, 117, 136, 170, 173, 191, 205, 223, 224, 225, 232, 235, 236
recreational, 20
rectus abdominis, 193
recurrence, ix, x, 107, 109, 143, 161

redistribution, 179, 180, 186, 238
reflexes, 184
rehabilitation, xi, 21, 125, 136, 163
reimburse, 170
relaxation, 58, 61, 62, 66, 69, 70
relaxation properties, 58
relevance, 67
reliability, 89, 168
relief, 6, 8, 24, 179, 208, 209
remission, 7
renal dysfunction, 30, 147, 159, 217
renal failure, 110, 152, 154, 215, 217
renin, 56, 183
repair, xii, 5, 11, 18, 78, 135, 140, 174, 192, 194, 203
requirements, xiii, 6, 7, 32, 106, 159, 191, 205, 239
resection, 13, 134, 193
resistance, 55, 69, 89, 126, 178, 179, 181, 183, 228
resolution, 3
resource utilization, 147, 239
resources, 23, 137
respiration, 2, 4, 180, 182, 185, 190, 191, 192, 194, 197, 200, 203, 235
respiratory failure, 2
respiratory rate, 126
response, xii, 7, 29, 32, 46, 56, 57, 58, 70, 72, 96, 98, 104, 168, 170, 176, 177, 178, 179, 209, 211, 216, 219, 258
restenosis, ix, 107, 108, 109, 164, 166
RH, 31, 118, 158
rhythm, xiii, 38, 188, 223, 224, 231
right atrium, 4, 10, 145, 149, 256
right ventricle, 2, 5, 40, 41, 46, 114, 144, 146, 149, 225
rings, 31, 118
risk factors, 19, 115, 116, 153, 185
risk profile, 108, 144, 157
risks, x, xiii, 22, 29, 108, 131, 143, 144, 176, 180, 217, 224
robotics, 29, 32, 105, 129, 135, 138, 140, 171
room temperature, 64, 112
root(s), 7, 8, 59
rubber, 100
Russia, 14, 27

# S

sadness, 17
safety, 51, 126, 130, 137, 152, 157, 165, 167, 168, 170, 234, 255
saturation, 40, 203, 205, 213
scar tissue, 18
science, 1
scoliosis, 125

scope, 22, 79, 80, 81, 86, 88, 105, 123, 132
second generation, 65
secrete, 54
security, 170
sedative, 1, 114, 182
sedative medication, 114, 182
seizure, 184
sensitivity, 57, 58, 183, 185
serum, 215, 228, 231
sex, 214
sexual activity, 186
shape, 18, 127
sheep, 50
shock, 3, 214, 215, 220
showing, xi, 21, 27, 56, 60, 163
side effects, vii, 25, 165, 174, 180
signs, 4, 110, 171, 199, 215, 223, 235
silhouette, 165
silk, 47, 88
Sinai, 9
skin, 8, 10, 84, 86, 87, 88, 149, 150, 152, 181, 182, 189, 190, 191, 192, 193, 206, 238
smooth muscle, 55, 56, 57, 58, 59, 177, 178
smooth muscle cells, 56, 59, 177, 178
societal cost, 136
sodium, 213
solution, 3, 11, 63, 64, 65, 70, 71, 73, 77, 89, 90, 91, 132, 139, 151, 181, 182, 198, 199, 213
South America, 256
SP, 160
spastic, 59, 62, 63
specialisation, 3
species, 5
spinal cord, 7, 184, 187
spinal cord injury, 184
spine, 3
sponge, 10, 195
SS, 31, 92, 118
St. Petersburg, 109
stability, viii, 30, 45, 49, 50, 51, 97, 98, 100, 103, 104, 127, 174, 176, 186, 191, 224, 225, 228, 256, 258
stabilization, viii, 29, 30, 32, 38, 43, 44, 45, 46, 47, 48, 49, 50, 51, 102, 123, 126, 136, 167, 176, 193, 199, 201, 225, 228, 237
stabilizers, 29, 38, 47, 48, 51, 99, 103, 122, 151, 212, 216
stable angina, 13, 18, 19, 20, 133
standard deviation, 172, 214, 215
staphylococci, 4
stasis, 85, 87
state, 98, 115, 176, 179, 217, 223
statistics, 16, 21

steel, 129
stenosis, x, 21, 22, 43, 48, 62, 65, 76, 89, 100, 108, 110, 111, 112, 116, 118, 133, 155, 156, 166, 178, 180, 187, 188, 215, 216
stent, ix, 30, 107, 108, 109, 115, 116, 138, 164, 169, 234
sterile, 9, 98, 182, 195, 199, 200, 204
sternum, 12, 90, 99, 101, 127, 144, 148, 190, 191, 192, 194, 195, 196, 199, 200, 202, 203
stimulation, 56, 71, 178, 180, 231
stimulus, 3, 5, 17, 23, 58
stomach, 8, 56, 151
stress, xi, 10, 22, 171, 173, 174, 175, 176, 177, 178, 186, 257, 258
stress response, xi, 173, 174, 175, 176, 186
stress test, 22, 171
stress testing, 171
stretching, 86, 194, 195, 197, 202, 203
stroke, xiii, 18, 30, 39, 40, 47, 105, 116, 131, 132, 147, 164, 221, 234, 237, 255, 257, 258
stroke volume, xiii, 39, 40, 47, 237, 255, 257
structure, 29, 54, 55, 56, 59, 140, 148, 186, 188
subcutaneous tissue, 190
subgroups, 19, 22, 97, 105, 206
success rate, 169
superior vena cava, 38, 46
supplementation, 209
suppository, 98
surgical intervention, 4, 6, 168, 217
surgical technique, 28, 51, 76, 144, 207
survival, xii, xiii, 14, 19, 20, 21, 22, 54, 66, 67, 91, 93, 106, 110, 117, 153, 154, 158, 161, 172, 207, 211, 221
survival rate, 20
suture, 2, 16, 18, 27, 29, 33, 41, 47, 49, 50, 88, 100, 102, 103, 104, 112, 127, 128, 149, 152, 192, 200
Swan-Ganz catheter, 39
Sweden, 12
swelling, 86
sympathectomy, 6, 7, 13, 175
sympathetic fibers, 177
sympathetic nervous system, 7
symptoms, ix, 5, 6, 9, 17, 18, 20, 107, 108, 109, 156
syndrome, 8, 114, 182, 193, 209, 220
syphilis, 5, 13
systolic blood pressure, 41, 102, 104, 149, 215, 256
systolic pressure, 4, 104

# T

tachycardia, 131, 177, 178, 229
tachypnea, 203
talc, 9

tantalum, 31, 109, 118
Task Force, 220
teams, x, 2, 21, 121, 125, 132, 134, 137
technological advancement, x, 38, 121
technology, vii, x, 1, 22, 23, 30, 76, 81, 88, 122, 125, 136, 137, 175
teeth, 177
temperature, 3, 56, 98, 181, 182, 213, 232, 235
tension, xii, 42, 48, 86, 100, 101, 102, 126, 128, 131, 151, 174, 191, 193, 194, 203, 234
territory, 11, 13, 103, 145, 147, 156, 165, 200, 201, 203, 256
theatre, 149
therapy, 6, 20, 21, 44, 63, 117, 155, 169, 170, 187, 213, 222, 237
thinning, 165
thoracotomy, 2, 18, 105, 109, 112, 114, 119, 123, 130, 133, 145, 147, 148, 150, 152, 153, 154, 155, 157, 158, 160, 161, 162, 167, 168, 171, 175, 189, 190, 191, 192, 193, 194, 197, 200, 202, 205, 208
thorax, 111, 124, 127, 182, 201, 203
thrombin, 234
thrombocytopenia, 187, 231
thrombolytic therapy, 215
thrombosis, 11, 14, 15, 169, 231, 234
thrombus, 5, 6, 15, 18
thymus, 150
thyroid, 7
thyroid gland, 7
thyrotoxicosis, 6, 7
time constraints, 85
time frame, 78
tissue, 39, 43, 48, 49, 56, 78, 81, 86, 87, 88, 102, 140, 195, 196, 228, 237, 238
tissue perfusion, 228
TLR, 172
tobacco, 96
tooth, 2
tourniquet, 33, 47, 49, 112
trachea, 4
tracheostomy, 126
tracks, 136
trade, 212, 219
trade-off, 212, 219
training, vii, 30, 42, 134, 135, 140
training programs, 135
trajectory, 136
transection, 168
transference, 87
transfusion, 30, 32, 106, 159, 191, 205, 206, 233, 239
transparency, 81
transplant, 12, 24, 25, 110

transplantation, 26, 57, 155
transport, 5
trauma, 48, 77, 89, 102, 122, 125, 128, 147, 169, 175, 177, 204, 205
treatment, ix, xi, 4, 6, 7, 13, 15, 18, 20, 21, 22, 24, 26, 30, 31, 50, 54, 68, 71, 72, 75, 90, 108, 118, 119, 125, 132, 140, 146, 155, 164, 169, 170, 173, 180, 184, 187, 206, 207, 212, 214, 228, 231
trial, 20, 21, 24, 67, 92, 117, 118, 137, 139, 159, 221, 222, 234, 236, 238, 239
tumor, 216
tumor necrosis factor, 216
turbulence, 15
Turkey, 173

## U

UK, 20
ultrasound, 38, 39, 40, 77, 86, 99, 104
uniform, viii, 53, 55, 60
United, 1, 2, 18, 25, 26, 28, 84, 109, 122, 143, 163, 218
United Kingdom, 1, 143, 163
United States, 2, 18, 25, 26, 28, 84, 109, 122, 218
unstable angina, 18, 21, 179
unwanted side effects, vii, 25
urinary bladder, 111
urinary retention, 184
urine, 228
urologist, 3
USA, 127, 149, 206, 213

## V

vacuum, 47, 176, 199
valve, 16, 122, 135, 166, 230, 257
variables, 29, 38, 39, 76, 78, 215
variations, 194
vascular endothelial growth factor (VEGF), 58
vascular surgery, 13
vasoactive intestinal peptide, 57, 68
vasoconstriction, 56, 57, 65, 68, 71, 72, 168, 177, 178
vasodilator, 58, 60, 65, 68, 70, 71, 91
vasopressin, 56, 57, 68, 69, 71, 183
vasospasm, 56, 57, 59, 61, 62, 63, 71, 72
ventilation, xi, 3, 23, 112, 114, 115, 124, 125, 126, 131, 152, 155, 165, 166, 167, 173, 177, 179, 180, 182, 183, 202, 204, 225, 233
ventricle, 2, 5, 9, 18, 41, 46, 47, 48, 102, 225, 229, 256, 257
ventricular fibrillation, 8, 9, 27

ventricular tachycardia, 231
vertebrae, 3
Viking, 5
vision, 5, 15, 88, 112, 122, 126, 150
visualization, 38, 47, 79, 80, 81, 82, 83, 86, 102, 111, 122, 126, 127, 213
vomiting, 177, 186

windows, 88
wires, 43, 47, 104, 148, 256
workload, 6, 7, 22
World War I, 4, 5, 8
worldwide, 28, 46
wound healing, 86
wound infection, 30, 78, 84, 85, 90, 93, 105, 108, 110, 116, 148

## W

waste, 187
water, 9
weakness, 184
wealth, 90

## X

xiphoid process, 151, 190, 191, 192, 193, 194
x-rays, 3